CHAPMAN & NAKIEL

AIDS TO RADIOLOGICAL DIFFERENTIAL DIAGNOSIS

Edited by

Stephen G Davies MA MB BChir MRCP FRCR
Consultant Radiologist,
Royal Glamorgan Hospital,
South Wales, UK,
Visiting Professor of Radiology,
University of Glamorgan

FIFTH EDITION

SAUNDERS

ELSEVIER

SAUNDERS
ELSEVIER

© Baillière Tindall 1990
© W B Saunders Company Limited 1995
© 2009, Elsevier Limited. All rights reserved.

First edition 1984
Second edition 1990
Third edition 1995
Fourth edition 2003
Fifth edition 2009
  Reprinted 2009, 2010, 2011, 2012

ISBN 9780702029790

British Library Cataloguing in Publication Data
A catalogue record for this book is available from the British Library

Library of Congress Cataloging in Publication Data
A catalog record for this book is available from the Library of Congress

The Publisher's policy is to use paper manufactured from sustainable forests

Printed in China

Preface to the first edition

During the period of study prior to taking the final Fellowship of the Royal College of Radiologists, or other similar radiological examinations, many specialist textbooks and the wealth of radiological papers are carefully scoured for lists of differential diagnoses of radiological signs. These will supplement the information already learned and enable that information to be used logically when analysing a radiograph. All this takes precious time when effort is best spent trying to memorize these lists rather than trying to find them within the massive texts or, even worse, trying to construct them oneself.

Consequently we decided to write a book which contains as many useful lists as one might reasonably be expected to know for a postgraduate examination. To make it manageable, we have omitted those lists and conditions which have limited relevance to routine radiological practice. In addition, many of the lists are constructed in terms of a 'surgical sieve' and by using this method we would hope that the lists are easier to remember. We have tried to present the conditions in some order of importance, although we realize that local patient selection and the geographical distribution of diseases will have a great influence in modifying the lists. The lists will, almost certainly, not be acceptable to all radiologists. However, the basic lists are supplemented with useful facts and discriminating features about each condition and these should enable the trainee to give a considered opinion of the radiograph. So that this added information can be kept concise and to avoid unnecessary repetition we have summarized the radiological signs of many important conditions separately in Part 2 of the book.

The book has no radiographs. We have assumed a basic knowledge of radiology in the reader and expect him or her to already be able to recognize the abnormal signs. A limited number of line drawings has been used to emphasize radiographic abnormalities.

The aim of the book is to assist with logical interpretation of the radiograph. It is not intended for use on its own because it is not a complete radiological textbook. Recourse will need to be made to the larger general and specialist texts and journals and the reading of them is still a prerequisite to passing the postgraduate examinations.

More exhaustive lists are to be found in Felson & Reeder's Gamuts in Radiology (Oxford: Pergamon Press, 1975) and Kreel's Outline of Radiology (London: Heinemann, 1971) and these books are to be commended.

Birmingham and Sheffield

Stephen Chapman
Richard Nakielny

Preface to the fifth edition

This new edition has been extensively revised in order to reflect developing radiological knowledge and evolving imaging techniques. Lists have been brought up to date and many new references added. A new chapter has been introduced for paediatrics. Readers familiar with earlier editions will recognize many of the established lists which have been brought up to date. In addition, new lists have been added in many of the chapters. I am greatly indebted to the contributors to this fifth edition who have carried out this review in such a detailed fashion.

I recognize that this book is a key source of information for preparation for radiological examinations. In addition I hope that established clinical radiologists will continue to refer to this book during the course of daily radiological practice long after they have completed their examinations.

Cardiff SGD
2009

Contents

Contents

Contributors

Aisling Butler FRCR MRCP
Consultant Radiologist
The Princess of Wales and Neath Port Talbot Hospitals
Abertawe Bro Morgannwg University NHS Trust
Wales, UK

Alistair D Calder FRCR
Consultant Paediatric Radiologist
Great Ormond Street Hospital for Children
London, UK

Nigel Cowan MA BM BCh PGDipLATHE FRCP FRCR
Consultant Radiologist
Department of Radiology
The Churchill Hospital
Oxford, UK

Colin Davies MB ChB FRCR
Consultant Radiologist
Department of Radiology
Royal Glamorgan Hospital
Llantrisant
South Wales, UK

Sujal R Desai MD MRCP FRCR
Consultant Radiologist
Department of Radiology
King's College Hospital
London, UK

Rebecca Greenhalgh MBBS AFRCSI FRCR
Department of Specialist X-Ray
University College Hospital
London, UK

Stephen Harden MA MB BS FRCS FRCR
Consultant Cardiothoracic Radiologist
Wessex Cardiothoracic Centre
Southampton, UK

Paul D Humphries BSc MRCP FRCR
Consultant Paediatric Radiologist
University College London Hospital NHS Trust
London, UK

Steven L J James FRCR
Consultant Radiologist
The Royal Orthopaedic Hospital NHS Foundation Trust
Birmingham, UK

Sarfraz Nazir MA BM BCh MRCS
Specialist Registrar Radiology
John Radcliffe Hospital
Oxford, UK

Simon P G Padley MBBS BSc MRCP FRCR
Consultant Radiologist and Honorary Senior Lecturer
Department of Radiology
Chelsea & Westminster Hospital
London, UK

Neil Stoodley BM BCh FRCS FRCR FRCPCH
Department of Neuroradiology
Frenchay Hospital
Bristol, UK

Stuart Taylor BSc MB BS MD MRCP FRCR
Consultant Radiologist and Senior Lecturer
Department of Specialist X-Ray
University College Hospital
London, UK

Explanatory notes

The 'surgical sieve' classification used in the longer lists is presented in order of commonness, e.g. when 'neoplastic' is listed first then this is the commonest cause as a group. Within the group of neoplastic conditions, number 1 is more common or as common as number 2. However, it does not necessarily follow that all the conditions in the first group are more common than those in subsequent groups, e.g. infective, metabolic, etc.

The groups entitled 'idiopathic' or 'others' are usually listed last even though the disease or diseases within them may be common. This has been done for the sake of neatness only.

In order that the supplementary notes are not unnecessarily repeated in several lists, those conditions which appear in several lists are denoted by an asterisk (*) and a summary of their radiological signs is to be found in Part 2 of the book. In this section conditions are listed alphabetically.

Abbreviations

ACE	Angiotensin-converting enzyme
ACTH	Adrenocorticotrophic hormone
AD	Autosomal dominant
AFP	Alpha-fetoprotein
AP	Anteroposterior
AR	Autosomal recessive
ASD	Atrial septal defect
AV	Atrioventricular
AVM	Arteriovenous malformation
AXR	Abdomen X-ray
CMCJ	Carpometacarpal joint
CMV	Cytomegalovirus
CNS	Central nervous system
CPA	Cerebellopontine angle
CSF	Cerebrospinal fluid
CT	Computerized tomography
CXR	Chest X-ray
DAI	Diffuse axonal injury
DCM	Dilated Cardiomyopathy
DIC	Disseminated intravascular coagulopathy
DIPJ	Distal interphalangeal joint
EDH	Extradural haemorrhage
FLAIR	Fluid-attenuated inversion recovery
GBM	Glioblastoma multiforme
GE	Gradient echo
HCG	Human chorionic gonadotrophin
HMPAO	Hexamethylpropyleneamineoxime
HOA	Hypertrophic osteoarthropathy
HCM	Hypertrophic cardiomyopathy
HRCT	High-resolution CT
HU	Hounsfield units
IAM	Internal auditory meatus
ICA	Internal carotid artery
IUCD	Intrauterine contraceptive device
IVC	Inferior vena cava
IVU	Intravenous urogram

LAT	Lateral
LV	Left Ventricle
MCA	Middle cerebral artery
MCPJ	Metacarpophalangeal joint
MIBG	Meta-iodo-benzyl-guanidine
MPA	Main pulmonary artery
MPS	Mucopolysaccharidosis
MRI	Magnetic resonance imaging
NEC	Necrotizing enterocolitis
NFT	Neurofibromatosis
PA	Posteroanterior
PAS	Periodic acid–Schiff (stain)
PD	Proton density
PDA	Patent ductus arteriosus
PET	Positron Emission Tomography
PIPJ	Proximal interphalangeal joint
PMF	Progressive massive fibrosis
PPH	Postpartum haemorrhage
RV	Right Ventricle
SAH	Subarachnoid haemorrhage
SDH	Subdural haemorrhage
SIJ	Sacroiliac joint
SLE	Systemic lupus erythematosus
SMA	Superior mesenteric artery
SOL	Space-occupying lesion
SPECT	Single photon emission computerized tomography
STIR	Short tau inversion recovery
SVC	Superior vena cava
SXR	Skull x-ray
TAPVD	Total anomalous pulmonary venous drainage
TB	Tuberculosis
TE	Echo time or time to echo
TGA	Transposition of the great arteries
TOF	Tracheo-oesophageal fistula
TR	Repetition time
T_1W	T_1-weighted
T_2W	T_2-weighted
US	Ultrasound
VMA	Vanillylmandelic acid
VSD	Ventricular septal defect
XR	X-linked recessive

Part 1

Bones

Steven James

1

1.1 GENERALIZED INCREASED BONE DENSITY

Myeloproliferative

1. **Myelosclerosis** – marrow cavity is narrowed by endosteal new bone. Patchy lucencies due to persistence of fibrous tissue. (Generalized osteopenia in the early stages due to myelofibrosis.) Hepatosplenomegaly.

Metabolic

1. **Renal osteodystrophy***.

Poisoning

1. **Fluorosis** – with periosteal reaction, prominent muscle attachments and calcification of ligaments and interosseous membranes. Changes are most marked in the innominate bones and lumbar spine.

Neoplastic (more commonly multifocal than generalized)

1. **Osteoblastic metastases** – most commonly prostate and breasts – see 1.18.
2. **Lymphoma***.
3. **Mastocytosis** – sclerosis of marrow containing skeleton with patchy areas of radiolucency. Urticaria pigmentosa. Can have symptoms and signs of carcinoid syndrome.

Idiopathic (more commonly multifocal than generalized)

1. Paget's disease*.

For those conditions with onset in the paediatric age group see 14.10.

1.2 SOLITARY SCLEROTIC BONE LESION

Developmental

1. Bone island (enostosis).
2. Fibrous dysplasia*.

Neoplastic

1. Metastasis – most commonly prostate or breast.
2. Lymphoma*.
3. Osteoma/osteoid osteoma/osteoblastoma*.
4. Healed or healing benign or malignant bone lesion – e.g. lytic metastasis following radiotherapy or chemotherapy, bone cyst, fibrous cortical defect, eosinophilic granuloma or brown tumour.
5. Primary bone sarcoma.

Vascular

1. Bone infarct.

Traumatic

1. Callus – especially a transverse density around a healing stress fracture.

Infective

1. Sclerosing osteomyelitis of Garré.

Idiopathic

1. Paget's disease*.

1.3 MULTIPLE SCLEROTIC BONE LESIONS

Developmental

1. **Fibrous dysplasia*.**
2. **Osteopoikilosis** – asymptomatic. 1–10mm, round or oval densities in the appendicular skeleton and pelvis. Ribs, skull and spine are usually exempt. Tend to be parallel to the long axis of the affected bones and are especially numerous near the ends of bones.
3. **Osteopathia striata** (Voorhoeve's disease) – asymptomatic. Linear bands of dense bone parallel with the long axis of the bone. The appendicular skeleton and pelvis are most frequently affected; skull and clavicles are spared.
4. **Tuberous sclerosis*.**

Neoplastic

1. **Metastases** (see 1.18) – most commonly prostate or breast.
2. **Lymphoma*.**
3. **Mastocytosis.**
4. **Multiple healed or healing benign or malignant bone lesions** – e.g. lytic metastases following radiotherapy or chemotherapy, eosinophilic granuloma and brown tumours.
5. **Multiple myeloma*** – sclerosis in up to 3% of cases.
6. **Osteomata** – e.g. Gardner's syndrome.
7. **Multifocal osteosarcoma*.**

Idiopathic

1. **Paget's disease*.**

Vascular

1. **Bone infarcts.**

Traumatic

1. **Callus** – around numerous fractures.

1.4 BONE SCLEROSIS WITH A PERIOSTEAL REACTION

Traumatic

1. **Healing fracture with callus.**

Neoplastic

1. **Metastasis.**
2. **Lymphoma*.**
3. **Osteoid osteoma/osteoblastoma*.**
4. **Osteosarcoma*.**
5. **Ewing's sarcoma*.**
6. **Chondrosarcoma*.**

Infective

1. **Osteomyelitis** – including Garré's sclerosing osteomyelitis and Brodie's abscess.
2. **Syphilis** – congenital or acquired.

Idiopathic

1. **Infantile cortical hyperostosis** (Caffey's disease) – in infants up to 6 months of age. Multiple bones involved at different times, most frequently mandible, ribs and clavicles; long bones less commonly; spine, hands and feet are spared. Increased density of bones is caused by massive periosteal new bone. In the long bones the epiphyses and metaphyses are spared.
2. **Melorheostosis** – cortical and periosteal new bone giving the appearance of molten wax flowing down a burning candle. The hyperostosis tends to extend from one bone to the next. Usually affects one limb but both limbs on one side may be affected. Sometimes it is bilateral but asymmetrical. Skull, spine and ribs are seldom affected.

Further Reading

Wenaden AE, Szyszko TA, Saifuddin A. Imaging of periosteal reactions associated with focal lesions of bone. Clin Radiol 2005;60(4):439–56.

1.5 SOLITARY SCLEROTIC BONE LESION WITH A LUCENT CENTRE

Neoplastic
1. Osteoid osteoma*.
2. Osteoblastoma*.

Infective
1. Brodie's abscess.
2. Syphilis, yaws and tuberculosis.

1.6 CONDITIONS INVOLVING SKIN AND BONE

Osteolytic bone lesions
1. Congenital
   (a) Neurofibromatosis*.
   (b) Basal cell naevus syndrome.
   (c) Angiodysplasias.
2. Acquired
   (a) Scleroderma*.
   (b) Rheumatoid arthritis*.
   (c) Gout*.
   (d) Leprosy.
   (e) Syphilis.
   (f) Actinomycosis.
   (g) Langerhans cell histiocytosis*.
   (h) Sarcoidosis*.
   (i) Mastocytosis.
   (j) Pancreatitis with osteonecrosis.

Osteosclerotic bone lesions
1. Congenital
   (a) Osteopoikilosis.
   (b) Osteopathia striata.
   (c) Melorrheostosis.
   (d) Gardner's syndrome.
2. Acquired
   (a) Reiter's syndrome*.
   (b) SAPHO* (Synovitis, Acne, Pustulosis, Hyperostosis, Osteitis).
   (c) Lymphoma*.
   (d) Sarcoidosis*.

(e) Haemangiomatosis.
(f) Lipoatrophic diabetes mellitus.

Mixed osteolytic/osteosclerotic bone lesions

1. Gaucher's disease.
2. Psoriatic arthritis*.
3. Sapho*.
4. Reiter's syndrome*.
5. Sarcoidosis*.
6. Pancreatic bone lesions.

Tumorous lesions

1. Maffucci's syndrome – enchondromatosis + haemangiomas.
2. Fibrous dysplasia*.
3. Haemangioma.

Further Reading
Earwaker JW, Cotton A. SAPHO: syndrome or concept? Imaging findings. Skeletal Radiol 2003;32(6):311–27.

1.7 COARSE TRABECULAR PATTERN

1. Paget's disease*
2. Osteoporosis (see 1.21) } Resorption of secondary trabeculae
3. Osteomalacia* } accentuates the remaining primary trabeculae.
4. Haemoglobinopathies – especially thalassaemia*.
5. Haemangioma – especially in a vertebral body.
6. Gaucher's disease.

1.8 SKELETAL METASTASES – MOST COMMON RADIOLOGICAL APPEARANCES

Lung
1. **Carcinoma** – lytic.
2. **Carcinoid** – sclerotic.

Breast
Lytic or mixed.

Genito-urinary
1. **Renal cell carcinoma** – lytic, expansile.
2. **Wilms' tumour** – lytic.
3. **Bladder (transitional cell)** – lytic, occasionally sclerotic.
4. **Prostate** – sclerotic.

Reproductive organs
1. **Cervix** – lytic or mixed.
2. **Uterus** – lytic.
3. **Ovary** – lytic.
4. **Testis** – lytic; occasionally sclerotic.

Thyroid
Lytic, expansile.

Gastrointestinal tract
1. **Stomach** – sclerotic or mixed.
2. **Colon** – lytic; occasionally sclerotic.
3. **Rectum** – lytic.

Adrenal
1. **Phaeochromocytoma** – lytic, expansile.
2. **Carcinoma** – lytic.
3. **Neuroblastoma** – lytic; occasionally sclerotic.

Skin
1. **Squamous cell carcinoma** – lytic.
2. **Melanoma** – lytic, expansile.

Further Reading

Schmidt GP, Schoenberg SO, Schmid R et al. Screening for bone metastases: whole-body MRI using a 32-channel system versus dual-modality PET-CT. Eur Radiol 2007;17(4):939–49.

Taira AV, Herfkens RJ, Gambhir SS et al. Detection of bone metastases: assessment of integrated FDG PET/CT imaging. Radiology 2007;243 (1):204–11.

1.9 SITES OF ORIGIN OF PRIMARY BONE NEOPLASMS

(A composite diagram modified from Madewell et al., 1981.)

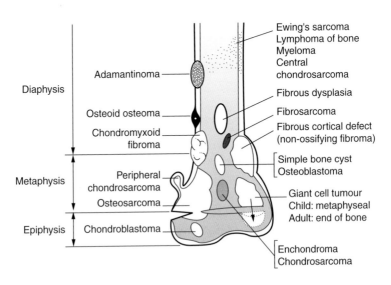

Further Reading

Madewell JE, Ragsdale BD, Sweet DE. Radiologic and pathologic analysis of solitary bone lesions. Radiol Clin North Am 1981;19:715–48.

1.10 PEAK AGE INCIDENCE OF PRIMARY BONE NEOPLASMS

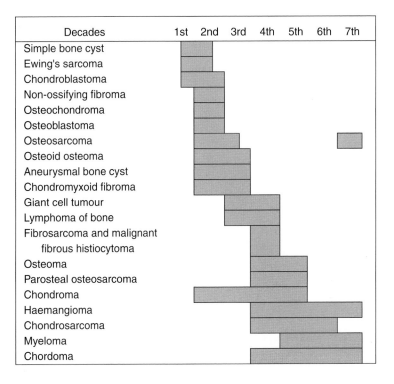

Decades	1st	2nd	3rd	4th	5th	6th	7th
Simple bone cyst							
Ewing's sarcoma							
Chondroblastoma							
Non-ossifying fibroma							
Osteochondroma							
Osteoblastoma							
Osteosarcoma							
Osteoid osteoma							
Aneurysmal bone cyst							
Chondromyxoid fibroma							
Giant cell tumour							
Lymphoma of bone							
Fibrosarcoma and malignant fibrous histiocytoma							
Osteoma							
Parosteal osteosarcoma							
Chondroma							
Haemangioma							
Chondrosarcoma							
Myeloma							
Chordoma							

1.11 LUCENT BONE LESION IN THE MEDULLA – WELL-DEFINED, MARGINAL SCLEROSIS, NO EXPANSION

Indicates a slowly progressing lesion.

1. **Geode** – a subarticular cyst. Other signs of arthritis. See 1.16.
2. **Healing benign or malignant bone lesion** – e.g. metastasis, eosinophilic granuloma or brown tumour.
3. **Brodie's abscess.**
4. **Benign bone neoplasms**
    (a) Simple bone cyst*.
    (b) Enchondroma*.
    (c) Chondroblastoma*.
5. **Fibrous dysplasia*.**

1.12 LUCENT BONE LESION IN THE MEDULLA – WELL-DEFINED, NO MARGINAL SCLEROSIS, NO EXPANSION

The absence of reactive bone formation implies a fast growth rate.

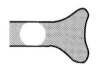

1. **Metastasis** – especially from breast, bronchus, kidney or thyroid.
2. **Multiple myeloma*.**
3. **Eosinophilic granuloma*.**
4. **Brown tumour of hyperparathyroidism*.**
5. **Benign bone neoplasms**
    (a) Enchondroma*.
    (b) Chondroblastoma*.

1.13 LUCENT BONE LESION IN THE MEDULLA – ILL-DEFINED

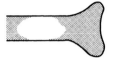

An aggressive pattern of destruction.

1. Metastasis.
2. Multiple myeloma*.
3. Osteomyelitis.
4. Lymphoma of bone.
5. Long bone sarcomas
    (a) Osteosarcoma*.
    (b) Ewing's sarcoma*.
    (c) Central chondrosarcoma*.
    (d) Fibrosarcoma and malignant fibrous histiocytoma.

Further Reading

Heyning FH, Kroon HM, Hogendoorn PC et al. MR imaging characteristics in primary lymphoma of bone with emphasis on non-aggressive appearance. Skeletal Radiol 2007;36(10):937–44.

Mellado Santos JM. Diagnostic imaging of pediatric hematogenous osteomyelitis: lessons learned from a multi-modality approach. Eur Radiol 2006;16(9):2109–19.

Tehranzadeh J, Wong E, Wang F et al. Imaging of osteomyelitis in the mature skeleton. Radiol Clin North Am 2001;39(2):223–50.

1.14 LUCENT BONE LESION IN THE MEDULLA – WELL-DEFINED, ECCENTRIC EXPANSION

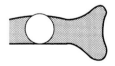

1. Giant cell tumour*.
2. Aneurysmal bone cyst*.
3. Enchondroma*.
4. Non-ossifying fibroma (fibrous cortical defect)*.
5. Chondromyxoid fibroma*.

1.15 LUCENT BONE LESION – GROSSLY EXPANSILE

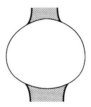

Malignant bone neoplasms

1. **Metastases** – renal cell carcinoma and thyroid; less commonly melanoma, bronchus, breast and phaeochromocytoma.
2. **Plasmacytoma*.**
3. **Central chondrosarcoma/lymphoma of bone/fibrosarcoma** – when slow growing may have this appearance.
4. **Telangiectatic osteosarcoma*.**

Benign bone neoplasms

1. **Aneurysmal bone cyst*.**
2. **Giant cell tumour*.**
3. **Enchondroma*.**

Non-neoplastic

1. **Fibrous dysplasia*.**
2. **Haemophilic pseudotumour** (see Haemophilia*) – especially in the iliac wing and lower limb bones. Soft-tissue swelling. ± Haemophilic arthropathy.
3. **Brown tumour of hyperparathyroidism*.**
4. **Hydatid.**

1.16 SUBARTICULAR LUCENT BONE LESION

Arthritides

1. **Osteoarthritis** – may be multiple 'cysts' in the load-bearing areas of multiple joints. Surrounding sclerotic margin. Joint-space narrowing, subchondral sclerosis and osteophytes.
2. **Rheumatoid arthritis*** – no sclerotic margin. Begins periarticularly near the insertion of the joint capsule. Joint-space narrowing and juxta-articular osteoporosis.
3. **Calcium pyrophosphate arthropathy** (see Calcium pyrophosphate dihydrate deposition disease*) – similar to osteoarthritis but frequently larger and with more collapse and fragmentation of the articular surface.
4. **Gout** – ± erosions with overhanging edges and adjacent soft-tissue masses.
5. **Haemophilia*.**

Neoplastic

1. **Metastases/multiple myeloma***
2. **Aneurysmal bone cyst*** – solitary.
3. **Giant cell tumour*** – solitary.
4. **Chondroblastoma*** – solitary.
5. **Pigmented villonodular synovitis***

Others

1. **Post-traumatic** – particularly in the carpal bones. Well-defined.
2. **Osteonecrosis** – with bone sclerosis, collapse and fragmentation. Preservation of joint space.
3. **Tuberculosis** – wholly epiphyseal or partly metaphyseal. Well-defined or ill-defined. No surrounding sclerosis.

Further Reading
Bullough PG, Bansal M. The differential diagnosis of geodes. Radiol Clin North Am 1988;26:1165–84.

1.17 LUCENT BONE LESION – CONTAINING CALCIUM OR BONE

Neoplastic

1. **Metastases** – especially from breast.
2. **Cartilage neoplasms**
   (a) Benign – enchondroma, chondroblastoma and chondromyxoid fibroma.
   (b) Malignant – chondrosarcoma.
3. **Bone (osteoid) neoplasms**
   (a) Benign – osteoid osteoma and osteoblastoma.
   (b) Malignant – osteosarcoma.
4. **Fibrous-tissue neoplasms**
   (a) Malignant – fibrosarcoma and malignant fibrous histiocytoma.

Others

1. **Fibrous dysplasia***.
2. **Osteoporosis circumscripta** (Paget's disease*).
3. **Avascular necrosis and bone infarction.**
4. **Osteomyelitis** – with sequestrum.
5. **Eosinophilic granuloma***.
6. **Intraosseous lipoma.**

1.18 'MOTH-EATEN BONE' IN AN ADULT

Multiple scattered lucencies of variable size with no major central lesion. Coalescence may occur later. Cancellous and/or cortical bone is involved.

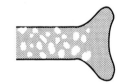

See also 14.12.

Neoplastic

1. **Metastases.**
2. **Multiple myeloma***.
3. **Leukaemia** – consider when there is involvement of an entire bone or a neighbouring bone with low signal on T_1W and high signal on T_2W and short tau inversion recovery (STIR) MRI.
4. **Long-bone sarcomas**
   (a) Ewing's sarcoma*.
   (b) Lymphoma of bone.

(c) Osteosarcoma*.
(d) Chondrosarcoma*.
(e) Fibrosarcoma and malignant fibrous histiocytoma.
5. **Langerhans cell histiocytosis***.

Infective

1. **Acute osteomyelitis.**

Further Reading

Tehranzadeh J, Wong E, Wang F et al. Imaging of osteomyelitis in the mature skeleton. Radiol Clin North Am 2001;39(2):223–50.

1.19 REGIONAL OSTEOPENIA

Decreased bone density confined to a region or segment of the appendicular skeleton.

1. **Disuse** – during the immobilization of fractures, in paralyzed segments and in bone and joint infections. Usually appears after 8 weeks of immobilization. The patterns of bone loss may be uniform (commonest), spotty (mostly periarticular), band-like (subchondral or metaphyseal) or endosteal cortical scalloping and linear cortical lucencies.
2. **Sudeck's atrophy** (reflex sympathetic dystrophy syndrome) – is mediated via a neurovascular mechanism and associated with post-traumatic and postinfective states, myocardial infarction, calcific tendinosis and cervical spondylosis. It most commonly affects the shoulder and hand and develops rapidly. Pain and soft-tissue swelling are clinical findings.
3. **Transient osteoporosis of the hip** – a severe, progressive osteoporosis of the femoral head and, to a lesser degree, of the femoral neck and acetabulum. Full recovery is seen in 6 months.
4. **Regional migratory osteoporosis** – pain, swelling and osteoporosis affect the joints of the lower limbs in particular. The migratory nature differentiates it from other causes. Marrow oedema in affected areas is seen as low signal on T_1W and high signal on T_2W MRI.

1.20 GENERALIZED OSTEOPENIA

1. **Osteoporosis** – diminished quantity of normal bone.
2. **Osteomalacia*** – normal quantity of bone but it has an excess of uncalcified osteoid.
3. **Hyperparathyroidism*** – increased bone resorption by osteoclasts.
4. **Diffuse infiltrative bone disease** – e.g. multiple myeloma and leukaemia.

Further Reading
Mayo-Smith W, Rosenthal DI. Radiographic appearance of osteopenia. Radiol Clin North Am 1991;29(1):37–47.

1.21 OSTEOPOROSIS

1. **Decreased bone density.**
2. **Cortical thinning** with a relative increase in density of the cortex and vertebral end-plates. Skull sutures are relatively sclerotic.
3. **Relative accentuation of trabecular stress lines** because of resorption of secondary trabeculae.
4. **Brittle bones** with an increased incidence of fractures, especially compression fractures of vertebral bodies, femoral neck and wrist fractures.

Endocrine

1. **Hypogonadism**
   (a) Ovarian – postmenopausal, Turner's syndrome*.
   (b) Testicular – eunuchoidism.
2. **Cushing's syndrome***.
3. **Diabetes mellitus.**
4. **Acromegaly***.
5. **Addison's disease.**
6. **Hyperthyroidism.**
7. **Mastocytosis** – mast cells produce heparin.

Disuse
Iatrogenic

1. **Steroids***.
2. **Heparin.**

Deficiency states
1. **Vitamin C** (scurvy*).
2. **Protein.**

Idiopathic
1. **In young people** – a rare self-limiting condition occurring in children of 8–12 years. Spontaneous improvement is seen.

Congenital
1. **Osteogenesis imperfecta*.**
2. **Turner's syndrome*.**
3. **Homocystinuria*.**
4. **Neuromuscular diseases.**
5. **Mucopolysaccharidoses.**
6. **Trisomy 13 and 18.**
7. **Pseudohypoparathyroidism and pseudopseudohypoparathyroidism*.**
8. **Glycogen storage diseases.**
9. **Progeria.**

Further Reading
Herman TE, McAlister WH. Inherited diseases in bone density in children. Radiol Clin North Am 1991;29(1):149–64.
Theodorou SJ, Theodorou DJ, Sartoris DJ. Osteoporosis: a global assessment of clinical and imaging features. Orthopedics 2005;28(11):1346–53.

1.22 OSTEOMALACIA AND RICKETS*

Vitamin D deficiency
1. **Dietary.**
2. **Malabsorption.**

Renal disease
1. **Glomerular disease** (renal osteodystrophy*).
2. **Tubular disease**
    (a) Renal tubular acidosis.
        (i) Primary – sporadic or hereditary.
        (ii) Secondary.
            – Inborn errors of metabolism, e.g. cystinosis, galactosaemia, Wilson's disease, tyrosinosis, hereditary fructose intolerance.
            – Poisoning, e.g. lead, cadmium, beryllium.

- Drugs, e.g. amphotericin B, lithium salts, outdated tetracycline, ifosfamide.
- Renal transplantation.

(b) Fanconi syndrome – osteomalacia or rickets, growth retardation, renal tubular acidosis (RTA), glycosuria, phosphaturia, aminoaciduria and proteinuria. It is most commonly idiopathic in aetiology but may be secondary to those causes of RTA given above.

(c) Vitamin D-resistant rickets (familial hypophosphataemia, X-linked hypophosphataemia) – short stature developing after the first 6 months of life, genu varum or valgum, coxa vara, waddling gait. Radiographic changes are more severe in the legs than the arms.

Hepatic disease

1. **Parenchymal failure.**
2. **Obstructive jaundice** – especially biliary atresia.

Vitamin D-dependent rickets – see below

Anticonvulsants

1. **Phenytoin and phenobarbitone.**

Tumour-associated

1. **Soft tissues** – haemangiopericytoma.
2. **Bone** – non-ossifying fibroma, giant cell tumour, osteoblastoma, osteosarcoma (and fibrous dysplasia, neurofibromatosis and melorrheostosis).

Conditions which mimic rickets/osteomalacia

1. **Hypophosphatasia*** – low serum alkaline phosphatase.
2. **Metaphyseal chondrodysplasia** (type Schmid) – normal serum phosphate, calcium and alkaline phosphatase differentiate it from other rachitic syndromes.

If the patient is less than 6 months of age then consider:

1. **Biliary atresia.**
2. **Metabolic bone disease of prematurity** – combined dietary deficiency and hepatic hydroxylation of vitamin D.
3. **Hypophosphatasia*.**
4. **Vitamin D-dependent rickets** – rachitic changes are associated with a severe myopathy in spite of adequate dietary intake of vitamin D.

Further Reading

Edmister KA, Sundaram M. Oncogenic osteomalacia. Semin Musculoskelet Radiol 2002;6(3):191–6.

Herman TE, McAlister WH. Inherited diseases in bone density in children. Radiol Clin North Am 1991;29(1):149–64.

1.23 PERIOSTEAL REACTIONS – TYPES

(Modified from Ragsdale et al., 1981.)

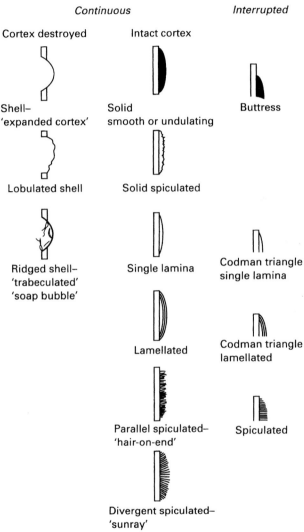

The different types are, in general, non-specific, having multiple aetiologies. However, the following comments can be made.

Continuous with destroyed cortex

This is the result of an expanding lesion. See 1.14 and 1.15.

Parallel spiculated ('hair-on-end')

1. Ewing's sarcoma*.
2. Syphilis.
3. Infantile cortical hyperostosis (Caffey's disease).

See 12.58 for causes in the skull vault.

Divergent spiculated ('sunray')

1. Osteosarcoma*.
2. Metastases – especially from sigmoid colon and rectum.
3. Ewing's sarcoma*.
4. Haemangioma*.
5. Meningioma.
6. Tuberculosis.
7. Tropical ulcer.

Codman angle (single lamina or lamellated)

1. Aggressive malignant tissue extending into soft tissue.
2. Infection – occasionally.

Further Reading

Ragsdale BD, Madewell JE, Sweet DE. Radiologic and pathologic analysis of solitary bone lesions. Part II: Periosteal reactions. Radiol Clin North Am 1981;19:749–83.

1.24 PERIOSTEAL REACTIONS – SOLITARY AND LOCALIZED

1. Traumatic.
2. Inflammatory.
3. Neoplastic
   (a) Malignant.
       (i) primary.
       (ii) secondary.
   (b) Benign – an expanding shell or complicated by a fracture.

Further Reading

Wenaden AE, Szyszko TA, Saifuddin A. Imaging of periosteal reactions associated with focal lesions of bone. Clin Radiol 2005;60(4):439–56.

1.25 PERIOSTEAL REACTIONS – BILATERALLY SYMMETRICAL IN ADULTS

1. **Hypertrophic osteoarthropathy** (HOA) – the condition can be caused by the conditions in section 1.27.
2. **Pachydermoperiostosis.**
3. **Vascular insufficiency** (venous, lymphatic or arterial).
4. **Thyroid acropachy.**
5. **Fluorosis.**
6. **Diffuse idiopathic skeletal hyperostosis** (DISH; Forestier Disease).

Further Reading

Pineda CJ, Sartoris DJ, Clopton P et al. Periostitis in hypertrophic osteoarthropathy: relationship to disease duration. Am J Roentgenol 1987;148:773–8.

Vanhoenacker FM. Thyroid acropachy: correlation of imaging and pathology. Eur Radiol 2001;11:1058–62.

1.26 PERIOSTEAL REACTIONS – BILATERALLY ASYMMETRICAL

1. **Metastases.**
2. **Osteomyelitis.**
3. **Arthritides** – especially Reiter's syndrome* and psoriatic arthropathy*.
4. **Osteoporosis** (q.v.)   } because of the increased
5. **Osteomalacia** (q.v.)   } liability to fractures.
6. **Non-accidental injury*.**
7. **Bleeding diatheses.**
8. **Hand-foot syndrome** (sickle-cell dactylitis) – see Sickle-cell anaemia*.

Further Reading

Jurriaans E, Singh NP, Finlay K et al. Imaging of chronic recurrent multifocal osteomyelitis. Radiol Clin North Am 2001;39(2):305–27.

1.27 HYPERTROPHIC OSTEOARTHROPATHY

Pulmonary

1. **Carcinoma of bronchus.**
2. **Lymphoma*.**
3. **Abscess.**
4. **Bronchiectasis** – frequently due to cystic fibrosis*.
5. **Metastases.**

Pleural

1. **Pleural fibroma** – has the highest incidence of accompanying HOA, although it is itself a rare cause.
2. **Mesothelioma.**

Cardiovascular

1. **Cyanotic congenital heart disease** – produces clubbing but only rarely a periosteal reaction.

Gastrointestinal

1. **Ulcerative colitis*.**
2. **Crohn's disease*.**
3. **Dysentery** – amoebic or bacillary.
4. **Lymphoma*.**
5. **Whipple's disease.**
6. **Coeliac disease.**
7. **Cirrhosis** – especially primary biliary cirrhosis.
8. **Nasopharyngeal carcinomas** (Schmincke's tumour).
9. **Juvenile polyposis.**

1.28 EXCESSIVE CALLUS FORMATION

1. **Steroid therapy and Cushing's syndrome*.**
2. **Neuropathic arthropathy*** – including congenital insensitivity to pain.
3. **Osteogenesis imperfecta*.**
4. **Non-accidental injury*.**
5. **Paralytic states.**
6. **Renal osteodystrophy*.**
7. **Multiple myeloma*.**

1.29 STRESS FRACTURES – SITES AND CAUSATIONS

(Modified from Daffner, 1978.)

Site	Activity
Lower cervical/upper thoracic spinous processes	Clay shovelling
Pars interarticularis	Ballet; heavy lifting; scrubbing floors
Obturator ring	Stooping; bowling; gymnastics
Ribs	Carrying heavy pack; coughing; golf
Coracoid process of scapula	Trap shooting
Humerus – distal shaft	Throwing a ball
Hamate	Golf; tennis; baseball
Ulna – coronoid	Pitching a ball
Ulna – shaft	Pitchfork worker; propelling a wheelchair
Femur – neck	Ballet; marching; long-distance running; gymnastics
Femur – shaft	Ballet; long distance running
Patella	Hurdling
Fibula – proximal shaft	Jumping; parachuting
Fibula – distal shaft	Long distance running
Tibia – proximal shaft	Running
Tibia – mid and distal shaft	Ballet; long distance running
Calcaneus	Jumping; parachuting; prolonged standing
Navicular	Marching; long distance running
Metatarsal – shaft	Marching; prolonged standing; ballet
Sesamoids of metatarsals	Prolonged standing

Further Reading

Daffner RH. Stress fractures: current concepts. Skeletal Radiol 1978;2:221–9.

Fayad LM, Kamel IR, Kawamoto S et al. Distinguishing stress fractures from pathologic fractures: a multimodality approach. Skeletal Radiol 2005; 34(5):245–59.

1.30 AVASCULAR NECROSIS

Toxic

1. **Steroids*** – probably does not occur with less than 2 years of treatment.
2. **Alcohol** – possibly because of fat emboli in chronic alcoholic pancreatitis.
3. **Immunosuppressives.**
4. **Anti-inflammatory drugs** – indomethacin and phenylbutazone.

Traumatic

1. **Idiopathic** – e.g. Perthes' disease and other osteochondritides.
2. **Fractures** – especially femoral neck, talus and scaphoid.
3. **Radiotherapy.**
4. **Heat** – burns.
5. **Fat embolism.**

Inflammatory

1. **Rheumatoid arthritis*** } in the absence of drugs
2. **Systemic lupus erythematosus*** } probably due to a vasculitis.
3. **Scleroderma*.**
4. **Infection** – e.g. following a pyogenic arthritis.
5. **Pancreatitis.**

Metabolic and endocrine

1. **Pregnancy.**
2. **Diabetes.**
3. **Cushing's syndrome*.**
4. **Hyperlipidaemias.**
5. **Gout*.**

Haemopoietic disorders

1. **Haemoglobinopathies** – especially sickle-cell anaemia*.
2. **Polycythaemia rubra vera.**
3. **Gaucher's disease.**
4. **Haemophilia*.**

Thrombotic and embolic

1. **Dysbaric osteonecrosis.**
2. **Arteritis.**

1.31 EROSIONS OF THE MEDIAL METAPHYSIS OF THE PROXIMAL HUMERUS

1. Normal variant.
2. Leukaemia.
3. Metastatic neuroblastoma.
4. Gaucher's disease.
5. Hurler's syndrome*.
6. Glycogen storage disease.
7. Niemann–Pick disease.
8. Hyperparathyroidism.
9. Rheumatoid arthritis.

1.32 EROSION OR ABSENCE OF THE OUTER END OF THE CLAVICLE

1. Rheumatoid arthritis*.
2. Post-traumatic osteolysis
3. Multiple myeloma*.
4. Metastasis.
5. Hyperparathyroidism*.
6. Cleidocranial dysplasia*.
7. Pyknodysostosis.

1.33 FOCAL RIB LESION (SOLITARY OR MULTIPLE)

Neoplastic

Secondary more common than primary. Primary malignant more common than benign.

1. **Metastases**
   (a) Adult male – bronchus, kidney or prostate most commonly.
   (b) Adult female – breast.
2. **Primary malignant**
   (a) Multiple myeloma/plasmacytoma*.
   (b) Chondrosarcoma*.
   (c) Askin tumour – uncommon tumour of an intercostal nerve causing rib destruction.

3. **Benign**
   (a) Osteochondroma*.
   (b) Enchondroma*.
   (c) Langerhans cell histiocytosis*.

Non-neoplastic

1. **Healed rib fracture.**
2. **Fibrous dysplasia.**
3. **Paget's disease*.**
4. **Brown tumour of hyperparathyroidism*.**
5. **Osteomyelitis** – bacterial, tuberculous or fungal.

Further Reading

Guttentag AR, Salwen JK. Keep your eyes on the ribs: the spectrum of normal variants and diseases that involve the ribs. Radiographics 1999;19:1125–42.

Omell GH, Anderson LS, Bramson RT. Chest wall tumours. Radiol Clin North Am 1973;11:197–214.

1.34 RIB NOTCHING – INFERIOR SURFACE

Arterial

1. **Coarctation of the aorta** – rib signs are unusual before 10 years of age. Affects 4th–8th ribs bilaterally; not the upper two if conventional. Unilateral and right-sided if the coarctation is proximal to the left subclavian artery. Unilateral and left-sided if associated with an anomalous right subclavian artery distal to the coarctation. Other signs include a prominent ascending aorta and a small descending aorta with an intervening notch, left ventricular enlargement and possibly signs of heart failure.
2. **Aortic thrombosis** – usually the lower ribs bilaterally.
3. **Subclavian obstruction** – most commonly after a Blalock operation (either subclavian-to-pulmonary artery anastomosis) for Fallot's tetralogy. Unilateral rib notching of the upper three or four ribs on the operation side.
4. **Pulmonary oligaemia** – any cause of decreased pulmonary blood supply.

Venous

1. **Superior vena caval obstruction.**

Arteriovenous

1. **Pulmonary arteriovenous malformation.**
2. **Chest wall arteriovenous malformation.**

Neurogenic

1. **Neurofibromatosis*** – 'ribbon ribs' may also be a feature.

Further Reading
Boone ML, Swenson BE, Felson B. Rib notching: its many causes. Am J
  Roentgenol 1964;91:1075–88.

1.35 RIB NOTCHING – SUPERIOR SURFACE

Connective tissue diseases
1. **Rheumatoid arthritis*.**
2. **Systemic lupus erythematosus*.**
3. **Scleroderma*.**
4. **Sjögren's syndrome.**

Metabolic
1. **Hyperparathyroidism*.**

Miscellaneous
1. **Neurofibromatosis*.**
2. **Restrictive lung disease.**
3. **Poliomyelitis.**
4. **Marfan's syndrome*.**
5. **Osteogenesis imperfecta*.**
6. **Progeria.**

1.36 WIDE OR THICK RIBS

1. **Chronic anaemias** – due to marrow hyperplasia.
2. **Fibrous dysplasia*.**
3. **Paget's disease*.**
4. **Healed fractures with callus.**
5. **Achondroplasia*.**
6. **Mucopolysaccharidoses.**

1.37 MADELUNG DEFORMITY

A deformity which comprises: (a) short distal radius which shows a dorsal and ulnar curve; (b) triangular shape of the distal radial epiphysis; (c) premature fusion of the ulnar side of the distal radial epiphysis; (d) dorsal subluxation of the distal ulna; (e) enlarged and distorted ulnar head; and (f) wedging of the triangular-shaped carpus between the distal radius and ulna.

1. **Isolated** – bilateral > unilateral. Asymmetrical. Predominantly adolescent or young adult women.
2. **Dyschondrosteosis** (Leri–Weil disease) – bilateral with mesomelic limb shortening. AD. Predominantly men.
3. **Diaphyseal aclasis.**
4. **Turner's syndrome*.**
5. **Post-traumatic.**
6. **Postinfective.**

1.38 CARPAL FUSION

Isolated

Tends to involve bones in the same carpal row (proximal or distal). More common in Afro-Caribbeans than Caucasians.

1. **Triquetral-lunate** – the most common site. Affects 1% of the population.
2. **Capitate-hamate.**
3. **Trapezium-trapezoid.**

Syndrome-related

Tends to exhibit massive carpal fusion affecting bones in different rows (proximal and distal).

1. **Acrocephalosyndactyly** (Apert's syndrome).
2. **Arthrogryposis multiplex congenita.**
3. **Ellis–van Creveld syndrome.**
4. **Holt–Oram syndrome.**
5. **Turner's syndrome*.**
6. **Symphalangism.**

Acquired

1. **Inflammatory arthritides** – especially juvenile idiopathic arthritis* and rheumatoid arthritis*.

2. Pyogenic arthritis.
3. Chronic tuberculous arthritis.
4. Post-traumatic.
5. Post-surgical.

Further Reading
Cope JR. Carpal coalition. Clin. Radiol 1974;25:261–6.

1.39 SHORT METACARPAL(S) OR METATARSAL(S)

As the sole or predominant abnormality.

1. **Idiopathic.**
2. **Post-traumatic** – iatrogenic, fracture, growth plate injury, thermal or electrical.
3. **Postinfarction** – e.g. sickle-cell anaemia*.
4. **Turner's syndrome*** – 4th ± 3rd and 5th metacarpals.
5. **Pseudohypoparathyroidism and pseudopseudohypoparathyroidism*** – 4th and 5th metacarpals.

Further Reading
Poznanski AK. The Hand in Radiologic Diagnosis, 2nd edn, Vol. 1. WB Saunders, Philadelphia, 1984, pp209–62.

1.40 ARACHNODACTYLY

Elongated and slender tubular bones of the hands and feet. The metacarpal index is an aid to diagnosis and is estimated by measuring the lengths of the 2nd, 3rd, 4th and 5th metacarpals and dividing by their breadths taken at the exact mid-points. These four figures are then added together and divided by 4.
Normal range 5.4–7.9.
Arachnodactyly range 8.4–10.4.
The metacarpal index is a poor discriminator between Marfan's syndrome and constitutional tall stature.

1. **Marfan's syndrome*** – although arachnodactyly is not necessary for the diagnosis.
2. **Homocystinuria*** – morphologically resembles Marfan's syndrome but 60% are mentally handicapped, they have a predisposition to arterial and venous thromboses and the lens of the eye dislocates downward rather than upward.

Further Reading

Eldridge R. The metacarpal index: a useful aid in the diagnosis of the Marfan syndrome. Arch Intern Med 1964;113:14–16.

Nelle M, Tröger J, Rupprath G et al. Metacarpal index in Marfan's syndrome and in constitutional tall stature. Arch Dis Child 1994;70:149–50.

1.41 DISTAL PHALANGEAL DESTRUCTION

NB. Because of reinforced Sharpey's fibres periosteal reaction is rare at this site.

Resorption of the tuft

1. **Scleroderma*.**
2. **Raynaud's disease.**
3. **Psoriatic arthropathy*** – can precede the skin changes.
4. **Neuropathic diseases** – diabetes mellitus, leprosy, myelomeningocoele, syringomyelia and congenital indifference to pain.
5. **Thermal injuries** – burns, frostbite and electrical.
6. **Trauma.**
7. **Hyperparathyroidism*.**
8. **Epidermolysis bullosa.**
9. **Porphyria** – due to cutaneous photosensitivity leading to blistering and scarring.
10. **Phenytoin toxicity** – congenitally in infants of epileptic mothers.
11. **Snake and scorpion venom** – due to tissue breakdown by proteinases.

Resorption of the mid-portion

1. **Polyvinyl chloride tank cleaners.**
2. **Acro-osteolysis of Hajdu and Cheney.**
3. **Hyperparathyroidism*.**

Periarticular

i.e. erosion of the distal interphalangeal joints

1. **Psoriatic arthropathy*.**
2. **Erosive osteoarthritis.**
3. **Hyperparathyroidism*.**
4. **Thermal injuries.**
5. **Scleroderma*.**
6. **Multicentric reticulohistiocytosis.**

Poorly defined lytic lesions

1. **Osteomyelitis** – mostly staphylococcal with diabetics at particular risk. Periosteal reaction is infrequent.
2. **Metastases** – bronchus is the most common primary site. Bone metastases to the hand are commonest in the terminal phalanx and may be the only metastasis to bone. The subarticular cortex is usually the last to be destroyed.
3. **Multiple myeloma***.
4. **Aneurysmal bone cyst*** – rare at this site. Marked thinning and expansion of cortex.
5. **Giant cell tumour*** – usually involving the base of the phalanx.
6. **Leprosy** – at any age, but 30% present before 15 years of age.

Well-defined lytic lesions

1. **Implantation dermoid/epidermoid cyst** – an expanding lesion. 1–20mm, with minimal sclerosis ± soft-tissue swelling.
2. **Enchondroma***.
3. **Sarcoidosis*** – associated 'lace-like' destruction of phalangeal shaft, subperiosteal erosion leading to resorption of terminal tufts and endosteal sclerosis.
4. **Glomus tumour** – soft-tissue swelling with disuse osteoporosis because of pain. Bone involvement is uncommon but there may be pressure erosion or a well-defined lytic lesion.
5. **Osteoid osteoma***.
6. **Fibrous dysplasia***.

Further Reading

Jones SN, Stoker DJ. Radiology at your fingertips; lesions of the terminal phalanx. Clin Radiol 1988;39:478–85.

1.42 FLUID-FLUID LEVELS IN BONE LESIONS ON CT AND MRI

Benign

1. Aneurysmal bone cyst*.
2. Chondroblastoma*.
3. Giant cell tumour*.
4. Simple bone cyst*.
5. Fibrous dysplasia*.

Malignant

1. Telangiectatic osteosarcoma*.
2. Malignant fibrous histiocytoma.
3. Any necrotic bone tumour.

1.43 INCREASED UPTAKE ON BONE SCANS

1. **Metastatic disease** – multiple, randomly scattered lesions especially in the axial skeleton.
2. **Joint disease** – commonly degenerative in the cervical spine, hips, hands and knees. Also inflammatory joint disease.
3. **Traumatic fractures**
   (a) Aligned fractures in ribs are traumatic.
   (b) Single lesions elsewhere – always ask if history of trauma.
   (c) Stress fractures.
4. **Post surgery** – after joint replacement. Increased uptake lasts 1 year.
5. **Paget's disease*** – diffuse involvement with much increased uptake often starting from bone end. Commonly affects the pelvis, skull, femur and spine. Involvement of the whole of the vertebra is typical.
6. **Superscan** – high uptake throughout the skeleton often due to disseminated secondary disease with poor or absent renal images but often with bladder activity.
7. **Metabolic bone disease** – high uptake in the axial skeleton, proximal long bones, with prominent calvarium and mandible. Faint or absent kidney images.
8. **Dental disease** – inflammation, recent extraction.
9. **Infection** – increased uptake in vascular and blood pool phases also.
10. See 1.44.

1.44 INCREASED UPTAKE ON BONE SCANS NOT DUE TO SKELETAL ABNORMALITY

Artefacts

These are common.

1. **Patient**
   (a) Beware of urine contamination.
   (b) Sweat – axillae.
   (c) Injection site.
   (d) Scars of recent operations.
   (e) Breast – accentuation of ribs at the lower border of the breast.
2. **Equipment**
   (a) Edge effect – increase in intensity at the edge of the field of view, especially in vertebrae.
   (b) Contamination of the collimator or crystal – check using a uniformity source.

Physiological variants

1. **Epiphyses in children.**
2. **Inferior angle of the scapula.**
3. **Calcification of cartilages** – especially those in the ribs and anterior neck.
4. **Bladder diverticulum.**
5. **Nipples** – especially confusing if at different heights.
6. **Renal pelvis.**

Soft-tissue uptake

1. **Calcification**
   (a) Myositis ossificans.
   (b) Soft-tissue osseous metaplasia.
   (c) Soft-tissue tumours with calcification.
   (d) Vascular calcification.
   (e) Calcific tendonitis.
   (f) Abscess.
2. **Others**
   (a) Acute infarction of the myocardium, cerebrum, skeletal muscle.
   (b) Malignant pleural effusion.
   (c) Inflammatory carcinoma of the breast.
   (d) Hepatic necrosis.
   (e) Hepatic metastases – colon, breast, oat-cell carcinoma.
   (f) Tumour uptake.

Visualization of normal organs

1. **Free pertechnetate** – thyroid, stomach, salivary glands.
2. **Colloid formation** – liver, spleen and sometimes lung.
3. **Study on the previous day.**

1.45 PHOTOPENIC AREAS (DEFECTS) ON BONE SCANS

1. **Artefacts** – the commonest cause.
   (a) External – metal objects such as coins, belts, lockets, buckles.
   (b) Internal – joint prosthesis, pacemakers.
2. **Avascular lesions** – for example cysts.
3. **Multiple myeloma*** – may show increased uptake.
4. **Metastases** – lytic: renal, thyroid, lung.
5. **Leukaemia** – may show increased uptake.
6. **Haemangiomas of the spine** – occasionally slightly increased uptake.
7. **Radiotherapy fields** – usually oblong in shape.

Spine

Steven James

2.1 SCOLIOSIS

Idiopathic

2% prevalence for curves $> 10°$.

1. **Infantile** – diagnosed before the age of 4 years. 90% are thoracic and concave to the right. More common in boys. 90% resolve spontaneously.
2. **Juvenile** – diagnosed between 4 and 9 years. More common in girls. Almost always progressive.
3. **Adolescent** – diagnosed between 10 years and maturity. More common in females. Majority are concave to the left in the thoracic region.

Congenital

Prognosis is dependent on the anatomical abnormality and a classification (see figure opposite) is, therefore, important.

Failure of Formation. A. Incarcerated hemivertebra. A straight spine with little tendency to progression. **B. Free hemivertebra.** May be progressive. **C. Wedge vertebra.** Better prognosis than a free hemivertebra. **D. Multiple hemivertebrae.** Failure of formation on the same side results in a severe curve. Hemivertebrae on opposite sides may compensate each other. **E. Central defect.** Butterfly vertebra.

Failure of Segmentation. A. Bilateral → block vertebra and a short spine, e.g. Klippel–Feil. **B. Unilateral unsegmented bar.** Severely progressive curve with varying degrees of kyphosis or lordosis depending on the position of the bar.

Mixed Defects. A. Unilateral unsegmented bar and a hemivertebra. Severely progressive. **B. Partially segmented incarcerated hemivertebra. C. Bilateral failure of segmentation incorporating a hemivertebra.**

Indicators of serious progression are:

(a) Deformity present at birth.
(b) Severe deformity of the chest wall.
(c) Unilateral unsegmented bars.
(d) Thoracic abnormality.

Associated abnormalities may occur – urinary tract (18%), congenital heart disease (7%), undescended scapulae (6%) and diastematomyelia (5%).

FAILURE OF FORMATION

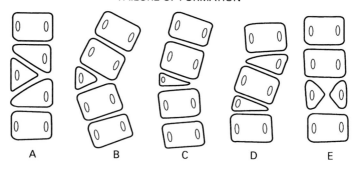

A   B   C   D   E

FAILURE OF SEGMENTATION

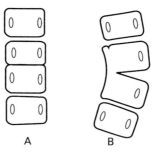

A   B

MIXED
e.g.

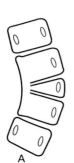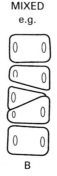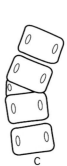

A   B   C

Neuropathic disorders

1. Tethered cord.
2. Syringomyelia.
3. Chiari malformations.
4. Diastematomyelia.
5. Meningocoele/myelomeningocoele.

Neuromuscular diseases

1. Myelomeningocoele.
2. Spinal muscular atrophy.
3. Friedreich's ataxia.
4. Poliomyelitis.
5. Cerebral palsy.
6. Muscular dystrophy.

Mesodermal and neuroectodermal diseases

1. **Neurofibromatosis*** – in up to 40% of patients. Classically a sharply angled short segment scoliosis with a severe kyphosis. The apical vertebrae are irregular and wedged with adjacent dysplastic ribs. 25% have a congenital vertebral anomaly.
2. **Marfan's syndrome*** – scoliosis in 40–60%. Double structural curves are typical.
3. **Homocystinuria*** – similar to Marfan's syndrome.
4. **Other skeletal dysplasias** – spondyloepiphyseal dysplasia congenita, spondyloepimetaphyseal dysplasia, pseudoachondroplasia, metatropic dwarfism, diastrophic dwarfism, Kniest disease, spondylocostal dysostosis.

Post radiotherapy

Wedged and hypoplastic vertebrae ± unilateral pelvic or rib hypoplasia.

Leg length discrepancy

A flexible lumbar curve, convex to the side of the shorter leg. Disparity of iliac crest level.

Painful scoliosis

1. **Osteoid osteoma*** – 10% occur in the spine. A lamina or pedicle at the apex of the curve will be sclerotic or overgrown.
2. **Osteoblastoma***.
3. **Intraspinal tumour** (see 2.16).
4. **Infection**.

Further Reading

Cassar-Pullicino VN, Eisenstein SM. Imaging in scoliosis: what, why and how? Clin Radiol 2002;57(7):543–562.

Hedequist D, Emans J. Congenital scoliosis: a review and update. J Pediatr Orthop 2007;7(1):106–116.

Van Goethem J, Van Campenhout A, van den Hauwe L et al. Scoliosis. Neuroimaging Clin N Am 2007;17(1):105–115.

2.2 SOLITARY COLLAPSED VERTEBRA

1. **Neoplastic disease**
   - **(a)** Metastasis – breast, bronchus, prostate, kidney and thyroid account for the majority of patients with a solitary spinal metastasis. The disc spaces are preserved until late. The bone may be lytic, sclerotic or mixed. ± destruction of a pedicle.
   - **(b)** Multiple myeloma/plasmacytoma* – a common site, especially for plasmacytoma. May mimic an osteolytic metastasis or be expansile and resemble an aneurysmal bone cyst.
   - **(c)** Lymphoma*.
2. **Osteoporosis** (q.v.) – generalized osteopenia. Coarsened trabecular pattern in adjacent vertebrae due to resorption of secondary trabeculae.
3. **Trauma.**
4. **Infection** – with destruction of vertebral end-plates and adjacent disc spaces.
5. **Langerhans cell histiocytosis*** – eosinophil granuloma is the most frequent cause of a solitary vertebra plana in childhood. The posterior elements are usually spared.
6. **Benign tumours** – haemangioma, giant cell tumour and aneurysmal bone cyst.
7. **Paget's disease*** – diagnosis is difficult when a solitary vertebra is involved. Neural arch is affected in most cases. Sclerosis and expansion. If other non-collapsed vertebrae are affected then diagnosis becomes much easier.

Further Reading

Laredo J-D, el Quessar A, Bossard P et al. Vertebral tumours and pseudotumours. Radiol Clin North Am 2001;39(1):137–163.

Varma R, Lander P, Assaf A. Imaging of pyogenic infectious spondylodiskitis. Radiol Clin North Am 2001;39(2):203–213.

2.3 MULTIPLE COLLAPSED VERTEBRAE

1. **Osteoporosis** (q.v.).
2. **Neoplastic disease** – wedge fractures are particularly related to osteolytic metastases and osteolytic marrow tumours, e.g. multiple myeloma, leukaemia and lymphoma. Altered or obliterated normal trabeculae. Disc spaces are usually preserved until late. Paravertebral soft-tissue mass is more common in myeloma than metastases.
3. **Trauma** – discontinuity of trabeculae, sclerosis of the fracture line due to compressed and overlapped trabeculae. Disc space usually preserved. The lower cervical, lower dorsal and upper lumbar spine are most commonly affected. Usually no soft-tissue mass. MRI usually shows the end-plates to be spared, c.f. pyogenic infection.
4. **Scheuermann's disease** – irregular end-plates and numerous Schmorl's nodes in the thoracic spine of children and young adults. Disc-space narrowing. Often progresses to a severe kyphosis. Secondary degenerative changes later.
5. **Infection** – destruction of end-plates adjacent to a destroyed disc.
6. **Langerhans cell histiocytosis*** – the spine is more frequently involved in eosinophilic granuloma and Hand–Schüller–Christian disease than in Letterer–Siwe disease. Most common in young people. The thoracic and lumbosacral spine are the usual sites of disease. Disc spaces are preserved.
7. **Sickle-cell anaemia*** – characteristic step-like depression in the central part of the end-plate.

Further Reading
James SL, Davies AM. Imaging of infectious spinal disorders in children and adults. Eur J Radiol 2006;58(1):27–40.
Laredo J-D, el Quessar A, Bossard P et al. Vertebral tumours and pseudotumours. Radiol Clin North Am 2001;39(1):137–163.

2.4 EROSION, DESTRUCTION OR ABSENCE OF A PEDICLE

1. **Metastasis**.
2. **Multiple myeloma***.
3. **Neurofibroma** – often causes erosion of adjacent pedicle or pedicles. Chronic intramedullary tumours, typically ependymoma, cause flattening of both pedicles at affected levels, with a widened interpedicular distance.
4. **Tuberculosis** – uncommonly. With a large paravertebral abscess.
5. **Benign bone tumour** – aneurysmal bone cyst or giant cell tumour.
6. **Congenital absence** – ± sclerosis of the contralateral pedicle.

2.5 SOLITARY DENSE PEDICLE

1. **Osteoblastic metastasis** – no change in size.
2. **Osteoid osteoma*** – some enlargement of the pedicle ± radiolucent nidus.
3. **Osteoblastoma*** – larger than osteoid osteoma and more frequently a lucency with a sclerotic margin rather than a purely sclerotic pedicle.
4. **Secondary to spondylolysis** – ipsilateral or contralateral.
5. **Secondary to congenitally absent or hypoplastic contralateral posterior elements.**

2.6 ENLARGED VERTEBRAL BODY

Generalized

1. **Gigantism.**
2. **Acromegaly*.**

Local (single or multiple)

1. **Paget's disease*.**
2. **Benign bone tumour**
   (a) Aneurysmal bone cyst* – typically purely lytic and expansile. Involves the anterior and posterior elements more commonly than the anterior or posterior elements alone. Rapid growth.
   (b) Haemangioma* – with a prominent vertical trabecular pattern.
   (c) Giant cell tumour* – involvement of the body alone is most common. Expansion is minimal.
3. **Hydatid** – over 40% of cases of hydatid disease in bone occur in vertebrae.

2.7 SQUARING OF ONE OR MORE VERTEBRAL BODIES

1. Ankylosing spondylitis*.
2. Paget's disease*.
3. Psoriatic arthropathy*.
4. Reiter's syndrome*.
5. Rheumatoid arthritis*.

2.8 BLOCK VERTEBRAE

1. **Klippel–Feil syndrome** – segmentation defects in the cervical spine, short neck, low hairline and limited cervical movement, especially rotation. The radiological appearance of the cervical spine resembles (1) above. C2–C3 and C5–C6 are most commonly affected. Other anomalies are frequently associated, the most important being:
   (a) Scoliosis > 20° in more than 50% of patients.
   (b) Sprengel's shoulder in 30%, ± an omovertebral body.
   (c) Cervical ribs.
   (d) Genito-urinary abnormalities in 66%; renal agenesis in 33%.
   (e) Deafness in 33%.
2. **Isolated congenital** – a failure of segmentation.
3. **Rheumatoid arthritis*** – especially juvenile onset rheumatoid arthritis and juvenile chronic arthritis with polyarticular onset. There may be angulation at the fusion site and this is not a feature of the congenital variety. The spinous processes do not fuse.
4. **Ankylosing spondylitis*** – squaring of anterior vertebral margins and calcification in the intervertebral discs and anterior and posterior longitudinal ligaments.
5. **Tuberculosis** – vertebral body collapse and destruction of the disc space, paraspinal calcification. There may be angulation of the spine.
6. **Operative fusion.**
7. **Post-traumatic.**

2.9 IVORY VERTEBRAL BODY

Single or multiple very dense vertebrae. The list excludes those causes where increased density is due to compaction of bone following collapse. If there is generalized involvement of the spine see 1.1.

1. Metastases.
2. Paget's disease*.
3. Lymphoma* – more frequent in Hodgkin's disease than the other reticuloses.
4. Low-grade infection.
5. Haemangioma.

2.10 ATLANTOAXIAL SUBLUXATION

When the distance between the posterior aspect of the anterior arch of the atlas and the anterior aspect of the odontoid process exceeds 3mm in adults and older children, or 5mm in younger children, or an interosseous distance that changes considerably between flexion and extension.

Trauma
Arthritides

1. **Rheumatoid arthritis*** – in 20–25% of patients with severe disease. Associated erosion of the odontoid may be severe enough to reduce it to a small spicule of bone.
2. **Psoriatic arthropathy*** – in 45% of patients with spondylitis.
3. **Juvenile idiopathic arthritis*** – most commonly in seropositive juvenile onset adult rheumatoid arthritis.
4. **Systemic lupus erythematosus***.
5. **Ankylosing spondylitis*** – in 2% of cases. Usually a late feature.

Congenital

1. **Down's syndrome*** – in 20% of cases. ± odontoid hypoplasia. May, rarely, have atlanto-occipital instability.
2. **Morquio's syndrome***.
3. **Spondyloepiphyseal dysplasia.**
4. **Congenital absence/hypoplasia of the odontoid process** – many have a history of previous trauma (NB. In children < 9 years it is normal for the tip of the odontoid to fall well below the top of the anterior arch of the atlas).

Infection
1. Retropharyngeal abscess in a child.

2.11 INTERVERTEBRAL DISC CALCIFICATION

1. **Degenerative spondylosis** – in the nucleus pulposus. Usually confined to the dorsal region.
2. **Alkaptonuria*.**
3. **Calcium pyrophosphate dihydrate deposition disease*.**
4. **Ankylosing spondylitis*.**
5. **Juvenile idiopathic arthritis*.**
6. **Haemochromatosis*.**
7. **Diffuse idiopathic skeletal hyperostosis** (DISH) – may mimic ankylosing spondylitis.
8. **Gout*.**
9. **Idiopathic** – a transient phenomenon in children. The cervical spine is most often affected. Clinically associated with neck pain and fever but may be asymptomatic. Persistent in adults.
10. **Following spinal fusion.**

Further Reading
Weinberger A, Myers AR. Intervertebral disc calcification in adults: a review. Semin Arthritis Rheum 1978;18:69–75.

2.12 BONY OUTGROWTHS OF THE SPINE

Syndesmophytes

Ossification of the annulus fibrosus. Thin, vertical and symmetrical. When extreme results in the 'bamboo spine'.

1. **Ankylosing spondylitis***.
2. **Alkaptonuria.**

AP

Paravertebral ossification

Ossification of paravertebral connective tissue which is separated from the edge of the vertebral body and disc. Large, coarse and asymmetrical.

1. **Reiter's syndrome***.
2. **Psoriatic arthropathy***.

AP

Claw osteophytes

Arising from the vertebral margin with no gap and having an obvious claw appearance.

1. **Stress response** – but in the absence of disc-space narrowing does not indicate disc degeneration.

Lateral

Traction spurs

Osteophytes with a gap between the end-plate and the base of the osteophyte and with the tip not protruding beyond the horizontal plane of the vertebral end-plate.

1. **Shear stresses across the disc** – more likely to be associated with a degenerative disc.

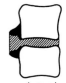

Lateral

Undulating anterior ossification

Undulating ossification of the anterior longitudinal ligament, intervertebral disc and paravertebral connective tissue.

1. **Diffuse idiopathic skeletal hyperostosis** (DISH).

Lateral

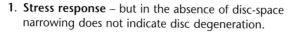

Further Reading

Jones MD, Pais MJ, Omiya B. Bony overgrowths and abnormal calcifications about the spine. Radiol Clin North Am 1988;26:1213–1234.

2.13 POSTERIOR SCALLOPING OF VERTEBRAL BODIES

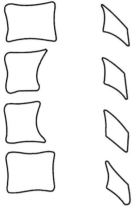

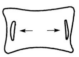

May be associated with flattening of the pedicles on the AP view

Scalloping is most prominent: (a) at either end of the spinal canal; (b) with large and slow growing lesions; and (c) with those lesions which originate during the period of active growth and bone modelling.

1. **Tumours in the spinal canal** – ependymoma (especially of the filum terminale and conus), dermoid, lipoma, neurofibroma and, less commonly, meningioma. Chronic raised intraspinal pressure distal to a tumour producing spinal block also causes extensive vertebral scalloping.
2. **Neurofibromatosis*** – scalloping is due to a mesodermal dysplasia and is associated with dural ectasia. Localized scalloping can also result from pressure resorption by a neurofibroma, in which case there may also be enlargement of an intervertebral foramen and flattening of one pedicle ('dumbbell tumour'). However, multiple wide thoracic intervertebral foramina are more likely owing to lateral meningocoeles than to local tumours.
3. **Acromegaly*** – other spinal changes include increased AP and transverse diameters of the vertebral bodies giving a spurious impression of decreased vertebral height, osteoporosis, spur formation and calcified discs.
4. **Achondroplasia*** – with spinal stenosis and anterior vertebral body beaks.

5. **Communicating hydrocephalus** – if severe and untreated.
6. **Syringomyelia** – especially if the onset is before 30 years of age.
7. **Other congenital syndromes**
    (a) Ehlers–Danlos } both associated with
    (b) Marfan's*   } dural ectasia.
    (c) Hurler's*.
    (d) Morquio's*.
    (e) Osteogenesis imperfecta*.

2.14 ANTERIOR SCALLOPING OF VERTEBRAL BODIES

1. **Aortic aneurysm** – intervertebral discs remain intact. Well-defined anterior vertebral margin.
   ± Calcification in the wall of the aorta.
2. **Tuberculous spondylitis** – with marginal erosions of the affected vertebral bodies. Disc-space destruction. Widening of the paraspinal soft tissues.
3. **Lymphadenopathy** – pressure resorption of bone results in a well-defined anterior vertebral body margin unless there is malignant infiltration of the bone.
4. **Delayed motor development** – e.g. Down's syndrome.

2.15 WIDENED INTERPEDICULAR DISTANCE

Most easily appreciated by comparison with adjacent vertebrae. ± flattening of the inner side of the pedicles.

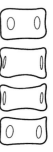

1. **Meningomyelocoele** – fusiform distribution of widened interpedicular distances with the greatest separation at the mid-point of the involved segment. Disc spaces are narrowed and bodies appear to be widened. Spinous processes and laminae are not identifiable. Facets may be fused into a continuous mass. Scoliosis (congenital or developmental) in 50–70% of cases ± kyphosis.
2. **Intraspinal mass** (see 2.16) – especially ependymoma.
3. **Diastematomyelia** – 50% occur between L1 and L3; 25% between T7 and T12. Widened interpedicular distances are common but not necessarily at the same level as the spur. The spur is visible in 33% of cases and extends from the neural arch forward. Laminar fusion associated with a neural arch defect at the same or adjacent level are important signs in predicting the presence of diastematomyelia. ± Associated meningocoele, neurenteric cyst or dermoid.
4. **Trauma**.

2.16 INTRASPINAL MASSES

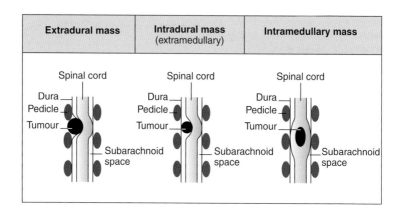

Extradural mass

1. **Prolapsed or sequestrated intervertebral disc** – occurs at all
   levels. Usually extradural, but occasionally penetrates dura,
   especially in thoracic region. May calcify, especially thoracic disc
   prolapse.
2. **Metastases, myeloma and lymphoma deposits** – common; look
   for associated vertebral infiltration. Most common sites of primary
   tumours are prostate, breast and lung. Thoracic spine is the most
   common site affected.
3. **Neurofibroma** – solitary, or multiple in neurofibromatosis. Lateral
   indentation of theca at the level of the intervertebral foramen.
4. **Neuroblastoma and ganglioneuroma** – tumours of childhood
   arising in adrenal or sympathetic chain, close to spine: direct
   invasion of spinal canal may occur.
5. **Meningioma** – may be extradural, but most are largely intradural
   (see below). Commonest site is thoracic, middle-aged females
   predominate.
6. **Haematoma** – may be due to trauma, dural AVM, anticoagulant
   therapy, some spontaneous. Long-segment, extradural mass on
   MRI, which may show signal characteristics of blood.
7. **Abscess** – usually secondary to disc or vertebral sepsis. Long
   segment extradural mass, with marginal enhancement on CT and
   MRI.
8. **Arachnoid cyst** – secondary to developmental dural defect.
   Uncommon, most spinal arachnoid cysts are intradural.

Intradural mass

1. **Meningioma** – as above commonly thoracic, mainly in middle-aged females. Occasional calcification.
2. **Neurofibroma** – usually extradural, but intradural neurofibromas occur, especially in cauda equina.
3. **Metastases** – from remote primary tumours, or due to CSF seeding in CNS tumours, e.g. pineal tumours, ependymoma, medulloblastoma and primitive neuroectodermal tumour (PNET). Lymphoma may also occur intradurally, particularly in lumbosacral canal.
4. **Subdural empyema.**

Intramedullary mass

1. **Ependymoma** – can occur anywhere in spinal canal, but commonest at conus and in lumbar canal (from filum terminale). Very slow-growing, and bone remodelling is often seen with expansion of the spinal canal. Best shown on MRI: high signal mass on T_2W images, low on T_1W, but with enhancement. Associated cord cavitation may occur.
2. **Astrocytoma** – commonest intramedullary tumour. Appearances similar to ependymoma, but faster growing, and bone changes not a feature.
3. **Dermoid** (including lipoma, teratoma) – most commonly seen in conus medullaris. Different tissue elements include lipomatous tissue: low attenuation on CT, bright on T_1W MRI, cystic spaces (low attenuation on CT, low signal on T_1W, high on T_2W MRI), and soft tissue (intermediate density on CT, and intermediate signal on T_1W MRI, enhancing after gadolinium).
4. **Infarct** – expanding in acute phase.
5. **Haematoma** – cord swelling only on CT, but features of blood on MRI.

Further Reading

Koeler KK, Rosenblum RS, Morrison AL. Neoplasms of the spinal cord and filum terminale: radiologic-pathologic correlation. Radiographics 2000;20:1721–1749.
Loughrey GJ, Collins CD, Todd SM et al. Magnetic resonance imaging in the management of suspected spinal canal disease in patients with known malignancy. Clin Radiol 2000;55:849–855.

3

Joints

Steven James

3.1 MONOARTHRITIS

1. **Trauma** – pointers to the diagnosis are: (a) the history, (b) the presence of a fracture, and (c) a joint effusion, especially a lipohaemarthrosis.
2. **Osteoarthritis.**
3. **Crystal-induced arthritis**
   (a) Gout*.
   (b) Calcium pyrophosphate dihydrate deposition disease*.
   (c) Calcium hydroxyapatite deposition disease.
4. **Rheumatoid arthritis*** – occasionally. Also juvenile idiopathic arthritis.
5. **Pyogenic arthritis** – commonest joints affected are the hip, knee and small joints of the hands and feet. 15% of those due to *Staphylococcus aureus* and 80% of those of gonococcal aetiology involve two or more joints. The joint may be radiographically normal at first presentation.
6. **Tuberculous arthritis** – Insidious onset with radiological changes present at the time of first examination. Erosions first develop at peripheral non-contact points of the joint.
7. **Pigmented villonodular synovitis*** – most commonly at the knee.
8. **Sympathetic** – a joint effusion can occur as a response to a tumour in the adjacent bone.
9. **Neuropathic arthropathy*.**
10. **Synovial chondromatosis.**
11. **Amyloidosis.**

Further Reading

Aliadadi P, Nikpoor N, Alparslan T. Imaging of neuropathic arthropathy. Semin Musculoskelet Radiol 2003;7:217–25.
Choi MH, MacKenzie JD, Dalinka MK. Imaging features of crystal-induced arthropathy. Rheum Dis Clin North Am 2006;32:427–46.

Learch TJ. Imaging of infectious arthritis. Semin Musculoskelet Radiol 2003;7:137–42.

Lin J, Jacobson JA, Jamadar DA et al. Pigmented villonodular synovitis and related lesions: the spectrum of imaging findings. Am J Roentgenol 1999;172:191–7.

Llauger J, Palmer J, Roson N et al. Nonseptic monoarthritis: imaging features with clinical and histopathologic correlation. Radiographics 2000;20: S263–78.

3

3.2 THE MAJOR POLYARTHRITIDES

Inflammatory		Chondropathic		Depositional
Periarticular (synovial) erosions		Subchondral erosions		Soft-tissue masses
Osteoporosis		Subchondral sclerosis		Extra-articular erosions
Tendon-related erosions		Osteophytes		– well defined
Periosteal reaction		Chondroalcinosis		– roofed
Syndesmophytes		Normal bone density		– mass-related
Malalignment				Normal bone density

Rheumatoid and its variants	*Seronegative*	*Degenerative*	*Metabolic*	
Symmetrical	Asymmetrical	Weight bearing joints,	Atypical distribution	
Small joints –	Large joints –	DIPJs and first CMCJs	Uniform cartilage loss	
esp. MCPJ and PIPJ	SIJs, spine and	Localized cartilage loss	Diffuse	
Osteoporosis	DIPJs of hand	Marginal calcification	chondrocalcinosis	
	Osteoporosis less marked		Large subchondral cysts	
	Periosteal reaction		Greater destruction	
	Syndesmophytes			

Rheumatoid arthritis	Ankylosing spondylitis	Osteoarthritis	Calcium pyrophosphate	Gout
Systemic lupus	Reiter's syndrome	Neuropathic	Haemochromatosis	Hypercholesteroalaemia
erythematosus	Psoriatic arthropathy	Haemophilic	Alkaptonuria	Reticulohistiocytosis
Scleroderma	Enteropathic arthritis		Hyperparathyroidism	Amyloidosis
Dermatomyositis	Juvenile idiopathic arthritis		Wilson's disease	

3.3 ARTHRITIS WITH OSTEOPOROSIS

1. Rheumatoid arthritis*.
2. Juvenile idiopathic arthritis.
3. Systemic lupus erythematosus*.
4. Pyogenic arthritis.
5. Tuberculous arthritis.
6. Reiter's syndrome* – in the acute phase.
7. Scleroderma*.
8. Haemophilia*.

3.4 ARTHRITIS WITH PRESERVATION OF BONE DENSITY

1. Osteoarthritis.
2. Calcium pyrophosphate arthropathy – see Calcium pyrophosphate dihydrate deposition disease*.
3. Gout*.
4. Psoriatic arthropathy*.
5. Ankylosing spondylitis.
6. Reiter's syndrome* – in chronic or recurrent disease.
7. Neuropathic arthropathy* – especially in the spine and lower extremities.
8. Pigmented villonodular synovitis*.

3.5 ARTHRITIS WITH A PERIOSTEAL REACTION

1. Juvenile idiopathic arthritis*.
2. Reiter's syndrome*.
3. Pyogenic arthritis.
4. Psoriatic arthropathy*.
5. Rheumatoid arthritis* – in less than 5% of patients.
6. Hypertrophic osteoarthropathy.
7. Haemophilia*.
8. AIDS-associated arthritis.

3.6 ARTHRITIS WITH PRESERVED OR WIDENED JOINT SPACE

1. **Early infective or inflammatory arthritis** – because of joint effusion.
2. **Psoriatic arthropathy*** – due to deposition of fibrous tissue.
3. **Acromegaly*** – due to cartilage overgrowth.
4. **Gout*.**
5. **Pigmented villonodular synovitis.**

3.7 ARTHRITIS WITH SOFT-TISSUE NODULES

1. **Gout*.**
2. **Rheumatoid arthritis*.**
3. **Pigmented villonodular synovitis*.**
4. **Multicentric reticulohistiocytosis.**
5. **Amyloidosis.**
6. **Sarcoidosis*.**

3.8 ARTHRITIS MUTILANS

A destructive arthritis of the hands and feet with resorption of bone ends and telescoping joints (main-en-lorgnette).

1. **Rheumatoid arthritis*.**
2. **Juvenile idiopathic arthritis*.**
3. **Psoriatic arthropathy*.**
4. **Diabetes.**
5. **Leprosy.**
6. **Neuropathic arthropathy*.**
7. **Reiter's syndrome*** – in the feet.

3.9 DIFFUSE TERMINAL PHALANGEAL SCLEROSIS

1. **Normal variant** – in 10% of normal individuals.
2. **Rheumatoid arthritis*** – most commonly in association with erosive arthropathy but may occur in its absence.
3. **Scleroderma*.**
4. **Systemic lupus erythematosus*.**
5. **Sarcoidosis*.**
6. **Sickle cell disease.**
7. **Werner syndrome.**

3.10 CALCIFIED LOOSE BODY (SINGLE OR MULTIPLE) IN A JOINT

1. **Detached osteophyte** – larger and more variable in size than synovial osteochondromata. Other signs of degenerative arthritis.
2. **Osteochondral fracture.**
3. **Osteochondritis dissecans** – most commonly the knee, talus and elbow. A corresponding defect in the parent bone may be visible.
4. **Neuropathic arthropathy*** – joint disorganization.
5. **Synovial osteochondromatosis** – knee most commonly; hip, ankle, wrist and shoulder less commonly. Multiple small nodules of fairly uniform size. Faintly calcified initially; later ossified. Secondary erosion of intracapsular bone, joint-space narrowing and osteophyte formation may occur later in the disease.

3.11 CALCIFICATION OF ARTICULAR (HYALINE) CARTILAGE (CHONDROCALCINOSIS)

1. **Calcium pyrophosphate dihydrate deposition disease*.**
2. **Hyperparathyroidism*.**
3. **Haemochromatosis*.**
4. **Alkaptonuria.**
5. **Acromegaly*.**
6. **Gout*.**
7. **Wilson's disease.**

3.12 SACROILIITIS

1. Changes initially in the lower and middle thirds of the joint and the iliac side is more severely affected than the sacral side.
2. Periarticular osteoporosis, superficial erosions and sclerosis of subchondral bone.
3. Further erosion leads to widening of the joint space.
4. Subchondral sclerosis progresses to bony ankylosis.
5. Eventual return of the bones to normal density.
   The most typical patterns of distribution are:

Bilateral symmetrical

1. **Ankylosing spondylitis*** – may be asymmetrical early in the disease.
2. **Inflammatory bowel disease** – ulcerative colitis, Crohn's disease and Whipple's disease. Identical appearances to ankylosing spondylitis.
3. **Psoriatic arthropathy*** – ankylosis is less frequent than in ankylosing spondylitis. Occurs in 30–50% of patients with arthropathy. Less commonly is asymmetrical or unilateral.
4. **Osteitis condensans ilii** – predominantly in young, multiparous women. A triangular segment of bone sclerosis on the inferior aspect of the iliac side of the joint is associated with a well-defined joint margin and a normal joint space.
5. **Hyperparathyroidism*** – subchondral bone resorption and joint-space widening only.
6. **Paraplegia** – joint-space narrowing and osteoporosis.

Bilateral asymmetrical

1. **Reiter's syndrome***.
2. **Psoriatic arthropathy*** – this pattern in 40% of cases.
3. **Rheumatoid arthritis*** – rare. Minimal sclerosis and no significant bony ankylosis.
4. **Gouty arthritis** (see Gout*) – large well-defined erosions with surrounding sclerosis.
5. **Osteoarthritis** – the articular margins are smooth and well defined. Joint-space narrowing, subchondral sclerosis and anterior osteophytes are observed.

Unilateral

1. **Infection.**

3.13 PROTRUSIO ACETABULI

1. **Rheumatoid arthritis*** – including juvenile idiopathic arthritis.
2. **Osteoporosis** (q.v.).
3. **Osteomalacia and rickets** (q.v.)*.
4. **Paget's disease***.
5. **Ankylosing spondylitis***.
6. **Osteoarthritis** – occasionally.
7. **Psoriatic arthropathy***.
8. **Trauma** – acetabular fractures.
9. **Familial or idiopathic**.
10. **Marfan's syndrome*** – 45% show evidence of protrusio acetabuli. Of these, 50% are unilateral and 90% have an associated scoliosis.

3.14 WIDENING OF THE SYMPHYSIS PUBIS

> 8mm at 7 years and over.

ACQUIRED

1. **Pregnancy** – resolves by the 3rd postpartum month.
2. **Trauma**.
3. **Osteitis pubis** – one or more months after parturition or pelvic surgery, especially prostatic surgery. It may also be observed as a chronic stress reaction in athletes. Symmetrical bone resorption with subchondral bony irregularity and sclerosis. Ankylosis may be a late finding.
4. **Osteolytic metastases**.
5. **Infection** – low-grade osteomyelitis shows similar radiological features to osteitis pubis.
6. **Ankylosing spondylitis*** and **rheumatoid arthritis*** – early in the disease.
7. **Hyperparathyroidism*** – due to subperiosteal bone resorption.

CONGENITAL

See 14.27.

3.15 FEMORAL HEAD AND NECK ABNORMALITIES

Coxa magna

The remodelled femoral head becomes wider and flatter.

1. **Developmental dysplasia of the hip.**
2. **Perthes' disease.**
3. **Septic arthritis.**

Coxa plana

Flattened femoral head.
1. **Avascular necrosis*** (see 1.30).

Coxa valga

In coxa valga the femoral angle is increased, so the femoral neck becomes more vertical. This angle is normally about 150° at birth but reduces to 120–130° by adulthood.

Idiopathic

Developmental
1. **Neuromuscular disorders.**
2. **Abductor muscle weakness.**
3. **Cleidocranial dysplasia*.**
4. **Diaphyseal aclasis** – multiple metaphyseal exostoses. Point away from the joint.
5. **Hunter's syndrome** – underdeveloped superior acetabular region, wide femoral neck.
6. **Multiple enchondromatosis.**
7. **Diastrophic dwarfism.**

Inflammatory
1. **Juvenile idiopathic arthritis.**
2. **Poliomyelitis.**

Traumatic
1. **Femoral neck fracture.**

Coxa vara

In coxa vara the femoral angle is reduced so the femoral neck becomes more horizontal.

Developmental
1. Neuromuscular disorders.
2. Developmental dysplasia of the hip.
3. Fibrous dysplasia*.
4. Cleidocranial dysplasia*.
5. Multiple epiphyseal dysplasia.
6. Osteogenesis imperfecta*.
7. Infantile (developmental) coxa vara
8. **Proximal femoral focal deficiency** – a disease spectrum relating to partial absence and shortening of the proximal portion of the femur. Congenital but not inherited.

Inflammatory
1. Rheumatoid arthritis*.

Traumatic
1. Slipped capital femoral epiphysis*.
2. Femoral neck fracture.

Vascular
1. Perthes' disease.
2. Avascular necrosis.

Metabolic
1. Renal osteodystrophy*.
2. Rickets*.
3. Paget's disease*.

3.16 EROSION (ENLARGEMENT) OF THE INTERCONDYLAR NOTCH OF THE DISTAL FEMUR

1. Juvenile idiopathic arthritis*.
2. Haemophilia*.
3. Psoriatic arthropathy*.
4. Tuberculous arthritis.
5. Rheumatoid arthritis*.

4

Respiratory tract

Sujal Desai and Simon Padley

4.1 UNEQUAL LUNG SIZE, LUCENCY AND VASCULARITY. WHICH IS THE ABNORMAL SIDE?

If vascularity is decreased, the lung is abnormal

If vascularity is normal or increased, the lung is probably normal

A small completely opaque hemithorax is abnormal

When the small hemithorax is completely opaque the diagnosis is total collapse or agenesis. Furthermore, the atelectasis can be presumed to be resorptive (i.e. secondary to obstruction) rather than compressive (i.e. from an overdistended contralateral lung). This is because, on the fully inspired film, an overexpanded lung will never compress the other lung to the extent of obliterating the costophrenic angle.

With inspiration – expiration, the lung changing least or not at all, is abnormal

Further Reading
Swischuk LE, John SD. Differential diagnosis in paediatric radiology, 2nd edn. Williams & Wilkins, Baltimore, 1995, pp7–11.

4.2 UNILATERAL HYPERTRANSRADIANT HEMITHORAX

The observer should exclude contralateral increased density, e.g. pleural effusion in a supine patient or pleural thickening.

Rotation

Poor technique Scoliosis } the hypertransradiant hemithorax is the side to which the patients is turned

Chest wall

1. **Mastectomy** – absent breast ± absent pectoral muscle shadows.
2. **Poliomyelitis** – atrophy of pectoral muscles ± atrophic changes in the shoulder girdle and humerus.
3. **Poland's syndrome** – unilateral congenital absence of pectoral muscles ± rib defects. Occurs in 10% of patients with syndactyly.

Pleura

1. **Pneumothorax** – note the lung edge and absent vessels peripherally.

Lung

1. **Compensatory emphysema** – following lobectomy (rib defects and opaque bronchial sutures indicate previous surgery) or lobar collapse.
2. **Airway obstruction** – air trapping on expiration results in increased lung volume and shift of the mediastinum to the contralateral side.
3. **Unilateral bullae** – vessels are absent rather than attenuated. May mimic pneumothorax.
4. **Swyer–James syndrome (McLeod's syndrome)** – the late sequela of childhood bronchiolitis (usually viral but non-viral organisms also implicated). On chest radiography, lung volume on affected side is either normal or slightly reduced but, importantly, there is air trapping on expiration. Ipsilateral hilar vessels are small. CT not infrequently shows bilateral disease with mosaic attenuation and bronchiectasis.
5. **Congenital lobar emphysema** – one-third present at birth. Marked overinflation of a lobe (most commonly left upper lobe followed by right upper lobe or right middle lobe). The ipsilateral lobes are compressed and there may be mediastinal displacement to the contralateral side.

Pulmonary vessels

1. **Pulmonary embolus** (see Pulmonary embolic disease*) – to a major pulmonary artery (at least lobar in size). The pulmonary artery is dilated proximally and the affected lung shows moderate loss of volume; N.B. small pulmonary emboli unlikely to result in any disparity.

4.3 BILATERAL HYPERTRANSRADIANT HEMITHORACES

With overexpansion of the lungs

1. **Emphysema** – with large central pulmonary arteries and peripheral arterial pruning. ± Bullae; centrilobular emphysema typically in mid/upper zones whereas panacinar emphysema commonly affects lower zones.
2. **Asthma** – during an acute episode or with chronic disease with 'fixed' airflow obstruction due to airway remodelling.
3. **Acute bronchiolitis** – particularly affects children in the first year of life. Overexpansion is due to small airways (bronchiolar) obstruction. May be associated with large airway mucosal thickening leading to bronchial wall thickening on plain radiography. Collapse and consolidation are not primary features of bronchiolitis.
4. **Tracheal, laryngeal or bilateral bronchial stenoses** (see 4.4).

With normal or small lungs

1. **Congenital heart disease producing oligaemia** – includes those conditions with right heart obstruction and right-to-left shunts. The hila are usually small except when there is post-stenotic dilatation of the pulmonary artery.
2. **Pulmonary artery stenosis** – if due to valvar stenosis, there is post-stenotic dilatation. 60% of congenital lesions have other associated cardiovascular abnormalities.
3. **Multiple pulmonary emboli**
4. **Primary pulmonary hypertension (PPH)**
5. **Schistosomiasis**
6. **Metastatic trophoblastic tumour**

identical radiological picture of big hilar vessels with peripheral pruning. History is most important. PP occurs predominantly in young females and may be familial. Schistosomiasis more usually presents as a diffuse reticulonodular pattern.

Further Reading

Frazier AA, Galvin JR, Franks TJ et al. Pulmonary vasculature: hypertension and infarction. Radiographics 2000;20:491–524.

4.4 BRONCHIAL STENOSIS OR OCCLUSION

In the lumen

1. **Foreign body** – air trapping is more common than atelectasis. The lower lobe is most frequently affected. The foreign body may be opaque. The column of air within the bronchus may be discontinuous: the 'interrupted bronchus sign'.
2. **Mucus plug.**
3. **Misplaced endotracheal tube.**
4. **Aspergillosis** – with thickened bronchial walls.
5. **Broncholithiasis.**

In the wall

1. **Bronchogenic carcinoma** – narrowing ± irregularity.
2. **Other bronchial tumours** – (e.g. carcinoid tumour) usually a smooth, rounded filling defect, convex toward the hilum. Main bulk of tumour may outside the lumen of the airway.
3. **Sarcoidosis.**
4. **Fibrosis** – e.g. tuberculosis and fungi. Can mimic carcinoma but usually produces a longer constriction.
5. **Bronchial atresia** – most commonly the apico-posterior segment of the left upper lobe.
6. **Fractured bronchus.**

Outside the wall

1. **Lymph nodes.**
2. **Mediastinal tumour** – smooth, eccentric narrowing.
3. **Enlarged left atrium.**
4. **Aortic aneurysm.**
5. **Anomalous origin of left pulmonary artery from right pulmonary artery** – producing compression of the right main bronchus as it passes over it, between the trachea and oesophagus to reach the left hilum. PA chest X-ray shows the right side of the trachea to be indented and the vessel is seen end-on between the trachea and oesophagus on the lateral view.

Further Reading

Franquet T, Muller NL, Gimenez A et al Spectrum of pulmonary aspergillosis: histologic, clinical, and radiologic findings. Radiographics 2001;21:825–37.

Lim-Dunham JE, Yousefzadeh DK. The interrupted bronchus: a fluoroscopic sign of bronchial foreign body in infants and children. Am J Roentgenol 1999;173:969–72.

Ward S, Morcos SK. Congenital bronchial atresia – presentation of three cases and a pictorial review. Clin Radiol 1999;54:144–8.

4.5 INCREASED DENSITY OF A HEMITHORAX

With central mediastinum

1. **Air space filling/opacification** – ± air bronchogram. Simply indicates displacement of air from the air spaces. May be due to infection but also oedema (see 4.14), aspiration, intra-alveolar blood, tumour (including disseminated adenocarcinoma, bronchoalveolar cell carcinoma and lymphoma).
2. **Pleural effusion** – when the patient is supine a small or moderate effusion gravitates posteriorly, producing a generalized increased density with an apical cap of fluid. Note that pulmonary vessels will be visible through the increased density. Erect or decubitus films confirm the diagnosis.
3. **Mesothelioma** – often associated with a pleural effusion which obscures the tumour. Encasement of the lung limits mediastinal shift (NB affected hemithorax may even be smaller). ± calcified pleural plaques (more commonly demonstrated at CT).

With mediastinal displacement away from the dense hemithorax

1. **Pleural effusion** (q.v.) – NB. A large effusion with no mediastinal shift implies underlying collapse which may indicate central obstruction.
2. **Diaphragmatic hernia** – on the right side with herniated liver; on the left side the hemithorax is not usually opaque because of air within the herniated bowel. The left hemithorax may be opaque in the early neonatal period when air has not yet had time to reach the herniated bowel.

With mediastinal displacement towards the dense hemithorax

1. **Collapse.**
2. **Post-pneumonectomy** – rib resection ± opaque bronchial sutures.
3. **Lymphangitis carcinomatosa** – unilateral disease is uncommon. Linear and nodular opacities ± ipsilateral hilar and mediastinal lymphadenopathy. Septal lines.
4. **Pulmonary agenesis and hypoplasia** – usually asymptomatic. Absent or hypoplastic pulmonary artery.
5. **Malignant pleural mesothelioma** – see above.

NB. 70% of unilateral diffuse lung opacities involve the right lung. Pneumonia, aspiration, pulmonary oedema, lymphangitis carcinomatosa and radiotherapy account for 90% (Youngberg 1977).

Further Reading
Youngberg AS. Unilateral diffuse lung opacity. Radiology 1977;123:277–82.

4.6 PULMONARY CYSTS

A pulmonary cyst is defined as a rounded circumscribed space surrounded by an epithelial or fibrous wall of variable thickness. More readily depicted at CT than plain chest radiography.

Post-infective

Cysts can appear during the first 2 weeks of the pneumonia and resolve within several months. Cysts may contain fluid levels

1. *Staphylococcus aureus* – a characteristic feature of childhood staphylococcal pneumonia, developing in 40-60% of cases.
2. *Streptococcus pneumoniae.*
3. *Escherichia coli.*
4. *Klebsiella pneumoniae.*
5. *Haemophilus influenzae.*
6. *Pneumocystis jiroveci* (NB formally *Pneumocystis carinii*) – usually multiple and in the upper parts of the lungs. Patients with cysts are more likely to suffer pneumothorax.
7. *Legionella pneumophila* (Legionnaire's disease).
8. **Hydatid.**

Post-traumatic

1. **Interstitial emphysema** – may be followed by thin-walled, air-containing cysts.

Congenital

1. **Congenital cystic adenomatoid malformation.**
2. **Intrapulmonary bronchogenic cyst.**
3. **Pulmonary sequestration.**

Neoplastic

1. **Following treatment of pulmonary metastases** – bladder cancer and germ cell tumours. May be visible only on CT.
2. **Hylanizing granulomas** – rare disorder of unknown aetiology but possible association with infection and autoimmunity. Multiple ill-defined/well defined nodules and cysts.
3. **Metastatic epithelioid sarcoma.**

Diffuse lung diseases:

1. **Langerhans' cell histiocytosis** (LCH) – Cysts, sometimes with bizarre (i.e. non-circular) outlines, in mid/upper zones. In 'early' disease multiple nodules which then cavitate. Relative sparing of lower zones and medial tips of middle lobe and lingula. Pulmonary LCH (but not other forms of LCH) is strongly linked to cigarette smoking.

2. **Lymphangioleiomyomatosis** (LAM) – Exclusively in female subjects of child-bearing age and related to mutation of TSC1 (chromosome 9). Smooth muscle proliferation around vessels, lymphatics and airways. Cysts are characteristic finding and more uniform in size than LCH. No zonal predilection (cf. LCH).

3. **Tuberose sclerosis** (TSC) – neurocutaneous disorder associated with mutations of TSC1 and TSC2 genes. Pathology of lung disease in TSC almost identical to LAM

4. **Neurofibromatosis** – Cystic lung disease and interstitial fibrosis are reported but some doubt exists and changes maybe simply represent smoking-related interstitial lung disease.

5. **Birt–Hogg–Dubé syndrome** – autosomal dominant multisystem disorder characterised by pulmonary cysts, cutaneous fibrofolliculomas and increased risk of renal tumours. Recurrent pneumothoraces due to lung involvement.

6. **Lymphocytic interstitial pneumonia** – rarely idiopathic; usually occurs in context of dysproteinaemias, HIV infection and connective tissue disorders (in particular rheumatoid arthritis, Sjögren's syndrome). Mechanism of cyst formation uncertain but may be due to partial obstruction of small airways.

7. **Subacute extrinsic allergic alveolitis** – possibly related to lymphocytic interstitial pulmonary infiltrate in subacute phase.

8. **End-stage idiopathic pulmonary fibrosis.**

9. **End-stage sarcoidosis.**

Further Reading

Ryu JH et al. Lack of evidence of association between neurofibromatosis and pulmonary fibrosis. Chest 2005;128:2381–6.

Silva CI. Diffuse lung cysts in lymphoid interstitial pneumonias: high-resolution CT and pathologic findings. J Thorac Imaging 2006;21:241–4.

Shibata Y. High-resolution CT findings in pulmonary hyalinizing granuloma. J Thorac Imaging 2007;22:374–7.

4.7 SLOWLY RESOLVING OR RECURRENT PNEUMONIA

1. **Bronchial obstruction** – e.g. due to a neoplasm or foreign body.
2. **Inappropriate antimicrobial therapy** – especially for tuberculosis, Klebsiella and mycoses.
3. **Recurrent aspiration** – secondary to a pharyngeal pouch, achalasia, systemic sclerosis, hiatus hernia, 'H' type tracheo-oesophageal fistula, paralytic/neuromuscular disorders, chronic sinusitis.
4. **Underlying lung pathology** – e.g. lung abscess, bronchiectasis (see 4.11)
   (a) Abscess.
   (b) Bronchiectasis – see 4.11.
5. **Impaired immunity** – e.g. prolonged corticosteroid or other immunosuppresive therapy, immunoglobulin deficiency, diabetes, cachexia, HIV-related.

Further Reading

Franquet T, Gimenez A, Roson N et al. Aspiration diseases: findings, pitfalls and differential diagnosis. Radiographics 2000;20:673–85.
Hansell DM. Bronchiectasis. Radiol Clin North Am 1998;36(1):107–28.
Parameswaran GI. Infection in high-risk populations. Infect Dis Clin North Am 2007;21;673–95.

4.8 PNEUMONIA WITH AN ENLARGED HILUM

Hilar lymph node enlargement may be secondary to the pneumonia or pneumonia may be secondary to bronchial obstruction by a hilar mass. Signs suggestive of a secondary pneumonia include segmental or lobar consolidation which is better defined than a primary pneumonia. Slow resolution. Recurrent consolidation in the same part of the lung. Associated volume loss or lobar collapse.

Secondary pneumonias

See 4.4, but note particularly 'Carcinoma of the bronchus'.

Primary pneumonias

1. **Primary tuberculosis** – lymph node enlargement is unilateral in 80% and involves the hilar (60%), or combined hilar and paratracheal (40%) nodes.
2. **Viral pneumonias.**

3. **Mycoplasma** – lymph node enlargement is common in children but rare in adults. May be unilateral or bilateral.
4. **Primary histoplasmosis** – in endemic areas. Hilar lymph node enlargement is common, particularly in children. During healing lymph nodes calcify and may cause bronchial obstruction, thereby initiating distal infection.
5. **Coccidioidomycosis** – in endemic areas. The pneumonic type consists of predominantly lower lobe consolidation which is frequently associated with hilar lymph node enlargement.

See also 4.24.

4.9 LOBAR PNEUMONIA

Consolidation involving the air spaces of an anatomically recognizable lobe. The entire lobe may not be involved and there may be a degree of associated collapse.

1. *Streptococcus pneumoniae* – the commonest cause. Usually unilobar. Cavitation rare. Pleural effusion is uncommon. Little or no collapse.
2. *Klebsiella pneumoniae* – often multilobar involvement. Great propensity for cavitation and lobar enlargement.
3. *Staphylococcus aureus* – especially in children. 40–60% of children develop pneumatocoeles. Effusion (empyema) and pneumothorax are also common. Bronchopleural fistula may develop. No lobar predilection.
4. **Tuberculosis** – in primary or post-primary tuberculosis, but more common in the former. Associated collapse is common. The right lung is affected twice as often as the left, and primary tuberculosis predilects the anterior segment of the upper lobe or the medial segment of the middle lobe.
5. *Streptococcus pyogenes* – affects the lower lobes predominantly. Often associated with pleural effusion.

4.10 CONSOLIDATION WITH BULGING OF FISSURES

Homogeneous or inhomogeneous air-space opacification with bulging of the bounding fissures.

1. **Infection with abundant exudates** – *Klebsiella pneumoniae* (Friedländer's pneumonia), *Streptococcus pneumoniae*, *Mycobacterium tuberculosis* and *Yersinia pestis* (plague pneumonia).
2. **Abscess** – when an area of consolidation breaks down. Organisms which commonly produce abscesses are *Staphylococcus aureus*, Klebsiella spp. and other Gram-negative organisms.
3. **Carcinoma of the bronchus** – this can fill and expand a lobe.

4.11 BRONCHIECTASIS

Radiological signs

Signs of bronchiectasis more reliably identified on CT than plain chest radiography particularly with 'mild' disease. More recently, multi-detector CT thought to be superior to HRCT for diagnosis.

Key signs (required for diagnosis):
Dilated non tapering airways: manifesting either as 'tramlines' (i.e. airways which are imaged in longitudinal section) or 'ring' opacities. In severe disease, large cystic spaces ± air-fluid levels may be present. NB In less severe disease plain chest radiograph of limited sensitivity and specificity

Ancillary signs (not diagnostic):
1. Volume loss in affected lobe(s).
2. Compensatory hyperexpansion.
3. Plugging of large and small airways leading to leading to tubular/ branching or small nodular opacities

Causes of bronchiectasis
More frequent:

1. **Immunodeficiency** – especially panhypogammaglobulinaemias and selective immunoglobulin deficiencies but also chronic granulomatous disease, HIV, Chédiak–Higashi syndrome.
2. **Cystic fibrosis**
3. **Idiopathic** – no apparent aetiology in up to one-third of patients with bronchiectasis.

Less frequent:

1. **Following childhood infections** – (e.g. secondary to measles and pertussis) less common cause in the antibiotic era in developed countries but continues to be an important factor in developing countries.
2. **Secondary to bronchial obstruction** – foreign body, neoplasm, broncholithiasis or bronchial stenosis.
3. **Chronic aspiration.**
4. **Congenital/Genetic anomalies**
   (a) Kartagener's syndrome – bronchiectasis with immobile cilia, dextrocardia and absent frontal sinuses. 5% of patients with dextrocardia will eventually develop bronchiectasis.
   (b) Williams–Campbell syndrome – bronchial cartilage deficiency.
   (c) Mounier–Kuhn syndrome – tracheobronchomegaly.
   (d) α1-antitrypsin deficiency.
   (e) Swyer–James or McLeod's syndrome (see 4.2).
5. **Collagen vascular diseases** – particularly rheumatoid arthritis, Sjögren's syndrome.
6. **Gastrointestinal disorders** – ulcerative colitis, coeliac disease.
7. **Immunological** – allergic bronchopulmonary aspergillosis, following organ (heart/lung) or bone marrow transplantation.

Further Reading

McGuinness G, Naidich DP. CT of airways disease and bronchiectasis. Radiol Clin North Am 2002;40(1):1–19.

Fraser RS, Müller NL, Colman N et al. Bronchiectasis and other bronchial abnormalities. In: Diagnosis of diseases of the chest, 4th edn. WB Saunders, Philadelphia, 1999, pp2265–97.

Hansell DM, Armstrong P, Lynch DA et al. Airways diseases. In: Imaging of diseases of the chest, 4th edn. Elsevier Mosby, Philadelphia, 2005.

4.12 AIR-SPACE FILLING/SHADOWING DISEASE

Sometimes termed alveolar shadowing but incorrect because the lung opacification is due to displacement of air from anatomically larger acini. The general term 'air-space' shadow or opacification is recommended. The signs of air-space disease are increased parenchymal density which obscures visibility of vessels and bronchial walls. Air bronchograms or bronchiologram may be visible.

Causes of air space opacification

(Note that any of the following may be unilateral and, in some instances, confined to a single lobe):

1. **Oedema** (see 4.13).
2. **Infection** – (see also 4.8–4.10)
   (a) Tuberculosis.
   (b) Histoplasmosis.
   (c) *Pneumocystis jirovecii*
   (d) Influenza – particularly in patients with mitral stenosis or who are pregnant.
   (e) Chicken pox (and other viral pneumonias) – may be confluent in the central areas of the lungs. ± Hilar lymph node enlargement.
3. **Haemorrhage** – e.g. idiopathic pulmonary haemosiderosis, anti-glomerular basement disease, microscopic polyangiitis, systemic lupus erythematosus, Behçet's syndrome, Wegener's granulomatosis, contusion, bleeding diatheses, Goodpasture's syndrome, idiopathic pulmonary haemosiderosis (in the acute stage), pulmonary infarction.
4. **Malignancy** – bronchoalveolar cell carcinoma (effusions are common; mediastinal lymph nodes are uncommon; diagnosis by sputum cytology or lung biopsy), disseminated adenocarcinoma or choriocarcinoma, lymphoma.
5. **Sarcoidosis*** – called 'air-space' sarcoidosis and occurring in up to 20%. Air space pattern is due to thickened interstitium and filling of air spaces by macrophages and granulomatous infiltration.
6. **Eosinophilic lung disease** – sometimes in the upper zones.
7. **Organizing pneumonia** – may be cryptogenic or response to other 'insult' (e.g. infection, drug-toxicity, connective tissue disease). Typically, multifocal air space opacities in periphery of mid/lower zones.

4.13 PULMONARY OEDEMA

Defined as an increase in extra-vascular lung water and traditionally regarded as being secondary to due to cardiogenic or non-cardiogenic causes.

Cardiogenic pulmonary oedema

Any cause of impaired left ventricular function

Non-cardiogenic pulmonary oedema

1. **Fluid overload** – excess i.v. fluids, renal failure and excess hypertonic fluids, e.g. contrast media.
2. **Cerebral disease** – cerebrovascular accident, head injury or raised intracranial pressure.
3. **Near drowning** – radiologically no significant differences between fresh-water and sea-water drowning.
4. **Aspiration** (Mendelson's syndrome).
5. **Radiotherapy** – several weeks following treatment. Ultimately has a characteristic straight edge as fibrosis ensues.
6. **Rapid re-expansion of lung following thoracocentesis.**
7. **Liver disease and other causes of hypoproteinaemia.**
8. **Transfusion reaction.**
9. **Drug-induced:**
    (a) Those which induce cardiac arrhythmias or depress myocardial contractility (contrast media can induce arrhythmias, alter capillary wall permeability and produce a hyperosmolar load).
    (b) Those which alter pulmonary capillary wall permeability, e.g. overdoses of heroin, morphine, methadone, cocaine, 'crack', dextropropoxyphene and aspirin. Hydrochlorothiazide, phenylbutazone, aspirin and nitrofurantoin can cause oedema as an idiosyncratic response. Interleukin-2 and tumour necrosis factor may cause increased permeability by an unknown pathophysiological process.
10. **Poisons:**
    (a) Inhaled (e.g. NO_2, SO_2, CO, phosgene, hydrocarbons and smoke).
    (b) Circulating – paraquat and snake venom.
11. **Mediastinal tumours** – producing venous or lymphatic obstruction.
12. **Acute respiratory distress syndrome** – may be primary (e.g. because of severe pneumonia, aspiration) or secondary (e.g. following non-thoracic sepsis or trauma); lungs radiographically normal in first 24 hours but progressive widespread opacification

with onset of interstitial and then frank intra-alveolar leak of haemorrhagic and oedema fluid.

13. **High altitude** (acute mountain sickness) – following rapid ascent to >3000 metres.

Further Reading

Gluecker T, Capasso P, Schnider P et al.Clinical and radiologic features of pulmonary edema. Radiographics 1999;19:1507–31.

Milne EN, Pistolesi M, Miniati M et al. The radiological distinction of cardiogenic and noncardiogenic edema. Am J Roentgenol 1985;144:879–94.

4.14 UNILATERAL PULMONARY OEDEMA

Pulmonary oedema on the same side as a pre-existing abnormality

1. **Prolonged lateral decubitus position.**
2. **Unilateral aspiration.**
3. **Pulmonary contusion.**
4. **Rapid thoracentesis of air or fluid.**
5. **Bronchial obstruction.**
6. **Systemic artery to pulmonary artery shunts** – e.g. Waterston (on the right side). Blalock–Taussig (left or right side) and Pott's procedure (on the left side).

Pulmonary oedema on the opposite side to a pre-existing abnormality

Oedema on the side opposite a lung with a perfusion defect.

1. **Congenital absence or hypoplasia of a pulmonary artery.**
2. **Macleod's syndrome.**
3. **Thromboembolism.**
4. **Unilateral emphysema.**
5. **Lobectomy.**
6. **Pleural disease.**

Further Reading

Calenoff L, Kruglik GD, Woodruff A. Unilateral pulmonary oedema. Radiology 1978;126:19–24.

4.15 SEPTAL LINES (KERLEY B LINES)

Due to thickening of the interlobular septa surrounding individual secondary pulmonary lobules. Interlobular septa contain lymphatics, venous radicals and interstitium. Thus, any cause of lymphatic or venous obstruction or infiltration or interstitial diseases might render interlobular septa visible. On chest radiography abnormal thickening of interlobular septa best appreciated in costophrenic angles; thickened interlobular septa more readily visible on CT.

Pulmonary venous pathology

1. **Left ventricular failure.**
2. **Mitral stenosis.**
3. **Pulmonary veno-occlusive disease.**

Lymphatic/interstitial disease

1. **Pneumoconioses** – surrounding tissues may contain a heavy metal, e.g. tin, which contributes to the density.
2. **Lymphangitic spread of tumours** (carcinomas, lymphoma or leukaemia).
3. **Sarcoidosis*** – septal lines are uncommon.
4. **Idiopathic bronchiectasis** – thickened interlobular septa may be a feature in around one-third of patients.
5. **Erdeim–Chester disease** – infiltration of pulmonary interstitium by histiocytes of non-Langerhans' type. Primarily a bone disorder but extraskeletal involvement in around 50%. Lung involvement in around one-third of patients. On chest radiography, reticulo-nodular infiltrate in mid/upper zones. On HRCT, smooth thickening of interlobular septa is characteristic, associated with ground-glass opacification and centrilobular nodules.
6. **Pulmonary haemorrhage.**
7. **Diffuse pulmonary lymphangiomatosis** – proliferation of lymphatic channels in pleura, interlobular septa and peri-bronchovascular connective tissue
8. **Congenital lymphangiectasia** – abnormal dilatation of lymphatic vessels (NB no increase in number of lymphatics [cf. lymphangiomatosis]). May be associated with extra-thoracic congenital anomalies (e.g. renal, cardiac). Usually fatal.
9. **Alveolar proteinosis** – smooth thickening of inter- (and intra-) lobular septa in geographical areas of ground-glass infiltration (i.e. the 'crazy-paving' pattern). Infiltration of air spaces and interstitium and air spaces by PAS positive macrophages.
10. **Alveolar microlithiasis.**
11. **Amyloidosis.**

Further Reading
Webb WR. Thin-section CT of the secondary pulmonary lobule: anatomy and the image – the 2004 Fleischner Lecture. Radiology 2006;239:322–38.

4.16 RETICULAR PATTERN WITH OR WITHOUT HONEYCOMBING

A reticular pattern (i.e. a lacework of fine or coarse criss-crossing lines) on chest radiography and CT generally indicates established interstitial lung disease. Honeycomb destruction (characterized on HRCT by irregular regions of low attenuation) may be present: note that honeycombing is more readily detected on HRCT than plain chest radiography. Thickening of interlobular septa (see also 4.15) also gives rise to reticular pattern. Distribution of reticular pattern (i.e. upper zone versus lower zone or central versus peripheral) may be discriminatory.

Reticular pattern – diffuse interstitial lung diseases

1. **Idiopathic pulmonary fibrosis (formerly cryptogenic fibrosing alveolitis)** most common idiopathic interstitial pneumonia. Associated with the histological/radiological pattern of usual interstitial pneumonia (UIP). Typical patient is male, aged 50–60 years and complaining of progressive dyspnoea. On chest radiography there is a reticular pattern in mid/lower zones. Predominant basal and sub-pleural reticular pattern with honeycombing is the characteristic finding at CT. Ancillary findings include ground-glass opacification (less extensive than reticular pattern), traction bronchiectasis/bronchiolectasis, mediastinal lymph node enlargement. Atypical HRCT findings in around one-third. Co-existent emphysema in upper zones (associated with preserved lung volumes). Increased incidence of lung cancer.

2. **Connective tissue diseases** (CTD) – fibrotic lung disease is common and most frequent cause of death. Variable patterns of interstitial lung disease including UIP, non-specific interstitial pneumonia (NSIP), lymphocytic interstitial pneumonia (LIP; see also 4.6) and diffuse alveolar damage. Variable prevalence in different CTDs: UIP pattern more prevalent than NSIP in rheumatoid arthritis; NSIP pattern more prevalent in systemic sclerosis and polymyositis. dermatomyositis; LIP most prevalent in rheumatoid arthritis and Sjögren's syndrome.

3. **Occupational lung disease**:
   (a) Asbestosis: basal and subpleural fibrosis almost indistinguishable from IPF on histopathology and radiology although fibrosis may be coarser in asbestosis than IPF and pleural abnormalities absent in IPF. Long latent period (>20 years) following exposure.
   (b) Hard metal pneumoconiosis: exposure to alloy of tungsten, carbon and cobalt ± other metals.
   (c) Paraquat poisoning: late phase of poisoning associated with pulmonary fibrosis.
4. **Sarcoidosis** – archetypal granulomatous fibrotic diffuse interstitial lung disease. Typically associated with symmetrical reticular pattern in upper zones. Calcified mediastinal and hilar lymph nodes.
5. **Extrinsic allergic alveolitis** – secondary to repeated exposure to a potentially wide variety of particulate (1–5μm diameter) organic antigens originating from animals, plants, drugs or bacteria/fungi. Lymphocytic infiltrate with plasma cells in acute phase followed by granulomatous inflammation and then fibrosis.
6. **'Cystic' lung diseases** – Because of the effects of anatomical superimposition on chest radiographs, the multiple cysts in disorders such as Langerhans' cell histiocytosis, lymphangioleiomyomatosis, tuberous sclerosis, etc. can manifest as a reticular pattern (see also 4.6). Relative preservation of lung volumes.
7. **Drug-induced lung disease** – nitrofurantoin, busulphan, cyclophosphamide, bleomycin and melphalan.
8. **Bone marrow transplantation** – airways disease (constrictive obliterative bronchiolitis) and upper zone fibrosis associated with recurrent small pneumothoraces.
9. **Miscellaneous causes of diffuse lung disease**:
   (a) Alveolar proteinosis – (see also 4.15).
   (b) Idiopathic pulmonary haemosiderosis.
   (c) Amyloidosis.

Reticular pattern – due to thickened interlobular septa

See 4.15.

Reticular pattern – due to perilobular infiltration

A variant pattern seen in organizing pneumonia.

Reticular pattern – due to parenchymal destruction leaving 'remnant' interlobular septa

Seen in α-1-antitrypsin deficiency related emphysema; seen in the lower zones.

Further Reading
Copley SJ, Wells AU, Muller NL et al. Thin-section CT in obstructive pulmonary disease: discriminatory value. Radiology 2002;223:812–9.
Souza CA. Idiopathic interstitial pneumonias: prevalence of mediastinal lymph node enlargement in 206 patients. AJR Am J Roentgenol 2006;186:995–9.
Sverzellati N. Small chronic pneumothoraces and pulmonary parenchymal abnormalities after bone marrow transplantation. J Thorac Imaging 2007;22:230–4.
Travis WD et al. ATS/ERS International multidisciplinary consensus classification of the idiopathic interstitial pneumonias. Am J Respir Crit Care Med 2002;165:277–304.

4

4.17 MULTIPLE PIN-POINT OPACITIES

Must be of very high atomic number to be rendered visible on plain chest radiography.

1. **Post lymphangiography** – iodized oil emboli. Contrast medium may be visible at the site of termination of the thoracic duct.
2. **Silicosis*** – usually larger than pin-point but can be very dense, especially in gold miners.
3. **Stannosis** – inhalation of tin oxide. Even distribution throughout the lungs. With Kerley A and B lines.
4. **Barytosis** – inhalation of barytes. Very dense, discrete opacities. Generalized distribution but bases and apices usually spared.
5. **Limestone and marble workers** – inhalation of calcium.
6. **Alveolar microlithiasis** – familial. Lung detail obscured by miliary calcifications. Few symptoms but may progress to cor pulmonale eventually. Pleura, heart and diaphragm may be seen as negative shadows.

4.18 MULTIPLE OPACITIES (0.5–2mm)

Soft-tissue density

1. **Miliary tuberculosis** – widespread and secondary to haematogeneous dissemination. Uniform size. Indistinct margins but discrete. No septal lines. Normal hila unless superimposed on primary tuberculosis.
2. **Fungal infection** – histoplasmosis, coccidioidomycosis, blastomycosis and *Cryptococcus* (torulosis). Similar appearance to miliary tuberculosis.
3. **Coal miner's pneumoconiosis*** – predominantly mid zones with sparing of the extreme bases and apices. Ill-defined and may be arranged in a circle or rosette. Septal lines.
4. **Sarcoidosis*** – predominantly mid zones. Ill-defined. Often with enlarged hila.
5. **Acute extrinsic allergic alveolitis*** – micronodulation in all zones, but predominantly basal; rarely seen on CXR or CT since patients who present with symptoms are managed as if for a febrile flu-like illness.

Greater than soft-tissue density

1. **Haemosiderosis** – secondary to chronic raised venous pressure (seen in 10–15% of patients with mitral stenosis), repeated pulmonary haemorrhage (e.g. Goodpasture's disease) or idiopathic. Septal lines. Smaller than miliary TB.
2. **Silicosis*** – relative sparing of bases and apices. Very well-defined and dense when due to inhalation of pure silica: ill-defined and of lower density when due to mixed dusts. Septal lines.
3. **Siderosis** – lower density than silica. Widely disseminated. Asymptomatic.
4. **Stannosis** – see 4.18.
5. **Barytosis** – see 4.18.

Further Reading

Hatipoglu ON. High resolution computed tomographic findings in pulmonary tuberculosis. Thorax 1996;51:397–402.

Miller WT (ed). Fungus disease of the chest. Semin Roentgenol 1996;31(1).

Kim KI et al. Imaging of occupational lung disease. Radiographics, 2001;21:1371–91.

4.19 MULTIPLE OPACITIES (2–5mm)

Remaining discrete

1. **Carcinomatosis** – breast, thyroid, sarcoma, melanoma, prostate, pancreas or bronchus (eroding a pulmonary artery). Variable sizes and progressive increase in size. ± Lymphatic obstruction.
2. **Lymphoma*** – usually with hilar or mediastinal lymph node enlargement.
3. **Sarcoidosis*** – predominantly mid zones. Often with enlarged hila.

Tending to confluence and/or varying in radiographic intensity over hours to days

1. **Multifocal pneumonia** – including aspiration pneumonia and tuberculosis.
2. **Pulmonary oedema** (see 4.13) – rapid fluid shifts can occur over a few hours in contrast to many other air space diseases.
3. **Intra-alveolar haemorrhage.**

4.20 SOLITARY PULMONARY NODULE

A nodule is defined as a rounded opacity that is reasonably well defined and measuring less than 3cm in diameter. A lesion greater than 3cm in diameter is termed a mass.

Granulomas

1. **Tuberculoma** – more common in the upper lobes and on the right side. Well defined; 0.5–4cm. 25% are lobulated. Calcification frequent. 80% have satellite lesions. Cavitation is uncommon and when present is small and eccentric. Usually persist unchanged for years.
2. **Histoplasmoma** – in endemic areas (Mississippi and the Atlantic coast of USA). More frequent in the lower lobes. Well-defined. Seldom larger than 3cm. Calcification is common and may be central, producing a target appearance. Cavitation is rare. Satellite lesions are common.
3. **Others** – e.g. coccidioidomycosis, cryptococcosis.

Malignant neoplasms

1. **Carcinoma of the bronchus** – usually greater than 2cm. Accounts for less than 15% of all solitary nodules at 40 years: almost 100% at 80 years. However, up to 38% of small (<1cm) nodules identified by

CT may be primary carcinoma of the bronchus. CXR appearances suggesting malignancy include:

(a) Recent appearance or rapid growth (review previous CXRs).
(b) Size greater than 4cm.
(c) The lesion crosses a fissure (although some fungus diseases also do so).
(d) Ill-defined margins.
(e) Umbilicated or notched margin (if present it indicates malignancy in 80%).
(f) Corona radiata (spiculation) (but also seen in PMF and granulomas).
(g) Peripheral line shadows.
(h) Calcification is rare (but seen in up to 10% at CT).

2. **Metastasis** – accounts for 3–5% of asymptomatic nodules. 25% of pulmonary metastases may be solitary. Most likely primaries are breast, sarcoma, seminoma and renal cell carcinoma. Predilection for the lung periphery. Calcification is rare but occurs with metastatic osteosarcoma, chondrosarcoma and some other rarer metastases. When considering the diagnosis of pulmonary metastases in children the following points must be borne in mind:

(a) In contrast to adults, it is highly unlikely that there will be an incidental finding of pulmonary metastatic disease.
(b) The majority of single lung nodules are benign and even in a child with known malignancy one-third of new lung nodules may be benign.
(c) Multiple lung nodules are more likely to be malignant than a single nodule.
(d) Therapy usually results in complete resolution of a metastatic nodule but occasionally there may be a residual scar.

3. **Alveolar cell carcinoma** – when localized, a mass is the most common presentation. More commonly ill-defined. Air bronchogram is common. No calcification. Pleural effusion in 5%. Mediastinal lymphadenopathy is much less common than with carcinoma of the bronchus.

4. **Rare malignant lung tumours** – pulmonary blastoma, pulmonary sarcoma, plasmacytoma, atypical carcinoid (see below).

Benign neoplasms

1. **Carcinoid tumour** – typical carcinoids account for majority (90%) and tend to be more benign than atypical (accounting for 10%) tumours, but spectrum of biological behaviour ranging from benign to small cell carcinoma. Typical carcinoids are generally central whereas atypical tend to be peripheral. May be associated with ectopic ACTH production (Cushing's syndrome).

2. **Hamartoma** – 96% occur over 40 years. 90% are intrapulmonary and usually within 2cm of the pleura. 10% produce bronchial stenosis. Usually less than 4cm diameter. Well-defined. Lobulated rather than smooth. Calcification in 30%, although incidence rises with the size of the lesion (in 75% when greater than 5cm). Calcification is 'pop-corn', craggy or punctate.

Infectious/inflammatory

1. **Pneumonia** – especially pneumococcal.
2. **Hydatid** – in endemic areas. Most common in the lower lobes and more frequent on the right side. Well-defined. 1–10cm. Solitary in 70%. May have a bizarre shape. Rupture results in the 'water lily' sign.
3. **Rounded atelectasis** – generally a sequela following an exudative (inflammatory) pleural effusion. Mass associated with adjacent smooth pleural thickening and parenchymal bands giving rise to 'comet tail' appearance.
4. **Wegener's granulomatosis** – Solitary nodules in up to one-third of patients but more commonly multiple (see below – 4.21).
5. **Sarcoidosis** – a solitary lung nodule (simulating malignancy) is rare but recognized.
6. **Organizing pneumonia** – can masquerade as (malignant) solitary pulmonary nodule.

Congenital

1. **Sequestration** – may be intralobar (more common; acquired abnormality probably secondary to chronic lung suppuration. No separate pleural covering. Venous drainage into pulmonary veins) or extralobar (rare; congenital lesion with separate pleural covering. Venous drainage into systemic circulation). Usually large (>6cm). Majority in the left lower lobe; next most common site is the right lower lobe, contiguous with the diaphragm. Well-defined, round or oval. Diagnosis confirmed by identification of the mass and its blood supply: increasingly possible with advent of multi-detector CT; MR angiography also of value in demonstration of anomalous vasculature MRI.
2. **Bronchogenic cyst** – Majority are mediastinal or hilar but occasional bronchogenic cysts are intrapulmonary (even more rarely: diaphragmatic, pleural, pericardial). Most intrapulmonary bronchogenic cysts are central (perihilar) and may have systemic arterial supply. Round or oval. Smooth-walled and well-defined.
3. **Intrapulmonary lymph node** – usually solitary, small (<2cm), well-defined and discovered incidentally at CT in mid/lower zones. Vast majority within 2cm of visceral pleura. Accounting for around 20% of all incidentally detected solitary nodules. Usually benign (even when detected in context of a known malignancy).

Vascular

1. **Haematoma** – peripheral, smooth and well-defined. 2–6cm. Slow resolution over several weeks.
2. **Arteriovenous malformation** – 66% are single. Well-defined, lobulated lesion. Feeding or draining vessels may be demonstrable. Calcification rare. Pulmonary angiography previously the gold-standard for diagnosis but now supplanted by multidetector CT.

Further Reading

Coley SC, Jackson JE. Pulmonary arteriovenous malformations. Clin Radiol 1998;53:396–404.

Erasmus JJ, Connolly JE, McAdams HP et al. Solitary pulmonary nodules: Part I. Morphologic evaluation for differentiation of benign and malignant lesions. Radiographics 2000;20:43–58.

Erasmus JJ, McAdams HP, Connolly JE. Solitary pulmonary nodules: Part II. Evaluation of the indeterminate nodule. Radiographics 2000;20:59–66.

Hoffman LV. Angioarchitecture of pulmonary arteriovenous malformations: characterization using volume-rendered 3-D CT angiography. Cardiovasc Intervent Radiol 2000;23:165–70.

Kang A et al. Multidetector CT angiography in pulmonary sequestration. J Comput Assist Tomogr 2006;30:926–32.

Oshiro Y et al. Intrapulmonary lymph nodes: thin-section CT features of 19 nodules. J Comput Assist Tomogr 2002;26:553–7.

Murphy J et al. Bronchiolitis obliterans organising pneumonia simulating bronchial carcinoma. Eur Radiol 1998;8:1165–9.

4.21 MULTIPLE PULMONARY NODULES (>5mm)

Neoplastic

1. **Metastases** – most commonly from breast, thyroid, kidney, gastrointestinal tract and testes. In children, Wilms' tumour, Ewing's sarcoma, neuroblastoma and osteosarcoma. Predilection for lower lobes and more common peripherally. Range of sizes. Well-defined. Ill-definition suggests prostate, breast or stomach. Hilar lymphadenopathy and effusions are uncommon.
2. **Multiple (synchronous) lung cancers.**

Infections

1. **Abscesses** – widespread distribution but asymmetrical. Commonly *Staphylococcus aureus*. Cavitation common. No calcification.
2. **Coccidioidomycosis** – in endemic areas. Well-defined with a predilection for the upper lobes. 0.5–3cm. Calcification and cavitation may be present.
3. **Histoplasmosis** – in endemic areas. Round, well-defined and few in number. Sometimes calcify. Usually unchanged for many years.
4. **Hydatid** – more common on the right side and in the lower zones. Well-defined unless there is surrounding pneumonia. Often 10cm or more. May rupture and show the 'water lily' sign.

Immunological

1. **Wegener's granulomatosis** – bilateral nodules or masses (± cavitation in 30–50% of cases) or unifocal/multifocal consolidation. Widespread distribution. Round and well-defined. No calcification. Cavitation.
2. **Rheumatoid nodules** – peripheral and more common in the lower zones. Round and well-defined. No calcification. Cavitation common.
3. **Caplan's syndrome** – well-defined. Develop rapidly in crops. Calcification and cavitation occur. Background stippling of pneumoconiosis.
4. **Sarcoidosis** – multiple nodules/masses, measuring up to 5cm, is an uncommon but recognized manifestation.
5. **Organizing pneumonia.**
6. **Amyloidosis** – Multiple nodules of varying size (calcified in up to 50%).

4

Vascular

1. **Arteriovenous malformations** – 33% are multiple. Well-defined. Lobulated. Tomography may show feeding or draining vessels. Calcification is rare.

Further Reading

Orseck MJ et al. Bronchiolitis obliterans organizing pneumonia mimicking multiple pulmonary metastases. Am Surg 2000;66:11–13.

Trousse D. Synchronous multiple primary lung cancer: an increasing clinical occurrence requiring multidisciplinary management. J Thorac Cardiovasc Surg 2007;133:1193–200.

4.22 LUNG CAVITIES

Infective, i.e. abscesses

1. *Staphylococcus aureus* – thick-walled with a ragged inner lining. No lobar predilection. Associated with effusion and empyema ± pyopneumothorax – almost invariable in children, not so common in adults. Pneumatocoeles. Multiple.
2. *Klebsiella pneumoniae* – thick-walled with a ragged inner lining. More common in the upper lobes. Usually single but may be multilocular ± effusion.
3. **Tuberculosis** – thick-walled and smooth. Upper lobes and apical segment of lower lobes mainly. Usually surrounded by consolidation. ± Fibrosis.
4. **Aspiration** – look for foreign body, e.g. tooth.
5. **Others** – Gram-negative organisms, actinomycosis, nocardiosis, histoplasmosis, coccidioidomycosis, aspergillosis, hydatid and amoebiasis.

Neoplastic

1. **Carcinoma of the bronchus** – thick-walled with an eccentric cavity. Predilection for the upper lobes. Found in 2–10% of carcinomas and especially if peripheral. More common in squamous cell carcinomas and may then be thin-walled.
2. **Metastases** – thin- or thick-walled. May only involve a few of the nodules. Seen especially in squamous cell, colon and sarcoma metastases.
3. **Hodgkin's disease** – thin- or thick-walled and typically in an area of infiltration. With hilar or mediastinal lymphadenopathy.

Vascular

1. **Infarction** – primary infection due to a septic embolus commonly results in cavitation. There may be secondary infection of an initially sterile infarct. An aseptic cavitating infarct may subsequently become infected: tertiary infection. Aseptic cavitation is usually solitary and arises in a large area of consolidation after about 2 weeks. If localized to a segment the commonest sites are apical or the posterior segment of an upper lobe or apical segment of lower lobe (cf. lower lobe predominance with non-cavitating infarction). Majority have scalloped inner margins and cross cavity band shadows. ± Effusion.

Abnormal lung

1. **Infected emphysematous bulla** – thin-walled. ± Air fluid level.
2. **Sequestrated segment** – thick- or thin-walled. 66% in the left lower lobe, 33% in the right lower lobe. ± Air fluid level. ± Surrounding pneumonia.
3. **Bronchogenic cyst** – in medial third of lower lobes. Thin-walled. ± Air fluid level. ± Surrounding pneumonia.

Granulomas

1. **Wegener's granulomatosis** – cavitation in some of the nodules. Thick-walled, becoming thinner with time. Can be transient.
2. **Rheumatoid nodules** – thick-walled with a smooth inner lining. Especially in the lower lobes and peripherally. Well-defined. Become thin-walled with time.
3. **Progressive massive fibrosis** – predominantly in the mid and upper zones. Thick-walled and irregular. Background nodularity.
4. **Sarcoidosis*** – thin-walled. In early disease due to a combination of central necrosis of areas of coalescent granulomas and a check-valve mechanism beyond partial obstruction of airways by endobronchial sarcoidosis.

Traumatic

1. **Haematoma** – peripheral. Air fluid level if it communicates with a bronchus.
2. **Traumatic lung cyst** – thin-walled and peripheral. Single or multiple. Unilocular or multilocular. Distinguished from cavitating haematomas as they present early, within hours of the injury.

Further Reading

John PR, Beasley SW, Mayne V. Pulmonary sequestration and related congenital disorders. A clinico-radiological review of 41 cases. Pediatr Radiol 1989;20:4–9.

Vourtsi A, Gouliamos A, Moulopoulos L et al. CT appearance of solitary and multiple cystic and cavitary lung lesions. Eur Radiol 2001;11:612–22.

Wilson AG, Joseph AE, Butland RJ. The radiology of aseptic cavitation in pulmonary infarction. Clin Radiol 1986;37:327–33.

4.23 NON-THROMBOTIC PULMONARY EMBOLI

1. **Septic embolism** – associated with indwelling venous catheters, tricuspid valve endocarditis and peripheral septic thrombophlebitis. Variable size, poorly marginated nodules, predominantly in the lower lobes, and which tend to form cavities.
2. **Catheter embolism** – catheter fragments are most common in the basilica vein and pulmonary arteries.
3. **Fat embolism** – 1–2 days post-trauma. Predominantly peripheral. Resolves in 1–4 weeks. Normal heart size. Pleural effusions uncommon. Neurological symptoms in up to 85% and skin abnormalities in 20–50%.
4. **Venous air embolism** – when iatrogenic, prognosis is affected by volume of air and speed of injection. Clinical effects are the result of right ventricular outflow obstruction or obstruction of pulmonary arterioles. CXR may be normal or show air in the main pulmonary artery, heart or hepatic veins, focal pulmonary oligaemia or pulmonary oedema.
5. **Amniotic fluid embolism** – rare. The majority of patients suffer cardiopulmonary arrest and the CXR shows pulmonary oedema.
6. **Tumour embolism** – common sources are liver, breast, stomach, kidney, prostate and choriocarcinoma. CXR is usually normal.
7. **Talc embolism** – in i.v. drug abusers.
8. **Iodinated oil embolism** – following contrast lymphangiography.
9. **Cotton embolism** – when cotton fibres adhere to angiographic catheters or guidewires and in i.v. drug abusers.
10. **Hydatid embolism.**

Further Reading

Rossi SE, Goodman PC, Franquet T. Nonthrombic pulmonary emboli. Am J Roentgenol 2000;174:1499–508.

4.24 PULMONARY CALCIFICATION OR OSSIFICATION

Localized calcification

1. **Tuberculosis** – demonstrable in 10% of those with a positive tuberculin test. Small central nidus of calcification. Calcification $\neq$ healed.
2. **Histoplasmosis** – in endemic areas, calcification due to histoplasmosis is demonstrable in 30% of those with a positive histoplasmin test. Calcification may be laminated, producing a target lesion. $\pm$ Multiple punctate calcifications in the spleen.
3. **Coccidioidomycosis.**
4. **Blastomycosis** – rare.

Calcification within a solitary nodule

Calcification within a nodule equates with a benign lesion. The exceptions are:

(a) Carcinoma engulfing a pre-existing calcified granuloma (eccentric calcification).
(b) Solitary calcifying/ossifying metastasis – osteosarcoma, chondrosarcoma, mucinous adenocarcinoma of the colon or breast, papillary carcinoma of the thyroid, cystadenocarcinoma of the ovary and carcinoid.
(c) $1°$ peripheral squamous cell or papillary adenocarcinoma.

Diffuse or multiple calcifications

1. **Infections**
   (a) Tuberculosis – healed miliary.
   (b) Histoplasmosis.
   (c) Varicella – following chicken pox pneumonia in adulthood. 1–3mm. Numbered in 10s.
2. **Chronic pulmonary venous hypertension** – especially mitral stenosis. Up to 8mm. Most prominent in mid and lower zones. $\pm$ Ossification.
3. **Silicosis** – in up to 20% of those showing nodular opacities.
4. **Metastases** – as above.
5. **Alveolar microlithiasis** – often familial. Myriad minute calcifications in alveoli which obscure all lung detail. Because of the lung's increased density, the heart, pleura and diaphragm may be evident as negative shadows.
6. **Metastatic due to hypercalcaemia** – chronic renal failure, $2°$ hyperparathyroidism and multiple myeloma*. Predominantly in the upper zones.
7. **Lymphoma following radiotherapy.**

Interstitial ossification

1. **Dendriform/disseminated pulmonary ossification.** Branching or nodular calcific densities extending along the bronchovascular distribution of the interstitial space. Seen in: long-term busulphan therapy, chronic pulmonary venous hypertension (e.g. due to mitral stenosis), idiopathic pulmonary fibrosis, asbestosis, following ARDS, chronic bronchitis.
2. **Idiopathic.**

Further Reading

Gevenois PA. Disseminated pulmonary ossification in end-stage pulmonary fibrosis: CT demonstration. Am J Roentgenol 1994;162:1303–4.

Jacobs AN, Neitzschman HR, Nicecm Jr. Metaplastic bone formation in the lung. Am J Roentgenol 1973;118:344–6.

Kuplic JB, Higley CS, Niewoehner DE. Pulmonary ossification associated with long-term busulfan therapy in chronic myeloid leukaemia. Case report. Am Rev Resp Dis 1972;106:759.

Lara JF. Dendriform pulmonary ossification, a form of diffuse pulmonary ossification: report of a 26-year autopsy experience. Arch Pathol Lab Med 2005;129:348–53.

Maile CW, Rodan BA, Godwin JD et al. Calcification in pulmonary metastases. Br J Radiol 1982;55:108–13.

4.25 UNILATERAL HILAR ENLARGEMENT

Lymph nodes

1. **Carcinoma of the bronchus** – the hilar enlargement may be due to the tumour itself or involved lymph nodes.
2. **Lymphoma*** – unilateral is very unusual; involvement is usually bilateral and asymmetrical.
3. **Infective**
   (a) Primary tuberculosis.
   (b) Histoplasmosis.
   (c) Coccidioidomycosis.
   (d) Mycoplasma.
   (e) Pertussis.
4. **Sarcoidosis*** – unilateral disease in only 1–5%.

Pulmonary artery

1. **Post-stenotic dilatation** – on the left side.
2. **Pulmonary embolus** (see Pulmonary embolic disease*) – massive to one lung. Peripheral oligaemia.
3. **Aneurysm** – in chronic pulmonary arterial hypertension. ± Egg-shell calcification.

Others

1. **Mediastinal mass** – superimposed on a hilum.
2. **Perihilar pneumonia** – ill-defined, ± air bronchogram.

See also 4.8.

Further Reading
Ko JP, Drucker A, Shepard J-O et al. CT depiction of regional nodal stations for
lung cancer staging. Am J Roentgenol 2000;174:775–82.

4.26 BILATERAL HILAR ENLARGEMENT

Due to lymph node enlargement or pulmonary artery enlargement.

Idiopathic

1. **Sarcoidosis*** – symmetrical and lobulated. Bronchopulmonary ±
unilateral or bilateral paratracheal lymphadenopathy.

Neoplastic

1. **Lymphoma*** – asymmetrical.
2. **Lymphangitis carcinomatosa/lymphomatosa.**

Infective

1. **Viruses** – most common in children.
2. **Primary tuberculosis** – rarely bilateral and symmetrical.
3. **Histoplasmosis.**
4. **Coccidioidomycosis.**

Vascular

1. **Pulmonary arterial hypertension** – see section 5.17.

Immunological

1. **Extrinsic allergic alveolitis*** – in mushroom workers.

Inhalational

1. **Silicosis*** – symmetrical.
2. **Chronic berylliosis** – only in a minority of cases. Symmetrical.

Further Reading
Baldwin DR, Lambert L, Pantin CF et al. Silicosis presenting as bilateral hilar
lymphadenopathy. Thorax 1996;51:1165–7.

4.27 'EGG-SHELL' CALCIFICATION OF LYMPH NODES

Defined as shell-like calcifications up to 2mm thick in the periphery of at least two lymph nodes in at least one of which, the ring of calcification must be complete and one of the affected lymph nodes must be at least 1cm in maximum diameter. Calcifications may be solid or broken. The central part of the lymph node may show additional calcifications.

1. **Silicosis*** – seen in approximately 5% of silicotics. Predominantly hilar lymph nodes but may also be observed in the nodal groups. Calcification more common in complicated pneumoconiosis. Lungs show multiple small nodular shadows or areas of massive fibrosis.
2. **Coal miner's pneumoconiosis*** – occurs in only 1% of cases. Associated pulmonary changes include miliary shadowing or massive shadows.
3. **Sarcoidosis*** – nodal calcification overall in approximately 5% of patients and is occasionally 'egg-shell' in appearance. Calcification appears about 6 years after the onset of the disease and is almost invariably associated with advanced pulmonary disease and in some cases with steroid therapy.
4. **Lymphoma following radiotherapy** – appears 1–9 years after radiotherapy.

Differential diagnosis

Note that determination of the anatomical location of calcification generally not problematic with multidetector CT

1. **Pulmonary artery calcification** – a rare feature of pulmonary arterial hypertension.
2. **Aortic calcification** – especially in the wall of a saccular aneurysm.
3. **Anterior mediastinal tumours** – teratodermoids and thymomas may occasionally exhibit rim calcification.

Further Reading

Gross BH, Schneider HJ, Proto AV. Eggshell calcification of lymph nodes: an update. Am J Roentgenol 1980;135:1265.
Jacobsen G, Felson B, Pendergrass EP et al. Eggshell calcification in coal and metal miners. Semin Roentgenol 1967;2:276–82.

4.28 DIFFUSE LUNG DISEASE WITH PRESERVED LUNG VOLUMES

1. Langerhans cell histiocytosis*.
2. Lymphangioleiomyomatosis/Tuberose sclerosis complex
3. Cystic fibrosis*.
4. Sarcoidosis* – obstruction of small airways is often a dominant finding in sarcoidosis.
5. Cryptogenic fibrosing alveolitis/Idiopathic pulmonary fibrosis with emphysema.

4.29 PLEURAL EFFUSION

Transudate (protein $<30g\ l^{-1}$)

1. Cardiac failure.
2. Hepatic failure.
3. Nephrotic syndrome.
4. Meigs syndrome.

Exudate (protein $>30g\ l^{-1}$)

1. Infection.
2. Malignancy.
3. Pulmonary infarction – see Pulmonary embolic disease*.
4. Collagen vascular diseases.
5. Subphrenic abscess.
6. Pancreatitis.

Haemorrhagic

1. Carcinoma of the bronchus.
2. Trauma.
3. Pulmonary infarction – see Pulmonary embolic disease*.
4. Bleeding disorders.

Chylous

1. Obstructed thoracic duct – due to trauma, malignant invasion or filariasis.

4.30 PLEURAL EFFUSION DUE TO EXTRATHORACIC DISEASE

1. **Pancreatitis** – acute, chronic or relapsing. Effusions are predominantly left-sided. Elevated amylase content.
2. **Subphrenic abscess** – with elevation and restriction of movement of the ipsilateral diaphragm and basal atelectasis or consolidation.
3. **Following abdominal surgery** – most often seen on the side of the surgery and larger after upper abdominal surgery. Disappears after 2 weeks.
4. **Meig's syndrome** – pleural effusion + ascites + benign pelvic tumour (most commonly an ovarian fibroma, thecoma, granulosa cell tumour or cystadenoma).
5. **Nephrotic syndrome.**
6. **Fluid overload** – e.g. due to renal disease.
7. **Cirrhosis.**

4.31 PLEURAL EFFUSION WITH AN OTHERWISE NORMAL CHEST X-RAY

Effusion may be the only abnormality or other signs may be obscured by the effusion.

Infective

1. **Primary tuberculosis** – more common in adults (40%) than children (10%). Rarely bilateral.
2. **Viruses and mycoplasma** – effusions occur in 10–20% of cases but are usually small.

Neoplastic

1. **Carcinoma of the bronchus** – effusion occurs in 10% of patients and a peripheral carcinoma may be hidden by the effusion.
2. **Metastases** – most commonly from breast; less commonly pancreas, stomach, ovary and kidney.
3. **Mesothelioma** – effusion in 90%; often massive and obscures the underlying pleural disease.
4. **Lymphoma*** – effusion occurs in 30% but is usually associated with lymphadenopathy or pulmonary infiltrates.

Immunological

1. **Systemic lupus erythematosus*** – effusion is the sole manifestation in 10% of cases. Usually small but may be massive. Bilateral in 50%. 35–50% of those with an effusion have associated cardiomegaly.

2. **Rheumatoid disease (see Rheumatoid arthritis*)** – observed in 3% of patients. Almost exclusively males. Usually unilateral and may predate joint disease. Tendency to remain unchanged for a long time.

Extrathoracic diseases
See 4.30.

Others
1. **Pulmonary embolus (see Pulmonary embolic disease*)** – effusion is a common sign and it may obscure an underlying area of infarction.
2. **Closed chest trauma** – effusion may contain blood, chyle or food (due to oesophageal rupture). The latter is almost always left-sided.
3. **Asbestosis*** – mesothelioma and carcinoma of the bronchus should be excluded but an effusion may be present without these complications. Effusion is frequently recurrent and usually bilateral. Usually associated with pulmonary disease.

Further Reading
Ng CS, Munden RF, Libshitz HI. Malignant pleural mesothelioma: the spectrum of manifestations on CT in 70 cases. Clin Radiol 1999;54:415–21.

4.32 PNEUMOTHORAX

1. **Spontaneous** – M:F, 8:1. Especially those of tall thin stature usually due to ruptured blebs or bullae. 20% are associated with a small pleural effusion.
2. **Iatrogenic** – following chest aspiration, artificial ventilation, lung biopsy or central line insertion.
3. **Trauma** – may be associated with rib fractures, haemothorax, surgical emphysema or mediastinal emphysema.
4. **Secondary to mediastinal emphysema** (see 4.33).
5. **Secondary to lung disease**
   (a) Emphysema.
   (b) 'Honeycomb lung' (q.v.).
   (c) Cystic fibrosis*.
   (d) Pneumonia.
   (e) Bronchopleural fistula, e.g. due to lung abscess or carcinoma.
   (f) Lung neoplasms – especially metastases from osteogenic sarcomas and other sarcomas.
6. **Pneumoperitoneum** – air passage through a pleuroperitoneal foramen.

4.33 PNEUMOMEDIASTINUM

Radiographic signs depend on air outlining normal anatomical structures. May be associated with a pneumothorax.

1. **Lung tear** – a sudden rise in intra-alveolar pressure, often with airway narrowing, causes air to dissect through the interstitium to the hilum and then to the mediastinum.
   (a) Spontaneous – the most common cause and may follow coughing or strenuous exercise.
   (b) Asthma – but usually not < 2 years of age.
   (c) Severe and protracted vomiting.
   (d) Vaginal delivery because of repeated Valsalva manoeuvres.
   (e) Artificial ventilation.
   (f) Chest trauma.
   (g) Foreign body aspiration – especially if < 2 years.
2. **Perforation of oesophagus**, trachea or bronchus – ruptured oesophagus is often associated with a hydrothorax or hydropneumothorax, usually on the left side.
3. **Perforation of a hollow abdominal viscus** – with extension of gas via the retroperitoneal space.

Further Reading
Burton EM, Riggs Jr W, Kaufman RA et al. Pneumomediastinum caused by foreign body aspiration in children. Pediatr Radiol 1989;20:45–7.
Fraser RG, Paré JAP, Paré PD et al. Pneumomediastinum. In: Diagnosis of Diseases of the Chest, 3rd edn. Vol. 4. WB Saunders, Philadelphia, pp2801–13.
Zylack CM, Standen JR, Barnes GR et al. Pneumomediastinum. Radiographics 2000;20:1043–57.

4.34 RIGHT-SIDED DIAPHRAGMATIC HUMPS

At any site
1. **Collapse/consolidation of adjacent lung.**
2. **Localized eventration.**
3. **Loculated effusion.**
4. **Subphrenic abscess.**
5. **Hepatic abscess.**
6. **Hydatid cyst.**
7. **Hepatic metastasis.**

Medially
1. **Pericardial fat pad.**
2. **Aortic aneurysm.**

3. **Pleuro-pericardial (spring water cyst).**
4. **Sequestrated segment.**

Anteriorly
1. **Morgagni hernia.**

Posteriorly
1. **Bochdalek hernia.**

Further Reading
Baron RL, Lee JKT, Melson GL. Sonographic evaluation of right
    juxtadiaphragmatic masses in children using transhepatic approach. J Clin
    Ultrasound 1980;8:156–8.
Kangerloo H, Sukov R, Sample F et al. Ultrasonic evaluation of
    juxtadiaphragmatic masses in children. Radiology 1977;125:785–7.
Khan AN, Gould DA. The primary role of ultrasound in evaluating right sided
    diaphragmatic humps and juxtadiaphragmatic masses: a review of 22 cases.
    Clin Radiol 1984;35:413–8.

4.35 UNILATERAL ELEVATED HEMIDIAPHRAGM

Causes above the diaphragm
1. **Phrenic nerve palsy** – smooth hemidiaphragm. No movement on respiration. Paradoxical movement on sniffing. The mediastinum is usually central. The cause may be evident on the x-ray.
2. **Pulmonary collapse.**
3. **Pulmonary infarction** – see Pulmonary embolic disease*.
4. **Pleural disease** – especially old pleural disease, e.g. haemothorax, empyema or thoracotomy.
5. **Splinting of the diaphragm** – associated with rib fractures or pleurisy.
6. **Hemiplegia** – an upper motor neuron lesion.

Diaphragmatic causes
1. **Eventration** – more common on the left side. The heart is frequently displaced to the contralateral side. Limited movement on normal respiration and paradoxical movement on sniffing. Stomach may show a partial volvulus.

Causes below the diaphragm
1. **Gaseous distension of the stomach or splenic flexure** – left hemidiaphragm only. May be transient.

2. **Subphrenic inflammatory disease** – subphrenic abscess, hepatic or splenic abscess and pancreatitis.

Scoliosis

The raised hemidiaphragm is on the side of the concavity.

Decubitus film

The raised hemidiaphragm is on the dependent side.

Differential diagnosis

1. **Subpulmonary effusion** – movement of fluid is demonstrable on a decubitus film. On the left side there is increased distance between the lung and stomach fundal gas.
2. **Ruptured diaphragm** – more common on the left. Barium meal confirms the diagnosis.

4.36 BILATERAL ELEVATED HEMIDIAPHRAGMS

General causes

1. **Poor inspiratory effort.**
2. **Obesity.**
3. **Muscular weakness and myopathy** – Myotonia, SLE.

Causes above the diaphragms

1. **Bilateral basal pulmonary collapse** – which may be secondary to infarction of subphrenic abscesses.
2. **Small lungs** – fibrotic lung disease, e.g. fibrosing alveolitis.

Causes below the diaphragms

1. **Ascites.**
2. **Pregnancy.**
3. **Pneumoperitoneum.**
4. **Hepatosplenomegaly.**
5. **Large intra-abdominal tumour.**
6. **Bilateral subphrenic abscesses.**

Differential diagnosis

1. **Bilateral subpulmonary effusions.**

4.37 PLEURAL CALCIFICATION

1. **Old empyema** ⎫ both may result in amorphous bizarre
2. **Old haemothorax** ⎬ plaques, often with a vacuolated
                        ⎪ appearance near the inner surface of
                        ⎪ greatly thickened pleura. Usually
                        ⎭ unilateral.
3. **Asbestos inhalation*** – small curvilinear plaques in the parietal pleura. More delicate than (1) and (2). Often multiple and bilateral and found over the domes of the diaphragms and immediately deep to the ribs. Observed in 10–15% of people exposed to asbestos but not before 20 years have elapsed. Not necessarily associated with asbestosis.
4. **Silicosis***.
5. **Talc exposure**.

4.38 LOCAL PLEURAL MASSES

1. **Loculated pleural effusion**.
2. **Metastases** – from bronchus or breast. Often multiple.
3. **Malignant mesothelioma** – nearly always related to asbestos exposure. The pleural thickening may be obscured by an effusion. Often contract hemithorax.
4. **Pleural fibroma (local benign mesothelioma)** – a smooth lobular mass, 2–15cm diameter, arising more frequently from the visceral pleura than the parietal pleura. May change position due to pedunculation. Forms an obtuse angle with the chest wall suggesting extrapulmonary location. Patients usually over 40 years of age and asymptomatic. When pleural fibroma is present there is a high chance of hypertrophic osteoarthropathy.

Differential diagnosis

1. **Extrapleural masses** – see 4.39.

Further Reading
Ng CS, Munden RF, Libshitz HI: Malignant pleural mesothelioma: the spectrum of manifestations on CT in 70 cases. Clin Radiol 1999;54:415–21.

4.39 RIB LESION WITH AN ADJACENT SOFT-TISSUE MASS

Neoplastic

1. **Bronchogenic carcinoma** – solitary site unless metastatic.
2. **Metastases** – solitary or multiple.
3. **Multiple myeloma*** – classically multiple sites and bilateral.
4. **Mesothelioma** – rib destruction occurs in 12%.
5. **Lymphoma***.
6. **Fibrosarcoma** – similar appearances to mesothelioma.
7. **Neurofibroma** – rib notching.

Infective

1. **Tuberculosis osteitis** – commonest inflammatory lesion of a rib but a rare manifestation of TB. Second only to malignancy as a cause of rib destruction. Clearly defined margins ± abscess.
2. **Actinomycosis** – usually a single rib and often associated with a lung mass due to consolidation.
3. **Nocardiosis**.
4. **Blastomycosis** – adjacent patchy or massive consolidation ± hilar lymphadenopathy.

Inflammatory

1. **Radiation osteitis**.

Metabolic

1. **Renal osteodystrophy**
2. **Cushing's syndrome**

} rib fractures and osteopenia associated with a subpleural haematoma.

Further Reading

Guttentag A, Salwen JK. Keep your eyes on the ribs: the spectrum of normal variants and diseases that involve ribs. Radiographics 1999;19:1125–42.

Steiner RM, Cooper MW, Brodovsky H. Rib destruction: a neglected finding in malignant mesothelioma. Clin Radiol 1982;33:61–5.

4.40 THE CHEST RADIOGRAPH FOLLOWING CHEST TRAUMA

Soft tissues
1. **Foreign bodies.**
2. **Surgical emphysema.**

Ribs
1. **Simple fracture**
2. **Flail chest**

may be associated with surgical emphysema, pneumothorax, extrapleural haematoma or haemothorax. First rib fractures (except stress fractures) have a high incidence of other associated injuries.

Sternum
1. **Fracture** – may be associated with a clinically unsuspected dorsal spine fracture.
2. **Sternoclavicular dislocation.**

Clavicles and scapulae
1. **Fracture** – scapular fractures are usually associated with other bony or intrathoracic injuries.

Spine
1. **Fracture** – when present, are multiple in 10% and non-contiguous in 80% of these. Thoracic spine injuries have a much higher incidence of neurological deficit than cervical or lumbar spine injuries.
2. **Cord trauma.**
3. **Nerve root trauma** – especially to the brachial plexus.

Pleura
1. **Pneumothorax** – simple (in 20–40% of patients with blunt chest trauma and 20% of patients with penetrating injuries) or tension. Signs of a small pneumothorax on a supine chest radiograph include a deep costophrenic sulcus, basal hyperlucency, a 'double' diaphragm, unusually clear definition of the right cardiophrenic angle or left cardiac apex and visualization of apical pericardial fat tags. CT is more sensitive than plain film radiography.
2. **Haemothorax** – in 25–50% of patients with blunt chest trauma and 60–80% of patients with penetrating wounds.

Lung

1. **Contusion** – non-segmental alveolar opacities which resolve in a few days.
2. **Haematoma** – usually appears following resolution of contusion. Round, well-defined nodule. Resolution in several weeks.
3. **Aspiration pneumonia**.
4. **Foreign body**.
5. **Pulmonary oedema** – following blast injuries or head injury (neurogenic oedema).
6. **Acute respiratory distress syndrome** – widespread air-space shadowing appearing 24–72 hours after injury.
7. **Fat embolism** – 1–2 days post-trauma. Resembles pulmonary oedema, but normal heart size and pleural effusions are uncommon. Resolves in 1–4 weeks. Neurological symptoms in up to 85% and skin abnormalities in 20–50%.

Trachea and bronchi

1. **Laceration or fracture** – initially surgical emphysema and pneumomediastinum followed by collapse of the affected lung or lobe.

Diaphragm

1. **Rupture** – in 3–7% of patients with blunt and 6–46% of patients with penetrating thoraco-abdominal trauma. Diagnosis may be delayed months or years. Plain film findings include herniated stomach or bowel above the diaphragm, pleural effusion, a supradiaphragmatic mass or a poorly visualized or abnormally contoured diaphragm. Probable equal incidence on both sides but rupture of the right hemidiaphragm is not so easily diagnosed.

Mediastinum

1. **Aortic injury** – 90% of aortic ruptures occur just distal to the origin of the left subclavian artery. The majority of patients with this complication die before radiological evaluation, especially when rupture involves the ascending aorta. Plain film radiographic abnormalities of aortic rupture are:
   - (a) Widening of the mediastinum (sensitivity 53–100%; specificity 1–60%).
   - (b) Abnormal aortic contour (sensitivity 53–100%; specificity 21–42%).
   - (c) Tracheal displacement to the right (sensitivity 12–100%; specificity 80–95%).
   - (d) Nasogastric tube displacement to the right of the T4 spinous process (sensitivity 9–71%; specificity 90–96%).

(e) Thickening of the right paraspinal stripe (sensitivity 12–83%; specificity 89–97%).

(f) Depression of the left mainstem bronchus > 40° below the horizontal (sensitivity 3–80%; specificity 80–100%).

(g) Loss of definition of the aortopulmonary window (sensitivity 0–100%; specificity 56–83%).

A normal chest radiograph has a 98% negative predictive value for traumatic aortic rupture.

2. **Mediastinal haematoma** – blurring of the mediastinal outline.
3. **Mediastinal emphysema** (see 4.33).
4. **Haemopericardium**.
5. **Oesophageal rupture**.

Further Reading

Desai SR. Acute respiratory distress syndrome: imaging of the injured lung. Clin Radiol 2002;57:8–17.

Groskin SA. Selected topics in chest trauma. Radiology 1992;183:605–17.

Patel NH, Stephens KE, Mirvis SE et al. Imaging of acute thoracic aortic injury due to blunt trauma: a review. Radiology 1998;209:335–48.

Reynolds J, Davis JT. Thoracic injuries. The radiology of trauma. Radiol Clin North Am 1966;4:383–402.

Tack D, Defrance P, Delcour C et al. The CT fallen lung-sign. Eur Radiol 2000;10:719–21.

Wintermark M, Wicky S, Schnyder P. Imaging of acute traumatic injuries of the thoracic aorta. Eur Radiol 2002;12:431–42.

4.41 DRUG-INDUCED LUNG DISEASE

Diffuse alveolar opacities

1. **Pulmonary oedema** – cocaine, cytosine arabinoside (Ara-C), heroin overdose, interleukin 2, morphine overdose, OKT3 (in association with fluid overload), sympathomimetics (ritodrine and terbutaline), salicylate overdose and tricyclic antidepressant overdose.
2. **Pulmonary haemorrhage** – anticoagulants and those drugs which produce an idiosyncratic thrombocytopenia, crack cocaine, penicillamine and quinidine.
3. **Allergic alveolitis** – pituitary snuff.

Focal alveolar opacities

1. **Phospholipidosis** – amiodarone.
2. **Pulmonary eosinophilia** – sulphonamides (sulphasalazine), nitrofurantoin, para-aminosalicylic acid and penicillin.
3. **Vasculitis** – ampicillin, penicillin and sulphonamides.

Diffuse interstitial opacities

1. **Acute interstitial reactions** – methotrexate, nitrofurantoin, procarbazine and drugs causing pulmonary oedema.
2. **Chronic interstitial reactions** – cytotoxic agents (BCNU, bleomycin, busulphan, cyclophosphamide, methotrexate and mitomycin-C).
3. **Non-cytotoxic agents** – amiodarone, gold salts and nitrofurantoin.

Bronchospasm

1. **β-blockers.**
2. **Histamine liberators** – iodine containing contrast media and morphine.
3. **Drugs as antigens** – antisera, penicillins and cephalosporins.
4. **Others** – aspirin, anti-inflammatory agents, paracetamol.

Hilar enlargement or mediastinal widening

1. **Phenytoin.**
2. **Steroids.**

Increased opportunistic infections

1. **Antimitotics.**
2. **Steroids.**
3. **Actinomycin C.**
4. **Drug-induced neutropenia or aplastic anaemia** – idiosyncratic or dose-related.

Further Reading

Aronchik JM, Gefter WB. Drug-induced pulmonary disorders. Semin Roentgenol 1995;30(1):18–34.

Ellis SJ, Cleverley JR, Muller NL. Drug-induced lung disease: high resolution CT findings. Am J Roentgenol 2000;175:1019–24.

Erasmus JJ, McAdams HP, Rossi SE. High-resolution CT of drug-induced lung disease. Radiol Clin North Am 2002;40(1):61–72.

Gefter WB, Aronchik JM, Miller WT Jr et al. Drug-induced chest disorders. In: A Categorical Course in Diagnostic Radiology. RSNA Scientific Assembly, RSNA, Chicago, pp167–80.

Rossi SE, Erasmus JJ, McAdams P et al. Pulmonary drug toxicity: radiologic and pathologic manifestations. Radiographics 2000;20:1245–59.

4.42 HIGH RESOLUTION CT – NODULES

These may be centrilobular, perilymphatic or random.

Centrilobular

The most peripheral nodules are >5mm from the pleural surfaces. They are often seen close to small vessels and are related to endobronchial and small airway disease. A 'tree in bud' appearance suggests endobronchial disease.

1. **Tuberculosis.**
2. **Endobronchial spread of tumour** – e.g. bronchoalveolar carcinoma.
3. **Hypersensitivity pneumonitis.**
4. **Bronchiolitis** – bronchiolitis obliterans, bronchiolitis obliterans organizing pneumonia, respiratory bronchiolitis.
5. **Diseases associated with bronchiectasis.**

Perilymphatic

Nodules will be seen closely related (i.e. <5mm) to the pleural surfaces, large vessels and bronchi, interlobular septa and centrilobular regions.

1. **Sarcoidosis*.**
2. **Lymphangitis carcinomatosa.**
3. **Silicosis*.**
4. **Coal miner's pneumoconiosis*.**
5. **Lymphoma*.**
6. **Lymphoid interstitial pneumonia.**
7. **Amyloidosis.**

Random

Nodules are seen randomly distributed in relationship to the secondary pulmonary lobule and thus also involve the pleural surfaces.

1. **Miliary tuberculosis.**
2. **Haematogenous metastasis.**
3. **Fungi.**
4. **Silicosis*.**
5. **Coal miner's pneumoconiosis.**
6. **Langerhans cell histiocytosis*.**

4.43 HIGH RESOLUTION CT – GROUND-GLASS OPACIFICATION

Defined as a hazy increase in lung parenchymal attenuation which does not obscure bronchial and vascular margins. It is important to stress that this CT pattern is wholly non-specific and can reflect partial air-space filling, interstitial infiltration (or a combination of the two), collapse of air spaces or an increased capillary blood volume.

1. **Infective** – e.g. *Pneumocystis carinii,* viral.
2. **Pulmonary oedema** – see 4.13.
3. **Pulmonary haemorrhage.**
4. **Diffuse interstitial lung disease** – idiopathic or otherwise
    (a) Non-specific interstitial pneumonia.
    (b) Usual interstitial pneumonia (NB ground-glass opacification less extensive than reticulation).
    (c) Desquamative interstitial pneumonia.
    (d) Respiratory bronchiolitis/respiratory bronchiolitis-associated interstitial lung disease.
    (e) Organizing pneumonia.
    (f) Acute interstitial pneumonia.
    (g) Lymphocytic interstitial pneumonia.
    (h) Sarcoidosis.
    (i) Extrinsic allergic alveolitis.
    (j) Alveolar proteinosis.
5. **Malignancy** – bronchoalveolar cell carcinoma, adenocarcinoma.

Further Reading

Hansell UDM et al. Fleischner Society: Radiology 2008;246:697–722.

Travis WD et al. ATS/ERS International multidisciplinary consensus classification of the idiopathic interstitial pneumonias. Am J Respir Crit Care Med 2002;165:277–304.

Webb WR, Müller NL, Naidich DP. High Resolution CT of the Lung. Lippincott Williams & Wilkins, Philadelphia, 2000.

4.44 HIGH RESOLUTION CT – MOSAIC ATTENUATION PATTERN

Purely descriptive term defined as a patchwork of regions of variable ('black' and 'grey') lung density. This pattern is seen in obliterative airways disease, vascular disease and infiltrative lung disease. When confronted with this pattern on CT the radiologist must first decide whether the black lung is normal or not. A disparity between the number/calibre of vessels in black and grey lung suggests that the black lung is abnormal, in which case the likely causes are small airways (constrictive obliterative bronchiolitis) or vascular (chronic pulmonary thromboembolic) disease: air-trapping on CT performed at end-expiration points to the former category. In patients with an infiltrative disease, there is no obvious discrepancy in the number/calibre of pulmonary vessels between regions of black and grey lung. Note that differentiation between different causes of mosaic attenuation is not always straightforward

Mosaic attenuation pattern – small airways disease (constrictive obliterative bronchiolitis)

1. **Idiopathic** – rare.
2. **Lower respiratory tract infection** – esp. viruses but also mycoplasma.
3. **Connective tissue diseases** – esp. rheumatoid arthritis, Sjögren's syndrome.
4. **Post-transplantation** – heart–lung, heart, bone marrow.
5. **Drugs** – penicillamine, *Sauropus androgynus*.
6. **Bronchiectasis.**
7. **Sarcoidosis.**
8. **Extrinsic allergic alveolitis.**
9. **Toxic fume inhalation.**

Mosaic attenuation pattern – vascular disease

1. **Chronic thromboembolic disease** – NOT a feature of acute pulmonary embolism.
2. **Pulmonary arterial hypertension.**
3. **Pulmonary artery tumours (sarcoma).**

Mosaic attenuation pattern – infiltrative disease

See 4.43 – causes of ground-glass opacification.

Further Reading
Bankier AA et al. Bronchiolitis obliterans in heart-lung transplant recipients: diagnosis with expiratory CT. Radiology 2001;218:533–9.

Dennie CJ et al. Intimal sarcoma of the pulmonary arteries seen as a mosaic pattern of lung attenuation on high-resolution CT. AJR Am J Roentgenol 2002;178:1208–10.

Desai SR, Hansell DM. Small airways disease: expiratory computed tomography comes of age. Clin Radiol 1997;52:332–7.

Sherrick AD. Mosaic pattern of lung attenuation on CT scans: frequency among patients with pulmonary artery hypertension of different causes. AJR Am J Roentgenol 1997;169:79–82.

Stern EJ et al. CT mosaic pattern of lung attenuation: etiologies and terminology. J Thorac Imaging 1995;10:294–7.

Webb WR, Müller NL, Naidich DP. High Resolution CT of the Lung, 3rd edn. Lippincott Williams & Wilkins, Philadelphia, 2001.

4.45 ANTERIOR MEDIASTINAL MASSES IN ADULTS

Anterior to the pericardium and trachea. Superiorly the retrosternal air space is obliterated. For ease of discussion it can be divided into three regions:

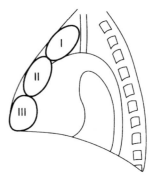

Region I

1. **Retrosternal goitre** – goitre extends into the mediastinum in 3–17% of cases. On a PA chest x-ray it appears as an inverted truncated cone with its base uppermost. It is well-defined, smooth or lobulated. The trachea may be displaced posteriorly and laterally, and may be narrowed. Calcification is common. CT shows the connection with the cervical thyroid. Relatively high attenuation compared with other mediastinal structures and other tumours. Uptake by ^{123}I is diagnostic when positive but the thyroid may be non-functioning.
2. **Tortuous innominate artery** – a common finding in the elderly.
3. **Lymph nodes** – due to reticuloses, metastases or granulomas.
4. **Thymic tumours** – are uncommon but occur in 15% of adult patients with myasthenia gravis. They are round or oval and smooth or lobulated. They may contain nodular or rim calcification. If the tumour contains a large amount of fat (thymolipoma) then it may be very large and soft and reach the diaphragm, leaving the superior mediastinum clear.
5. **Aneurysm of the ascending aorta.**

Region II

1. **Germinal cell neoplasms** – including dermoids, teratomas, seminomas, choriocarcinomas, embryonal carcinomas and endodermal sinus tumours. More than 80% are benign and they occur with equal incidence to thymic tumours. Usually larger than thymomas (but not thymolipomas). Round or oval and smooth. They usually project to one or other side of the mediastinum on the PA view. Calcification, especially rim calcification, and fragments of bone or teeth may be demonstrable, the latter being diagnostic.
2. **Thymic tumours** – see above.
3. **Sternal tumours** – metastases (breast, bronchus, kidney and thyroid) are the most common. Of the primary tumours, malignant (chondrosarcoma, myeloma, reticulum cell sarcoma and lymphoma) are more common than benign (chondroma, aneurysmal bone cyst and giant cell tumour).

Region III (anterior cardiophrenic angle masses)

1. **Pericardiac fat pad** – especially in obese people. A triangular opacity in the cardiophrenic angle on the PA view. It appears less dense than expected because of the fat content. CT is diagnostic. Excessive mediastinal fat can be due to steroid therapy.
2. **Diaphragmatic hump** – or localized eventration. Commonest on the anteromedial portion of the right hemidiaphragm. A portion of liver extends into it and this can be confirmed by ultrasound or isotope examination of the liver.
3. **Morgagni hernia** – through the defect between the septum transversum and the costal portion of the diaphragm. It is almost invariably on the right side but is occasionally bilateral. It usually contains a knuckle of colon or, less commonly, colon and stomach. Appears solid if it contains omentum and/or liver. Ultrasound and/or barium studies will confirm the diagnosis.
4. **Pericardial cysts** – either a true pericardial cyst ('spring water' cyst) or a pericardial diverticulum. The cyst is usually situated in the right cardiophrenic angle and is oval or spherical. CT confirms the liquid nature of the mass.

Further Reading

Buckley JA, Stark P. Intrathoracic mediastinal thyroid goiter: imaging manifestations. Am J Roentgenol 1999;173:471–5.

Drevelegas A, Palladas P, Scordalaki A. Mediastinal germ cell tumours: a radiologic-pathologic review. Eur Radiol 2001;11:1925–32.

Landwehr P, Schulte O, Lackner K. MR imaging of the chest: mediastinum and chest wall. Eur Radiol 1999;9:1737–44.

4.46 MIDDLE MEDIASTINAL MASSES IN ADULTS

Between the anterior and posterior mediastinum and containing the heart, great vessels and pulmonary roots. Causes of cardiac enlargement are excluded.

1. **Lymph nodes** – the paratracheal, tracheobronchial, bronchopulmonary and/or subcarinal nodes may be enlarged. This may be due to neoplasm (most frequently metastatic bronchial carcinoma), reticuloses (most frequently Hodgkin's disease), infection (most commonly tuberculosis, histoplasmosis or coccidioidomycosis) or sarcoidosis.
2. **Carcinoma of the bronchus** – arising from a major bronchus.
3. **Aneurysm of the aorta** – CT scanning after i.v. contrast medium or, if this is not available, aortography is diagnostic. Peripheral rim calcification is a useful sign if present.
4. **Bronchogenic cyst** – see 14.40.

Further Reading
Landwehr P, Schulte O, Lackner K. MR imaging of the chest: mediastinum and chest wall. Eur Radiol 1999;9:1737–44.

4.47 POSTERIOR MEDIASTINAL MASSES IN ADULTS

For ease of discussion it can be divided into three regions:

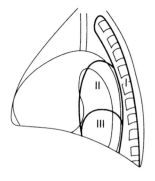

Region I (paravertebral)

1. **Reticuloses, myeloma and metastases** – bone destruction with preserved discs.
2. **Extramedullary haemopoiesis** – with splenomegaly ± bone changes of specific disease entities, e.g. haemolytic anaemias.
3. **Abscess** – with disc space and vertebral body destruction.
4. **Ganglioneuroma** – see 14.40.

Region II

1. **Dilated oesophagus** – especially achalasia. Contains mottled gas shadows ± an air fluid level. Diagnosis is confirmed by barium swallow.
2. **Aorta** – unfolded, dilated or ruptured.

Region III

1. **Hiatus hernia** – often contains an air fluid level which is projected through the cardiac shadow on a penetrated PA view.

Further Reading
Landwehr P, Schulte O, Lackner K. MR imaging of the chest: mediastinum and chest wall. Eur Radiol 1999;9:1737–44.

4

4.48 CT MEDIASTINAL MASS CONTAINING FAT

1. **Teratodermoid** – well-defined soft-tissue mass containing fat and calcification.
2. **Diaphragmatic hernia** – bowel, liver, kidney or stomach may also be present. Anterior (Morgagni) hernias are usually on the right, and posterior (Bochdalek) hernias usually on the left. Linear soft-tissue densities representing omental vessels help to distinguish hernias which only contain omental fat from pericardial fat pads.
3. **Lipoma** – relatively rare. Can occur anywhere in the mediastinum.
4. **Liposarcoma** – can contain calcification, and may also appear as a soft-tissue mass with no visible fat, due to excess soft-tissue component of the sarcoma.
5. **Thymolipoma** – occurs in children and young adults. Accounts for 2–9% of thymic tumours. Usually asymptomatic.
6. **Mediastinal lipomatosis** – associated with Cushing's, steroid treatment and obesity.
7. **Hamartoma**.
8. **Chylolymphatic cyst** – fat/fluid level in cyst.
9. **Neurofibroma** – can have a negative CT attenuation due to myelin content.

Further Reading
Phillips GWL, Serapati A, Young AE. Chylolymphatic-mesenteric cyst: a diagnostic appearance on computed tomography. Br J Radiol 1988;61:413–4.
Reed DH. The changing mediastinum. Br J Radiol 1988;61:695–6.
Shirkhoda A, Chasen MH, Eftekhari F et al. MR Imaging of mediastinal thymolipoma. J Comput Assist Tomogr 1987;11:364–5.

4.49 CT MEDIASTINAL CYSTS

1. **Congenital**
   (a) Bronchogenic cyst – usually subcarinal or right paratracheal site. 50% homogeneous water density, 50% soft-tissue density due to mucus or milk of calcium content. Occasional calcification in cyst wall, and air in cyst if communicating with airway.
   (b) Enteric cyst – para-oesophageal site.
   (c) Neuroenteric cyst – associated anomaly of spine.
2. **Pericardial cyst** – usually cardiophrenic angle.
3. **Thymic cyst** – can develop following radiotherapy for Hodgkin's.
4. **Cystic tumours**
   (a) Lymphangioma.
   (b) Teratoma.
   (c) Teratodermoid.
5. **Pancreatic pseudocyst** – can track up into mediastinum.
6. **Meningocoele** – 75% association with neurofibromatosis.
7. **Chronic abscess.**
8. **Old haematoma.**

Further Reading

Aviv RI, McHugh K, Hunt J. Angiomatosis of bone and soft tissue: a spectrum of disease from diffuse lymphangiomatosis to vanishing bone disease in young patients. Clin Radiol 2001;56:184–90.

Charruau L, Parrens M, Jougon J et al. Mediastinal lymphangioma in adults: CT and MR imaging features. Eur Radiol 2000;10:1310–4.

DuMontier C, Graviss ER, Silberstein MJ et al. Bronchogenic cysts in children. Clin Radiol 1985;36:431–6.

Nakata H, Sato Y, Nakayama T et al. Bronchogenic cyst with high C.T. numbers: analysis of contents. J Comput Assist Tomogr 1986;10:360–2.

4.50 CT THYMIC MASS

Normal shape of thymus is an arrowhead with maximum length <2cm and maximum width <1.8cm if age <20 years, and 1.3cm if age >20 years. However, measurements are misleading, and a multilobular appearance or focal alteration in shape is abnormal at any age. Fatty involution occurs after the age of 30.

1. **Thymoma** – occurs in 15% of those with myasthenia gravis (usually occurring in the fourth decade) and 40% of these will be malignant. If malignant it is usually locally invasive and can extend along pleura to involve diaphragm and even spread into abdomen. Can contain calcification.
2. **Thymic hyperplasia**
   (a) Lymphoid – occurs in 65% of those with myasthenia gravis. Only medulla enlarges and this is not sufficient to be visible on CT.
   (b) True hyperplasia – occurs in myasthenia gravis, post-chemotherapy rebound, Graves thyrotoxicosis, Addison's and acromegaly. Thymus increases in size but is normal in shape.
3. **Germ cell tumour** – teratodermoid, benign and malignant teratomas.
4. **Lymphoma*** – thymus is infiltrated in 35% of Hodgkin's disease but there is always associated lymphadenopathy.
5. **Thymolipoma** – usually children or young adults. Asymptomatic.

Further Reading
Heron CW, Husband JE, Williams MP. Hodgkin's disease: CT of the thymus. Radiology 1988;167:647–51.
Moore NR. Imaging in myasthenia gravis. Clin Radiol 1989;40:115–6.
Williams MP. Problems in radiology: CT assessment of the thymus. Clin Radiol 1989;40:113–4.

4.51   VENTILATION PERFUSION MISMATCH

Mismatched perfusion defects

Perfusion defect greater than ventilation defect.

1. **Pulmonary embolus** – especially if multiple and segmental.
2. **Bronchial carcinoma** – but more commonly matched.
3. **Tuberculosis** – typically affecting an apical segment.
4. **Vasculitis** – polyarteritis nodosa, systemic lupus erythematosus, etc.
5. **Tumour embolus.**
6. **Fat embolus.**
7. **Post-radiotherapy.**
8. **Pulmonary hypertension.**

Mismatched ventilation defects

Bronchial obstruction with normal blood supply. Ventilation defect greater than perfusion defect.

1. **Chronic obstructive airways disease.**
2. **Pneumonia.**
3. **Carcinoma** – the rarest appearance with bronchial carcinoma.
4. **Lung collapse** – of any cause.
5. **Pleural effusion.**

Further Reading
Carvandho P, Lavender JP. Incidence and aetiology of the reverse (V/Q) mismatch defect. Nucl Med Commun 1988;9:167.

4.52   MULTIPLE MATCHED VENTILATION/ PERFUSION DEFECTS

See 4.51.

1. **Chronic bronchitis.**
2. **Pulmonary infarct** (do not confuse with the mismatched perfusion defect of embolus).
3. **Asthma or acute bronchitis** – may also show mismatched ventilation or perfusion defects.
4. **Collagen vascular disease.**
5. **Lymphangitis carcinomatosa.**
6. **Pulmonary hypertension.**
7. **Sarcoidosis.***
8. **Intravenous drug abuse.**

Further Reading
Benson ML, Balseiro J. Multiple matched ventilation-perfusion defects in illicit drug use. Semin Nucl Med 1993;23:180–3.

5

Cardiovascular system

Stephen Harden

5.1 GROSS CARDIOMEGALY ON CHEST X-RAY

1. **Ischaemic heart disease** and other cardiomyopathies.
2. **Pericardial effusion** – (globular or flask-shaped heart, crisp cardiac outline).
3. **ASD.**
4. **Multivalve disease** – (particularly regurgitation).
5. **Congenital heart disease** – notably Ebstein's anomaly (congenital displacement of the septal and posterior leaflets of the tricuspid valve towards the apex of the RV producing atrialization of the RV and complex tricuspid regurgitation).

5.2 RIGHT ATRIAL ENLARGEMENT

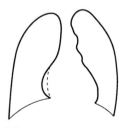

PA
Prominent right heart border

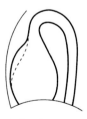

Lateral
Prominent anterosuperior part of cardiac shadow

Secondary to RV failure

Volume loading

1. Tricuspid regurgitation.
2. ASD.
3. AVSD.
4. Anomalous pulmonary venous return.

Pressure loading

1. Tricuspid stenosis.
2. Tricuspid valve obstruction from tumour or thrombus.

5.3 RIGHT VENTRICULAR ENLARGEMENT

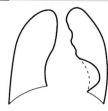

PA
Prominent left heart
border
Elevated apex

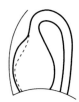

Lateral
Prominent anterior part
of cardiac shadow

Volume loading

1. Tricuspid regurgitation.
2. Pulmonary regurgitation.
3. ASD.
4. VSD.
5. Anomalous pulmonary venous drainage.

Pressure loading

1. **Pulmonary hypertension** (which may be secondary to LV failure).
2. **Pulmonary stenosis.**
3. **Acute PE** (right heart strain in massive embolus).

5.4 LEFT ATRIAL ENLARGEMENT

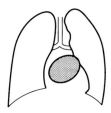

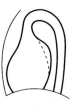

PA
1 Prominent left atrial appendage
2 'Double' right heart border
3 Increased density due to left atrium
4 Splaying of carina and elevated left main bronchus

Lateral
1 Prominent posterosuperior part of cardiac shadow
2 Prominent left atrial impression on oesophagus during barium swallow

Volume loading
1. Mitral regurgitation.
2. VSD.
3. PDA.

Pressure loading
1. Left ventricular failure.
2. Mitral stenosis.
3. Mitral valve obstruction due to tumour, e.g. myxoma.

5.5 LEFT VENTRICULAR ENLARGEMENT

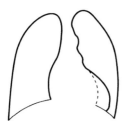 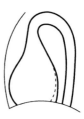

PA
1 Prominent left heart border
2 Rounding of left heart border
3 Apex displaced inferiorly

Lateral
Prominent posteroinferior
part of cardiac shadow

Myocardial disease

1. **Ischaemic heart disease.**
2. **Cardiomyopathy,** e.g. dilated cardiomyopathy (DCM).

Volume loading

1. **Aortic regurgitation.**
2. **Mitral regurgitation.**
3. **PDA.**

Pressure loading

1. **Hypertension.**
2. **Aortic stenosis.**

Further Reading for 5.1–5.5

Baron MG. Plain film diagnosis of common cardiac anomalies in the adult. Radiol Clin North Am 1999;37:401–19.

Baron MG, Book WM. Congenital heart disease in the adult: 2004. Radiol Clin North Am 2004;42:675–90.

Gross GW, Steiner RM. Radiographic manifestations of congenital heart disease in the adult patient. Radiol Clin North Am 1991;29:293–318.

5.6 CARDIAC CALCIFICATION

Valves

1. **Aortic valve calcification** (bicuspid aortic valve, degenerative aortic sclerosis, previous rheumatic fever).
2. **Mitral calcification** (rheumatic fever, degenerative annular calcification).
3. **Pulmonary calcification** (pulmonary stenosis, rheumatic fever).
4. **Tricuspid calcification** (rare; rheumatic fever, endocarditis, ASD).
5. **Homograft calcification.**

Intracardiac calcification

1. **Calcified thrombus.**
2. **Calcified tumour,** mostly myxomas.

Myocardium

1. **Post-infarction.**
2. **LV aneurysm.**
3. **Previous rheumatic fever.**

Pericardium

1. **Previous pericarditis,** e.g. TB, rheumatic fever.
2. **Previous trauma,** e.g. haemopericardium, cardiac surgery.
3. **Renal failure.**
4. **Asbestos-related pleural plaques** overlying the pericardium.

Coronary arteries

1. **Atheroma** (the amount correlates with the patient's cardiovascular risk profile independent of other risk factors).
2. **Chronic renal failure** (often heavy diffuse calcification which is partly related to advanced atheroma).

Further Reading
Gowda RM, Boxt LM. Calcifications of the heart. Radiol Clin North Am 2004;42:603–17.
Greenland P et al. ACCF/AHA 2007 Clinical expert consensus document on coronary artery calcium scoring by CT in global cardiovascular risk assessment and in evaluation of patients with chest pain. J Am Coll Cardiol 2007;49:378–402.

5.7 MYOCARDIAL DISEASES

LV generalized myocardial thickening

1. **Hypertension.**
2. **Aortic stenosis.**
3. **Myocardial infiltration,** e.g. amyloid.

RV thickening

1. **Pulmonary hypertension.**
2. **RV outflow tract obstruction.**
3. **Pulmonary stenosis.**

Focal myocardial thickening

1. **Hypertrophic cardiomyopathy** (HCM). The classical form affects the base of the interventricular septum, causing obstruction of the left ventricular outflow tract. The next most common form is apical HCM.

Myocardial thinning

1. **Generalized** in LV dilatation due to ischaemic heart disease or DCM.
2. **Focal** LV thinning from previous infarction. May also be associated with focal calcification or focal fat deposition.

Fatty lesions

1. **Lipoma.**
2. **Lipomatous hypertrophy** of the interatrial septum (normal variant associated with obesity and steroid use).
3. **Fatty replacement** of a myocardial infarct.
4. **Fatty infiltration** into the RV free wall (arrhythmogenic right ventricular dysplasia or ARVD).

5.8   PERICARDIAL DISEASES

Pericardial thickening
1. **Previous pericarditis** (infection, connective tissue diseases).
2. **Previous trauma** including surgery.

Pericardial effusion
1. **Transudate** from left ventricular failure, hypoalbuminaemia, renal failure.
2. **Exudate** from collagen vascular diseases, infections, e.g. TB or viral, chronic renal failure myocardial infarction.
3. **Haemopericardium** from acute aortic dissection, trauma including surgery, acute myocardial infarction, tumour (primary, local tumour invasion, metastases, lymphoma).
4. **Chylous** (malignancy, cardiothoracic surgery).

Further Reading
Kim JS, Kim HH, Yoon Y. Imaging of pericardial diseases. Clin Radiol 2007;62:626–31.

5.9   CARDIAC MASSES

1. **Thrombus** (ventricular after acute MI and in aneurysms, atrial in AF particularly the left atrial appendage).
2. **Benign tumours.** The commonest are myxomas which occur most frequently in the atria. There is often a pedicle attaching the mass to the region of the fossa ovalis. Other benign tumours include lipomas and fibromas.
3. **Malignant tumours.** Primary malignant tumours are rare but tend to be sarcomas, particularly angiosarcomas and rhabdomyosarcomas. Metastases are the commonest form of cardiac tumour (melanoma has a predilection).

Further Reading
Shapiro LM Cardiac tumours: diagnosis and management. Heart 2001;85: 218–22.

5.10 DELAYED HYPERENHANCEMENT ON CARDIAC MRI

1. **Myocardial infarction.** The distribution is subendocardial or full thickness.
2. **Cardiomyopathy,** due to sarcoid, myocarditis, HCM, DCM, ARVD. The distribution is not that of infarction and is mid-myocardial or subepicardial.
3. **Amyloid** diffuse hyperenhancement can be seen with extensive cardiac infiltration.

Further Reading
Jackson E et al. Ischaemic and non-ischaemic cardiomyopathies – a review of cardiac MR appearances with delayed hyperenhancement. Clin Radiol 2007;62:395–403.

5.11 MALIGNANT CORONARY ARTERY ANOMALIES IN THE ADULT

1. **Aberrant right coronary artery** arising from the left sinus and passing between the aorta and the MPA.
2. **Aberrant left coronary artery** arising from the right sinus and passing between the aorta and the MPA.

Further Reading
Kim SY et al. Coronary artery anomalies: classification and ECG-gated multi-detector row CT findings with angiographic correlation. Radiographics 2006; 26: 317–333.

5.12 CAUSES OF A PERFUSION DEFECT ON A CARDIAC SPECT SCAN

1. **Inducible ischaemia.**
2. **Infarction.**
3. **Hibernating myocardium** (often reduced activity at stress and at rest).
4. **Breast-related artefact** (particularly anterior defects).
5. **Inferior wall defects** may result from diaphragmatic motion or the increased distance of this wall from the camera.
6. **Apical thinning.**

5.13 ACUTE AORTIC SYNDROMES

Aortic dissection

1. Classified as type A if it involves the aorta proximal to the left subclavian artery and type B if it involves only the aorta distal to the left subclavian artery.
2. X-ray signs include widening of the mediastinum, ill-defined mediastinal outline, left pleural effusion or pleural cap, displaced intimal calcification.
3. CT signs include the dissection flap with flow in the true ± the false lumen, mediastinal haemorrhage, haemopericardium, haemothorax, mural haematoma. There may be no contrast opacification of the right coronary artery if it is involved with the dissection.

Intramural haematoma

1. Blood collects in the media of the arterial wall with no intimal tear.
2. Tends to occur in hypertensive patients and in blunt trauma.
3. Increased attenuation in the aortic wall most visible on non-contrast CT.
4. May resolve spontaneously but can proceed to aortic dissection.

Penetrating aortic ulcer

1. Focal ulceration of the aortic wall at the site of intimal atherosclerotic plaques, particularly in the descending aorta.
2. Progressive erosion can lead to intramural haematoma.
3. May proceed to aneurysm formation or aortic dissection.

Aortic transection

1. Post-traumatic, particularly high speed deceleration injuries.
2. Usually occurs at the isthmus in the proximal descending aorta due to tethering by the ligamentum arteriosum.
3. X-ray signs include widening and ill-definition of the mediastinal contour, left apical cap and left pleural effusion. The chest x-ray may be normal.
4. CT signs are often subtle. The normal circular contour of the lumen of the aortic isthmus is lost and there may be a pseudoaneurysm. Mediastinal haemorrhage is usually present. May proceed to dissection. Extravasation of contrast is a poor prognostic sign.

Further Reading
Macura KJ et al. Pathogenesis in acute aortic syndrome: aortic dissection, intramural haematoma and penetrating atherosclerotic aortic ulcer. Am J Roentgenol 2003;181:309–16.
Vilacosta I, San Roman JA. Acute aortic syndrome. Heart 2001;85: 365–8.

5.14 AORTIC ARCH ANOMALIES

The figure shows the double aortic arch that exists early in embryonic life. Part of this ring atrophies.

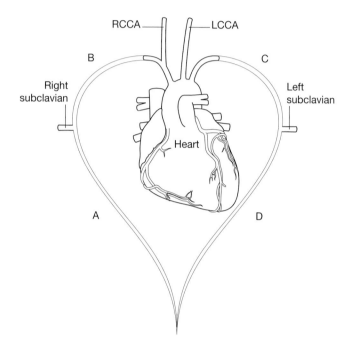

1. **If segment A atrophies,** this produces the normal arrangement of the head and neck vessels from a left-sided aortic arch.
2. **If segment B atrophies,** there is a left-sided arch with an aberrant right subclavian artery.
3. **If segment C atrophies,** the aortic arch is right-sided with an aberrant left subclavian artery. This is associated with a low (~12%) incidence of congenital heart disease including Fallot's tetralogy and coarctation.
4. **If segment D atrophies,** the aortic arch is right-sided with mirror image branching of the head and neck vessels. This is associated with a high incidence (~98%) of congenital heart disease, particularly Fallot's tetralogy.

5.15 THORACIC AORTIC ANEURYSM

Ascending aortic aneurysm
1. **Post-stenotic dilatation** from aortic stenosis.
2. **Atheroma.**
3. **Cystic medial necrosis** which is seen in Marfan's, Ehlers–Danlos and with bicuspid aortic valves.
4. **Syphilis.**

Descending aortic aneurysm
1. **Atheroma.**
2. **Aortic dissection** involving the descending thoracic aorta.
3. **Previous trauma** with missed transection.

Further Reading
Isselbacher EM. Thoracic and abdominal aortic aneurysms. Circulation 2005;111:816–28.

5.16 PULMONARY ARTERIAL ENLARGEMENT

The figure shows a flow chart for the analysis of increased pulmonary arterial size.

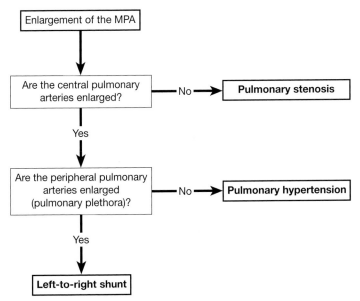

5.17 PULMONARY HYPERTENSION

1. **Pulmonary venous hypertension** (LVF, mitral stenosis).
2. **Chronic lung disease** (COPD, CF, bronchiectasis).
3. **Chronic PE.**
4. **Chronic left-to-right shunt.**
5. **Vasculitis.**
6. **Primary pulmonary hypertension** (young adult females).

Further Reading
Ley S et al. Assessment of pulmonary hypertension by CT and MR imaging. Eur
  Radiol 2004;14:359-368.

5.18 PULMONARY VENOUS ENLARGEMENT

May be accompanied by perihilar haze, Kerley B and other
interstitial lines, perihilar consolidation.

1. **LV failure.**
2. **Atrial or mitral valve level obstruction** (mitral stenosis, mitral valve
   obstruction).
3. **Pulmonary veno-occlusive disease.**
4. **Constrictive pericarditis.**

Abdomen and gastrointestinal tract

Stuart Taylor and Rebecca Greenhalgh

6.1 PNEUMOPERITONEUM

Radiological signs

1. **Plain film** (sensitivity 50–70%)
   (a) Erect – free gas under diaphragm or liver. Can detect 10ml of air. Can take 10 min for all gas to rise.
   (b) Supine – gas outlines both sides of bowel wall, which then appears as a white line. In infants a large volume of gas will collect centrally, producing a rounded, relative translucency over the central abdomen. The falciform ligament may also be outlined by free gas.
2. **CT** (greater sensitivity than plain film). **Suspected perforation**
   (a) Focal bowel wall thickening ± discontinuity in bowel wall.
   (b) Extra-luminal +ve oral contrast.
   (c) Extra-luminal gas.
      (i) Large volume – usually upper GI, post endoscopy or secondary to obstruction.
      (ii) Lesser sac – usually gastric or duodenal (rarely oesophagus or transverse colon).
      (iii) Ligamentum teres – often gastric or duodenal.
      (iv) Mesenteric folds – usually small bowel or colon (very rarely gastric).
      (v) Retroperitoneal (duodenum ascending/descending colon, rectum, lower sigmoid).

Causes

1. **Perforation**
   (a) Peptic ulcer – 30% do not have free air visible.
   (b) Inflammation – diverticulitis, appendicitis, toxic megacolon, necrotizing enterocolitis.
   (c) Infarction.

 (d) Malignant neoplasms.
 (e) Obstruction.
 (f) Pneumatosis coli – the cysts may rupture.
2. **Iatrogenic (surgery: peritoneal dialysis)** – may take 3 weeks to reabsorb (faster in obese and children). Free air may be seen on CT up to 14 days post-surgery.
3. **Pneumomediastinum** – see 4.33.
4. **Introduction per vaginam** – e.g. douching.
5. **Pneumothorax** – due to a congenital pleuroperitoneal fistula.
6. **Idiopathic.**

Further Reading

Furuka A, Sakoda M, Yamasaki M et al. Gastrointestinal tract perforation: CT diagnosis of presence, site, and cause. Abdom Imaging 2005;30:524–34.

6.2   GASLESS ABDOMEN

Adult

1. **High obstruction** (e.g. gastric outflow obstruction, congenital atresia).
2. **Ascites.**
3. **Pancreatitis (acute)** – due to excess vomiting.
4. **Fluid-filled bowel** – closed-loop obstruction, total active colitis, mesenteric infarction (early), bowel wash-out.
5. **Large abdominal mass** – pushes bowel laterally.
6. **Normal.**

6.3 PHARYNGEAL/OESOPHAGEAL POUCHES AND DIVERTICULA

Upper third

1. **Zenker's diverticulum** – posteriorly, usually on left side, between the fibres of the inferior constrictor and cricopharyngeus. Can cause dysphagia, regurgitation, aspiration and hoarseness ± an air/fluid level.
2. **Lateral pharyngeal pouch and diverticulum** – through the unsupported thyrohyoid membrane in the anterolateral wall of the upper hypopharynx. Pouches are common and patients are asymptomatic. Diverticula are uncommon and are seen in patients with chronically elevated intrapharyngeal pressure, e.g. glass blowers and trumpeters.
3. **Lateral cervical oesophageal pouch and diverticulum** – through the Killian–Jamieson space. Pouches are transient; diverticula are persistent. Patients are usually asymptomatic. The opening is below the level of cricopharyngeus.

Middle third

1. **Traction** – at level of carina. May be related to fibrosis after treatment for TB. Asymptomatic.
2. **Developmental** – failure to complete closure of tracheo-oesophageal communication.
3. **Intramural** – very rare. Multiple, tiny flask-shaped outpouchings. 90% have associated strictures, mainly in the upper third of the oesophagus.

Lower third

1. **Epiphrenic.**
2. **Ulcer** – peptic or related to steroids, immunosuppression and radiotherapy.
3. **Mucosal tears** – Mallory–Weiss syndrome, post-oesophagoscopy.
4. **After Heller's operation.**

Further Reading
Rubesin SE. The pharynx. Structural disorders. Radiol Clin North Am 1994;32 (6):1083–101.
Schwartz EE, Tucker J, Holt GP. Cervical dysphagia: pharyngeal protrusions and achalasia. Clin Radiol 1981;32:643–50.

6.4 OESOPHAGEAL ULCERATION

In addition to ulceration there may be non-specific signs of oesophagitis:

1. Thickening of longitudinal folds (>2mm), which may be slightly scalloped.
2. Thickening of transverse folds resembling small bowel mucosal folds.
3. Reduced or absent peristalsis.

Inflammatory

1. **Reflux oesophagitis** – ± hiatus hernia. Signs characteristic of reflux oesophagitis are:
   (a) A gastric fundal fold crossing the gastro-oesophageal junction and ending as a polypoid protuberance in the distal oesophagus.
   (b) Erosions – dots or linear streaks of barium in the distal oesophagus.
   (c) Ulcers which may be round or, more commonly, linear or serpiginous.
2. **Barrett's oesophagus** – to be considered in any patient with oesophageal ulceration or stricture but especially if the abnormality is in the body of the oesophagus (although strictures are more common in the lower oesophagus). Hiatus hernia in 75–90%. Usually endoscopic diagnosis.
3. **Candida oesophagitis** – predominantly in immunosuppressed patients. Early: small, plaque-like filling defects, often orientated in the long axis of the oesophagus. Advanced: cobblestone mucosal surface ± luminal narrowing. Ulceration is uncommon. Tiny bubbles along the top of the column of barium – the 'foamy' oesophagus. Patients with mucocutaneous candidiasis or oesophageal stasis due to achalasia, scleroderma etc. may develop chronic infection which is characterized by a lacy or reticular appearance of the mucosa ± nodular filling defects.
4. **Viral** – herpes and CMV occurring mostly in immunocompromised patients. May manifest as discrete ulcers, ulcerated plaques or mimic Candida oesophagitis. Discrete ulcers on an otherwise normal background mucosa are strongly suggestive of a viral aetiology.
5. **Caustic ingestion** – ulceration is most marked at the sites of anatomical hold-up and progresses to a long, smooth stricture.
6. **Radiotherapy** – ulceration is rare. Altered oesophageal motility is frequently the only abnormality.
7. **Crohn's disease*** – aphthoid ulcers and, in advanced cases, undermining ulcers, intramural tracking and fistulae.
8. **Drug-induced** – due to prolonged contact with tetracycline, quinidine and potassium supplements.
9. **Behçet's disease**.
10. **Intramural diverticulosis**.

Neoplastic

1. **Carcinoma.**
2. **Leiomyosarcoma and leiomyoma.**
3. **Lymphoma*.**
4. **Melanoma.**

Further Reading

Chen MY, Frederick MG. Barrett esophagus and adenocarcinoma. Radiol Clin North Am 1994;32(6):1167–81.

Canon CL, Morgan DE, Einstein DM et al. Surgical approach to gastro-oesophageal reflux disease: what the radiologist needs to know. Radiographics 2005;25(6):1485–99.

Sam JW, Levine MS, Rubesin SE et al. The 'foamy' esophagus: a radiographic sign of Candida esophagitis. Am J Roentgenol 2000;174:999–1002.

Yee J, Wall SD. Infectious esophagitis. Radiol Clin North Am 1994;32(6):1135–45.

6.5 OESOPHAGEAL STRICTURES – SMOOTH

Inflammatory

1. **Peptic** – the stricture develops relatively late. Most frequently at the oesophagogastric junction and associated with reflux and a hiatus hernia. Less commonly, more proximal in the oesophagus and associated with heterotopic gastric mucosa (Barrett's oesophagus). ± Ulceration.
2. **Scleroderma*** – reflux through a wide open cardia may produce stricture. Oesophagus is the commonest internal organ to be affected. Peristalsis is poor, cardia wide open and the oesophagus dilated (contains air in the resting state).
3. **Corrosives** – acute: oedema, spasm, ulceration and loss of mucosal pattern at 'hold-up' points (aortic arch and oesophagogastric junction). Strictures are typically long and symmetrical, may take several years to develop and are more likely to be produced by alkalis than acid.
4. **Iatrogenic** – prolonged use of a nasogastric tube. Stricture in distal oesophagus probably secondary to reflux.

Neoplastic

1. **Carcinoma** – squamous carcinoma may infiltrate submucosally. The absence of a hiatus hernia and the presence of an extrinsic soft-tissue mass should differentiate it from a peptic stricture but a carcinoma arising around the cardia may predispose to reflux.
2. **Mediastinal tumours** – carcinoma of the bronchus and lymph nodes. Localized obstruction ± ulceration and an extrinsic soft-tissue mass.
3. **Leiomyoma** – narrowing due to a smooth, eccentric, polypoid mass. ± Central ulceration.

Others

1. **Achalasia** – 'rat-tail' tapering may mimic a stricture; this occurs below the diaphragm. Considerable oesophageal dilatation with food in the lumen.
2. **Skin disorders** – epidermolysis bullosa, pemphigus.

6.6 OESOPHAGEAL STRICTURES – IRREGULAR

Neoplastic

1. **Carcinoma** – increased incidence in achalasia, Plummer–Vinson syndrome, Barrett's oesophagus, coeliac disease, asbestosis, lye ingestion and tylosis. Mostly squamous carcinomas; adenocarcinoma becoming more common. Appearances include:
   (a) Irregular filling defect – annular or eccentric.
   (b) Extraluminal soft-tissue mass on CT or MRI.
   (c) Shouldering.
   (d) Ulceration.
   (e) Proximal dilatation.
2. **Leiomyosarcoma**.
3. **Carcinosarcoma** – big polypoid tumour ± pedunculated. Better prognosis than squamous carcinoma.
4. **Lymphoma*** – usually extension from gastric involvement.

Inflammatory

1. **Reflux** – rarely irregular.
2. **Crohn's disease*** – rare.

Iatrogenic

1. **Radiotherapy** – rare, unless treating an oesophageal carcinoma. Dysphagia after radiotherapy is usually due to a motility disorder. Acute oesophagitis may occur with a dose of 50–60 Gy (5000–6000 rad).
2. **Fundoplication**.

6.7 TERTIARY CONTRACTIONS IN THE OESOPHAGUS

Unco-ordinated, non-propulsive contractions.

1. **Reflux oesophagitis.**
2. **Presbyoesophagus** – impaired motor function due to muscle atrophy in the elderly. Occurs in 25% of people over 60 years.
3. **Obstruction at the cardia** – from any cause.
4. **Neuropathy**
   (a) Early achalasia – before dilatation occurs.
   (b) Diabetes.
   (c) Alcoholism.
   (d) Malignant infiltration.
   (e) Chagas' disease.

Further Reading
Summerton SL. Radiographic evaluation of esophageal function. Gastrointest Endosc Clin N Am 2005;15(2):231–42.

6

6.8 STOMACH MASSES AND FILLING DEFECTS

Primary malignant neoplasms

1. **Carcinoma** – most polypoidal carcinomas are 1–4cm in diameter. (Any polyp greater than 2cm in diameter must be considered to be malignant.) Endoscopic USS accurate in local staging for early disease. CT superior for more advanced disease.
2. **Lymphoma*** – 1–5% of gastric malignancy. Usually non-Hodgkin's. It can be ulcerative, infiltrative and/or polypoid. Often cannot be distinguished from carcinoma, but extension across the pylorus is suggestive of a lymphoma. Mucosa-associated lymphoid tissue (MALT) lymphoma is strongly associated with *Helicobacter pylori* infection. CT – marked hyopattenuating wall thickening; mean 3–5cm. Whole stomach involved in 50%. Most (not all) have adjacent lymphadenopathy.
3. **Gastrointestinal stromal tumour (GIST).** KIT +ve. Most common in stomach but also small bowel, colon, mesentery. Variable size and malignant potential. Large tumours hyperenhancing and often heterogeneous on CT/MRI. Ulceration and fistulation common. 50% have metastasis at presentation (liver peritoneum, lung). May enlarge with treatment-reduced enhancement suggest response.

Polyps

1. **Hyperplastic** – accounts for 80–90% of gastric polyps. Usually multiple, small (<1cm in diameter) and occur randomly throughout stomach but predominantly affect body and fundus. Associated with chronic gastritis. Rarely can be very large (3–10cm).

2. **Adenomatous** – usually solitary, 1–4cm in diameter, sessile and occur in antrum. High incidence of malignant transformation (particularly if >2cm in size) and carcinomas elsewhere in stomach (because of dysplastic epithelium). Associated with pernicious anaemia.
3. **Hamartomatous** – characteristically multiple, small and relatively spare the antrum. Occur in 30% of Peutz–Jeghers syndrome, 40% of familiar polyposis coli and Gardner's syndrome.

Submucosal neoplasms

Smooth, well-defined filling defect, with a re-entry angle.

1. **Leiomyoma** – commonest by far. Can be very large with a substantial exogastric component. Central ulceration and massive haematemesis may occur.
2. **Lipoma** – can change shape with position of patient and may be relatively mobile on palpation.
3. **Neurofibroma** – NB Leiomyomas and lipomas are more common, even in patients with generalized neurofibromatosis.
4. **Metastases** – Frequently ulcerate: 'bull's-eye' lesion (q.v.). Usually melanoma, but bronchus, breast, lymphoma, Kaposi's sarcoma and any adenocarcinoma may metastasize to stomach. Breast primary often produces a scirrhous reaction in the distal part of the stomach which is indistinguishable from linitis plastica (q.v.).

Extrinsic indentation

1. **Pancreatic tumour/pseudocyst.**
2. **Splenomegaly/hepatomegaly.**
3. **Retroperitoneal tumours.**

Others

1. **Nissen fundoplication** – may mimic a distorted mass in the fundus.
2. **Bezoar** – 'mass' may be mobile. Tricho- (hair) or phyto- (vegetable matter).
3. **Lymphoid hyperplasia** – innumerable, 1–3 mm diameter, round nodules in the antrum or antrum and body. Association with *H. pylori* gastritis.
4. **Pancreatic 'rest'** – ectopic pancreatic tissue causes a small filling defect, usually on the inferior wall of the antrum, and resembles a submucosal tumour. Central 'blob' of barium ('bull's-eye' or target lesion) in 50%.

Further Reading

An SK, Han JK, Kim YH et al. Gastric mucosa-associated lymphoid tissue lymphoma: spectrum of findings at double contrast gastrointestinal examination with pathologic correlation. Radiographics 2001;21:1491–504.

Gore RM. Gastric cancer. Clinical and pathologic features. Radiol Clin North Am 1997;35(2):295–310.

King DM. The radiology of gastrointestinal stromal tumours (GIST). Cancer Imaging 2005;15(5):150–6.

6.9 THICK STOMACH FOLDS/WALL

Thickness greater than 1cm. CT assessment of non-distended stomach remains limited.

Inflammatory

1. **Gastritis** – localized or generalized fold thickening ± associated with inflammatory nodules (<1cm , mostly in the antrum), erosions and coarse areae gastricae.
2. **Zollinger–Ellison syndrome** – suspect if post-bulbar ulcers. Ulceration in both first and second parts of duodenum is suggestive, but ulceration distal to this is virtually diagnostic. Thick folds and small bowel dilatation may occur in response to excess acidity. Due to gastrinoma of non-beta cells of pancreas (no calcification, moderately vascular). 50% malignant – metastases to liver. (10% of gastrinomas may be ectopic – usually in medial wall of the duodenum.)
3. **Pancreatitis (acute).**
4. **Crohn's disease*** – mild thickening of folds with aphthoid ulceration may occur in up to 40% of Crohn's.

Infiltrative/neoplastic

1. **Lymphoma*** – usually non-Hodgkin's lymphoma and may be primary or secondary.
2. **Carcinoma** – irregular folds with rigid wall.
3. **Pseudolymphoma** – benign reactive lymphoid hyperplasia. 70% have an ulcer near the centre of the area affected.
4. **Eosinophilic gastroenteritis.**

Others

1. **Ménétrier's disease** – smooth folds predominantly on greater curve. Rarely extend into antrum. No rigidity or ulcers. 'Weep' protein sufficient to cause hypoproteinaemia (effusion, oedema, thick folds in small bowel). Commonly achlorhydric: cf. Zollinger–Ellison syndrome.
2. **Varices** – occur in fundus and usually associated with oesophageal varices.

Further Reading

An SK, Han JK, Kim YH et al. Gastric mucosa-associated lymphoid tissue lymphoma: spectrum of findings at double contrast gastrointestinal examination with pathologic correlation. Radiographics 2001;21:1491–504.
Mendelson RM, Fermoyle S. Primary gastrointestinal lymphomas: a radiological-pathological review. Part 1: Stomach, oesophagus and colon. Australas Radiol 2005;49(5):353–64.

6.10 LINITIS PLASTICA

Neoplastic

1. **Gastric carcinoma.**
2. **Lymphoma*.**
3. **Metastases** – particularly breast.
4. **Local invasion** – pancreatic carcinoma.

Inflammatory

1. **Corrosives** – can cause rigid stricture of antrum extending up to the pylorus.
2. **Radiotherapy** – can cause rigid stricture of antrum with some deformity. Mucosal folds may be thickened or effaced. Large antral ulcers can also occur.
3. **Granulomata** – Crohn's disease, TB.
4. **Eosinophilic enteritis** – commonly involves gastric antrum (causing narrowing and nodules) in addition to small bowel. Blood eosinophilia. Occasionally spares the mucosa, so needs full thickness biopsy for confirmation.

6.11 'BULL'S-EYE' (TARGET) LESION IN THE STOMACH

Ulcer on apex of a nodule.

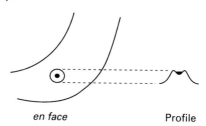

en face   Profile

1. **Submucosal metastases** – may be multiple
   (a) Melanoma – commonest.
   (b) Lymphoma*.
   (c) Carcinoma – breast, bronchus, pancreas.
   (d) Carcinoid.
2. **Leiomyoma.**
3. **Pancreatic 'rest'** – ectopic pancreatic tissue. Usually on inferior wall of antrum. A central 'blob' of barium is seen in 50% – collects in primitive duct remnant. Can also occur in duodenum, jejunum, Meckel's diverticulum, liver, gallbladder and spleen.
4. **Neurofibroma** – may be multiple. Other stigmata of neurofibromatosis.

6.12 DECREASED/ABSENT DUODENAL FOLDS

1. **Scleroderma** (often with dilatation)*.
2. **Crohn's disease***.
3. **Strongyloides**.
4. **Cystic fibrosis***.
5. **Amyloidosis**.

6.13 DUODENAL MURAL/FOLD THICKENING OR MASS

Neoplastic

1. **Adenocarcinoma** (50–70% small bowel carcinoma occurs in duodenum or proximal jejunum). Polypoidal mass or asymmetric wall thickening on CT. 50% have metastasis at presentation.
2. **Lipoma**
3. **Brunner gland Hamartoma** (10% of benign duodenal tumours). Usually D1. No malignant potential. 1–12cm sessile or pedunculated filling defect.
4. **Adenoma** (malignant potential; associated with familial adenomatous polyposis).
5. **GIST** (unusual in duodenum – usually D2, D3; large size, heterogeneous rim enhancement and local invasion suggest malignant transformation).
6. **Leiomyoma**.
7. **Lymphoma** (usually non Hodgkin's, T cell; CT-segmental non obstructing mural thickening or extrinsic mass with or without aneurysmal dilatation).
8. **Neuroendocrine tumour** (2–3% occur in duodenum; polypoidal or mass with rapid contrast enhancement and wash out on CT).
9. **Metastasis** (most common melanoma, breast and lung).

Inflammatory/infiltrative

1. **Duodenitis/ulcer** (usually D1 related to *H. pylori*. Focal wall thickening and avid enhancement on CT. May see large ulcer cavity).
2. **Crohn's disease** (mural thickening on CT/MRI ± layered contrast enhancement). Mild signs occur in duodenum in up to 40%, but severe involvement only occurs in 2%. Cap and proximal half of second part of duodenum predominantly affected.
3. **Cystic dystrophy** (possible secondary to heterotopic pancreatic tissue in duodenal wall – D2). Presents with weight loss, pain and

6

obstruction. Well defined duodenal wall cysts on CT/MRI/USS often with delayed mural enhancement due to fibrosis ± signs of chronic pancreatitis. Inflammatory changes in acute episode.

4. **Groove pancreatitis** (segmental inflammation between the head of pancreas and duodenum).
5. **Varices.**
6. **Diverticulum** (up to 23%; may be large).
7. **Duplication** (less than 5% of intestinal duplications; thin walled cyst on CT/MRI often with no luminal communication).
8. **Infiltration** (eosinophilic gastroenteritis, mastocytosis [dense bones], Whipple's, amyloid).
9. **Haematoma.**
10. **Ischaemia** (widespread changes can occur in vasculitis secondary to radiotherapy, collagen diseases and Henoch–Schönlein purpura).
11. **Infestations** (e.g. Giardia, worms).

See also 6.17 and 6.18.

Further Reading

Wei CJ, Chiang JH, Lin WC et al. Tumor and tumor-like lesions of duodenum: CT and barium imaging features. Clin Imaging 2003;27:89–96.
Zissin R, Osadchy A, Gayer G et al. Pictorial review. CT of duodenal pathology. Br J Radiol 2002;75:78–84.

6.14 DILATED SMALL BOWEL

Calibre: proximal jejunum >3.5cm (4.5cm if small bowel enema)
mid-small bowel >3.0cm (4.0cm if small bowel enema)
ileum >2.5cm (3.0cm if small bowel enema).

Normal folds

1. **Mechanical obstruction** – ± dilated large bowel, depending on level of obstruction. CT 78–100% sensitivity for high grade obstruction (less in sub-acute). Small bowel faeces sign non-specific but may indicate point of obstruction.
2. **Paralytic ileus** – dilated small and large bowel.
3. **Coeliac disease, tropical sprue, dermatitis herpetiformis** – can produce identical signs. Dilatation is the hallmark, and correlates well with severity, but it is relatively uncommon. ± Dilution and flocculation of barium. See 6.16.
4. **Scleroderma.**
5. **Iatrogenic** – postvagotomy and gastrectomy may produce dilatation due to rapid emptying of stomach contents. Dilatation may also occur proximal to a small bowel loop.

Thick folds

1. **Ischaemia**.
2. **Crohn's disease*** – combination of obstructive and inflammatory changes.
3. **Radiotherapy**.
4. **Lymphoma***.
5. **Zollinger–Ellison syndrome** – ileus due to excess acidity.
6. **Extensive small bowel resection** – compensatory dilatation and thickening of folds.
7. **Amyloidosis**.

Further Reading

Maglinte DD, Kelvin FM, Sandrasegaran K et al. Radiology of small bowel obstruction: contemporary approach and controversies. Abdom Imaging 2005;30(2):160–78.

Sinha R, Verma R. Multidetector row computed tomography in bowel obstruction. Part 1. Small bowel obstruction. Clin Radiol 2005;60(10):1058–67.

6

6.15 STRICTURES IN THE SMALL BOWEL

1. **Adhesions** – angulation of bowel which is constant in site. Normal mucosal folds.
2. **Crohn's disease*** – ± ulcers and altered mucosal pattern.
3. **Ischaemia** – ulcers are rare. Evolution is more rapid than Crohn's ± long strictures.
4. **Radiation enteritis** – see 6.16.
5. **Tumours**
   (a) Lymphoma* – usually secondary to contiguous spread from lymph nodes. Primary disease may occur and is nearly always due to non-Hodgkin's lymphoma.
   (b) Carcinoid – although the appendix is the commonest site, these never metastasize. Of those occurring in small bowel, 90% are in ileum (mostly distal 2 feet), and 30% are multifocal. A fibroblastic response to infiltration produces a stricture ± mass. It is the commonest primary malignancy of small bowel, but only 30% metastasize (more likely if >2cm diameter) or invade. Carcinoid syndrome only develops with liver metastases – see 6.21.
   (c) Carcinoma – if duodenal lesions are included this is the most common primary malignancy of the small bowel and the duodenum is the most frequent site. Ileal lesions are rare (unless associated with Crohn's disease). Short segment annular stricture with mucosal destruction, ulcerating or polypoidal lesion. High incidence of second primary tumours.

(d) Sarcoma – lymphosarcoma or leiomyosarcoma. Thick folds with an eccentric lumen. Leiomyosarcomas may present as a large mass displacing bowel loops with a large barium-filled cavity.

(e) Metastases – usual sites of origin are malignant melanoma, ovary, pancreas, stomach, colon, breast, lung and uterus. Rounded deformities of the bowel wall with flattened mucosal folds. In patients with gynaecological malignancies, duodenal or jejunal obstructions are most likely due to metastases; most radiation-induced strictures are in the ileum.

6. **Enteric coated potassium tablets**.

Further Reading

Paulsen SR, Huprich JE, Fletcher JG et al. CT enterography as a diagnostic tool in evaluating small bowel disorders: review of clinical experience with over 700 cases. Radiographics 2006;26(3):641–57.

Ramachandran I, Sinha R, Rajesh A et al. Multidetector row CT of small bowel tumours. Clin Radiol 2007;62(7):607–14.

6.16 THICKENED FOLDS IN NON-DILATED SMALL BOWEL – SMOOTH AND REGULAR

Fold thickness: jejunum > 2.5 mm
                 ileum   > 2.0 mm

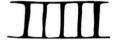

Vascular

1. **Intramural haematoma**
   Homogeneous high attenuation wall on CT.
   (a) Trauma – commonest in duodenum, since fixed to posterior abdominal wall ('stacked coin' appearance).
   (b) Bleeding diathesis – commonly localized to a few loops.
2. **Ischaemia**
   (a) Acute – embolus, Henoch–Schönlein purpura. Can produce ileus. May perforate. Ulcers rare.
   (b) Chronic – vasculitis (collagen, radiotherapy), atheroma, fibromuscular dysplasia. Presents with postprandial pain, and malabsorption.

Radiotherapy

1. **Acute** – thickening of valvulae conniventes and poor peristalsis. Ulceration is rare.
2. **Chronic** – latent period of up to 25 years. Most common signs are submucosal thickening of valvulae conniventes and/or mural thickening. Stenoses, adhesions, sinuses and fistulae may also occur.

(The absence of ulceration, cobblestoning and asymmetry differentiate it from Crohn's disease.) May show homogeneous enhancement on contrast-enhanced CT.

Oedema

1. **Adjacent inflammation** – focal.
2. **Hypoproteinaemia** – e.g. nephrotic, cirrhosis, protein-losing enteropathy. Generalized.
3. **Venous obstruction** – e.g. cirrhosis, Budd–Chiari syndrome, constrictive pericarditis.
4. **Lymphatic obstruction** – e.g. lymphoma, retroperitoneal fibrosis, primary lymphangiectasia (child with leg oedema).
5. **Angioneurotic**.

Early infiltration

1. **Amyloidosis** – gastrointestinal tract commonly involved. Primary amyloid tends to produce generalized thickening, whereas secondary amyloid produces focal lesions. Malabsorption is unusual.
2. **Eosinophilic enteritis** – focal or generalized. Gastric antrum frequently involved. No ulcers. Blood eosinophilia. Occasionally spare mucosa – therefore need full thickness biopsy for diagnosis.

Coeliac disease

Thickening of folds is not common, and is probably a functional abnormality rather than true fold thickening. ± Jejunal dilatation.

Abetalipoproteinaemia

Rare, inherited. Malabsorption, acanthocytosis, and CNS abnormality. ± Dilated bowel.

Further Reading

Ledermann HP, Borner N, Strunk H et al. Bowel wall thickening on transabdominal sonography. Am J Roentgenol 2000;174:107–17.
Rogalla P. CT of the small intestine. Eur Radiol 2005;15(Suppl 4):D142–8.

6.17 THICKENED FOLDS IN NON-DILATED SMALL BOWEL – IRREGULAR AND DISTORTED

Fold thickness: jejunum <2.5mm
ileum <2.0mm.

Localized

Inflammatory

1. **Crohn's disease*** – occurs before aphthoid ulcers.
2. **Zollinger–Ellison syndrome** – predominantly proximal small bowel. Dilatation may occur.

Neoplastic

1. **Lymphoma***.
2. **Metastases** – particularly melanoma, breast, ovary and gastrointestinal tract.
3. **Carcinoid** – commonest primary malignant small bowel tumour. 90% in the ileum and mostly in the distal 60cm. It is more common in the appendix, where it is a benign tumour.

Infective

1. **Tuberculosis** – can look identical to Crohn's disease, but predominant caecal involvement may help to distinguish it. Less than 50% have pulmonary tuberculosis.

Widespread

Infiltrative

1. **Amyloidosis**.
2. **Eosinophilic enteritis**.
3. **Mastocytosis** – may have superimposed small nodules, urticaria pigmentosa and sclerotic bone lesions.
4. **Whipple's disease** – flitting arthralgia, lymphadenopathy and sacroiliitis.

Inflammatory

1. **Crohn's disease***.

Infestations

1. **Giardiasis** – associates with hypogammaglobulinaemia and nodular lymphoid hyperplasia.
2. **Strongyloides** – ± absent folds in chronic cases.

Stomach abnormality with thickened small bowel mucosal folds

1. Lymphoma/metastases.
2. Zollinger–Ellison syndrome.
3. Ménétrier's disease.
4. Amyloidosis.
5. Eosinophilic enteritis.

Further Reading

Hara AK, Leighton JA, Sharma VK et al. Imaging of small bowel disease: comparison of capsule endoscopy, standard endoscopy, barium examination, and CT. Radiographics 2005;25(3):697–711.

Maglinte DD, Sandrasegaran K, Lappas JC. CT enteroclysis: techniques and applications. Radiol Clin North Am 2007;45(2):289–301.

6.18 SMALL BOWEL MURAL THICKENING ON CROSS SECTIONAL IMAGING – DIFFERENTIATION BY CONTRAST ENHANCEMENT

Summary of small bowel fold patterns

Dilated small bowel		Non-dilated small bowel with thickened folds	
Normal folds	Thick folds	Regular folds	Irregular folds
• Mechanical obstruction • Paralytic ileus • Coeliac disease • Scleroderma	• Ischaemia • Crohn's disease • Radiotherapy • Lymphoma • Zollinger-Ellison syndrome	• Intramural haematoma • Radiotherapy • Oedema	

Irregular folds:

Localized	Widespread
• Crohn's disease • Zollinger-Ellison syndrome • Lymphoma • Metastases • Carcinoid • Tuberculosis	• Amyloidosis • Eosinophilic enteritis • Crohn's disease • Giardiasis

Normal mural thickness 1–2mm (distended bowel), 3–4mm (collapsed bowel).

Avid contrast enhancement

(Similar to adjacent venous enhancement)

1. **Ischaemia** ('shock bowel' – often reversible).
2. **Acute inflammatory bowel disease** (often with dilated vasa recta).
3. **Malignancy.**

Moderate homogeneous contrast enhancement

(Similar to muscle)

1. **Chronic inflammatory bowel disease.**
2. **Chronic ischaemia.**
3. **Chronic radiation enteritis.**
4. **Malignancy** (including lymphoma).

Heterogeneous enhancement

1. **Malignancy.**
2. **GIST.**
3. **Endometriosis.**
4. **Lymphoma** (rare pattern of enhancement).

Layered enhancement

Halo sign
– almost always reflects a non-malignant process
– double halo (higher attenuation outer layer with low attenuation inner layer, or higher attenuation inner layer with lower attenuation outer layer).

Target sign (3 layers – higher attenuation inner and outer layer with lower attenuation middle layer).

1. **Inflammatory bowel disease.**
2. **Ischaemia** (arterial and venous).
3. **Vasculitis** (e.g. SLE).
4. **Angioedema.**
5. **Infection.**
6. **Radiation enteritis.**
7. **Graft versus host disease.**
8. **Haemorrhage.**

Reduced enhancement

1. **Ischaemia.**

6.19 SMALL BOWEL MURAL THICKENING ON CROSS SECTIONAL IMAGING – DIFFERENTIATION BY LENGTH OF INVOLVEMENT

Focal ($\leq$5cm)

Malignant

1. Adenocarcinoma, lymphoma.
2. GIST.
3. Metastasis.

Inflammatory

1. Perforation.
2. Crohn's disease.
3. Diverticulitis.
4. Endometriosis.

Segmental (6–40cm)

1. Haemorrhage.
2. Lymphoma.
3. Crohn's disease.
4. Infection.
5. Ischaemia (usually SMA embolus).
6. Vasculitis.
7. Radiation.

Diffuse (>40cm)

1. Hypoalbuminaemia.
2. Intestinal ischaemia (proximal SMA embolus).
3. Vasculitis.
4. Angioedema.
5. Graft-versus-host disease.
6. Infectious enteritis.

Further Reading

Macari M, Megibow AJ, Balthazar EJ. A pattern approach to the abnormal small bowel: observations at MDCT and CT enterography. Am J Roentgenol 2007;188:1344–55.

Wittenberg J, Harisinghani MG, Jhaveri K et al. Algorithmic approach to CT diagnosis of the abnormal bowel wall. Radiographics 2002;22:1093–107.

6.20 MULTIPLE NODULES IN THE SMALL BOWEL

Inflammatory

1. **Nodular lymphoid hyperplasia** – nodules 2–4mm with normal fold thickness. Associated with hypogammaglobulinaemia (IgA and IgM). Produces malabsorption, and there is a high incidence of intestinal infections (particularly giardiasis, but Strongyloides and Candida may also occur). Can also affect the colon, where it may be an early sign of Crohn's disease (in adults).
2. **Crohn's disease*** – 'cobblestone' mucosa but other characteristic signs present.

Infiltrative

1. **Whipple's disease** – ± myriad of tiny (<1mm) nodules superimposed on thick folds.
2. **Waldenström's macroglobulinaemia** – ± myriad of tiny (<1mm) nodules. Folds usually normal, but may occasionally be thick.
3. **Mastocytosis** – nodules a little larger and folds usually thick.

Neoplastic

1. **Lymphoma*** – can produce diffuse nodules (2–4mm) of varying sizes. Ulceration in the nodules is not uncommon.
2. **Polyposis**
   (a) Peutz–Jeghers' syndrome – AD. Buccal pigmentation. Multiple hamartomas (± intussusception) 'carpeting' the small bowel. Can also involve the colon (30%) and stomach (25%). Not in themselves premalignant, but associated with carcinoma of stomach, duodenum and ovary.
   (b) Gardner's syndrome – predominantly in the colon. Occasionally has adenomas in small bowel.
   (c) Canada–Cronkhite syndrome – predominantly stomach and colon, but may affect the small bowel.
3. **Metastases** – on antimesenteric border. Particularly melanoma, breast, gastrointestinal tract and ovary. (Rarely bronchus and kidney.) ± Ascites.

Infective

1. **Typhoid** – hypertrophy of 'Peyer's patches'.
2. **Yersinia** – ± nodules in terminal ileum.

6.21 LESIONS IN THE TERMINAL ILEUM

Inflammatory

1. **Crohn's disease*.**
2. **Ulcerative colitis*** – 10% of those with total colitis have 'backwash' ileitis for up to 25cm causing granular mucosa, ± dilatation. No ulcers.
3. **Radiation enteritis** – submucosal thickening of mucosal folds, mural thickening, symmetrical stenoses, adhesions, sinuses and fistulae. Ulceration and cobblestoning are not seen.

Infective

1. **Tuberculosis** – can look identical to Crohn's disease. Continuity of involvement with caecum and ascending colon can occur. Longitudinal ulcers are uncommon. Less than 50% have pulmonary TB. Caecum is predominantly involved – progressive contraction of caecal wall opposite the ileocaecal valve, and cephalad retraction of the caecum with straightening of the ileocaecal angle.
2. **Yersinia** – 'cobblestone' appearance and aphthoid ulcers. No deep ulcers and spontaneous resolution, usually within 10 weeks, distinguishes it from Crohn's disease.
3. **Actinomycosis** – very rare. Predominantly caecum. ± Associated bone destruction with periosteal reaction.
4. **Histoplasmosis** – very rare.

Neoplastic

1. **Lymphoma*** – may look like Crohn's disease.
2. **Carcinoid** – appendiceal carcinoid tumours are the most common and are usually benign. Most ileal carcinoids originate in the distal ileum and are invariably malignant if >2cm. Radiological signs reflect the primary lesion [annular fibrotic stricture (± obstruction); intraluminal filling defect(s)], the mesenteric secondary mass (stretching of loops; rigidity and fixation), interference with the blood supply to the ileum by the secondary mass (thickening of mucosal folds) or the effects of fibrosis (sharp angulation of a loop; stellate arrangement of loops). The caecum may be involved and strictures may be multifocal.
3. **Metastases** – no ulcers.

Ischaemia

A rare site. Thickened folds, 'cobblestone' appearance and 'thumb printing', but rapid progression of changes helps to discriminate it from Crohn's disease.

6

Further Reading

Hara AK, Leighton JA, Sharma VK et al. Imaging of small bowel disease: comparison of capsule endoscopy, standard endoscopy, barium examination, and CT. Radiographics 2005;25(3):697–711.

Silva AC, Beaty SD, Hara AK et al. Spectrum of normal and abnormal CT appearances of the ileocecal valve and cecum with endoscopic and surgical correlation. Radiographics 2007;27(4):1039–54.

6.22 COLONIC POLYPS

Sensitivity of CT virtual colonoscopy likely superior to barium enema.

Adenomatous

1. **Simple tubular adenoma, tubulovillous adenoma, villous adenoma** – these three form a spectrum both in size and degree of dysplasia. Villous adenoma is the largest, shows the most severe dysplasia and has the highest incidence of malignancy. Signs suggestive of malignancy are:

   (a) Size: <5mm   0% malignant
               5mm–1cm   1% malignant
               1–2cm   10% malignant
               > 2cm   50% malignant.

   (b) Sessile – base greater than height.

   (c) 'Puckering' of colonic wall at base of polyp.

   (d) Irregular surface.

   Villous adenomas are typically fronded, sessile and are poorly coated by barium because of their mucous secretion. May cause a protein-losing enteropathy or hypokalaemia.

2. **Familial polyposis coli and Gardner's syndrome** – AD.

Both conditions may represent a spectrum of the same disease. Multiple adenomas of the colon which are more numerous in the distal colon and rectum. Colonic carcinoma develops in early adulthood (in 30% by 10 years after diagnosis and in 100% by 20 years). Associated with mesenteric fibromatosis – a non-calcified soft-tissue mass which may displace bowel loops and produce mucosal irregularity from local invasion. US reveals a hypoechoic or hyperechoic mass and CT a homogeneous mass of muscle density, dental abnormalities, osteomas and gastric small bowel hamartomatous and adenomatous polyps. 60% of those who present with colonic symptoms already have a carcinoma. The carcinoma is multifocal in 50%.

Hyperplastic

1. **Solitary/multiple** – most frequently found in rectum.
2. **Nodular lymphoid hyperplasia** – usually children. Filling defects are smaller than familial polyposis coli.

Hamartomatous

1. **Juvenile polyposis** – ± familial. Children under 10 years. Commonly solitary in the rectum.
2. **Peutz–Jeghers syndrome** – AD. 'Carpets' small bowel, but also affects colon and stomach in 30%. Increased incidence of carcinoma of stomach, duodenum and ovary.

Inflammatory

1. **Ulcerative colitis*** – polyps can be seen at all stages of activity of the colitis (no malignant potential): acute – pseudopolyps (i.e. mucosal hyperplasia); chronic – sessile polyp (resembles villous adenoma); quiescent – tubular/filiform ('wormlike') and can show a branching pattern. Dysplasia in colitic colons is usually not radiologically visible. When visible it appears as a solitary nodule, several separate nodules (both non-specific) or as a close grouping of multiple adjacent nodules with apposed, flattened edges (the latter appearance being associated with dysplasia in 50% of cases).
2. **Crohn's disease*** – polyps less common than in ulcerative colitis.

Infective

1. **Schistosomiasis** – predominantly involves rectum. ± Strictures.
2. **Amoebiasis**.

Others

1. **Canada–Cronkhite syndrome** – not hereditary. Predominantly affects stomach and colon, but can occur anywhere in bowel. Increased incidence of carcinoma of colon. Other features are alopecia, nail atrophy and skin pigmentation.
2. **Turcot's syndrome** – AR. Increased incidence of CNS malignancy.

6

6.23 COLONIC STRICTURES

Neoplastic

1. **Carcinoma** – mucosal destruction and 'shouldering'. Often shorter than 6cm.
2. **Lymphoma*.**

Inflammatory

Tend to be symmetrical, smooth and tapered.

1. **Ulcerative colitis*** – usually requires extensive involvement for longer than 5 years. Commonest in sigmoid colon. May be multiple. Beware malignant complications – these are commonly irregular, annular strictures (30% are multiple). Risk factors are: total colitis, length of history (risk starts at 10 years and increases by 10% per decade), epithelial dysplasia on biopsy.
2. **Crohn's disease*** – strictures occur in 25% of colonic Crohn's disease, and 50% of these are multiple.
3. **Pericolic abscess** – can look malignant, but relative lack of mucosal destruction.
4. **Radiotherapy** – occurs several years after treatment. Commonest site is rectosigmoid colon, which appears smooth and narrow, and rises vertically out of pelvis due to thickening of surrounding tissue.

Ischaemia

Infarction heals by stricture formation relatively rapidly.
Commonest site is splenic flexure, but 20% occur in other sites.
It can be extensive and has tapering ends.

Infective

1. **Tuberculosis** – commonest in ileocaecal region. Short, 'hour-glass' stricture.
2. **Amoeboma** – more common in descending colon. Occurs in 2–8% of amoebiasis and is multiple in 50%. Rapid improvement after treatment with metronidazole.
3. **Schistosomiasis** – commonly rectosigmoid region. Granulation tissue forming after the acute stage (oedema, fold-thickening and polyps) may cause a stricture.
4. **Lymphogranuloma venereum** – sexually transmitted Chlamydia. Late complications are strictures which are characteristically long and tubular, and affect the rectosigmoid region. Fistulae may occur.

Extrinsic masses

Inflammatory, tumours (primary and secondary), and endometriosis.

Further Reading

Dachman AH, Lefere P, Gryspeerdt S et al. CT colonography: visualization methods, interpretation, and pitfalls. Radiol Clin North Am 2007;45(2):347–59.

Rollandi GA, Biscaldi E, DeCicco E. Double contrast barium enema: technique, indications, results and limitations of a conventional imaging methodology in the MDCT virtual endoscopy era. Eur J Radiol 2007;61(3):382–7.

Thoeni RF, Cello JP. CT imaging of colitis. Radiology 2006;240(3):623–38.

6.24 COLITIS ON CROSS-SECTIONAL IMAGING

Sign of inflammatory colitis on CT/MRI are often non specific. The following is a guide only.

Diffuse

1. **Ulcerative colitis** (UC).
2. **CMV.**
3. *E. coli.*
4. **Pseudomembranous colitis** (*Clostridium difficile* toxin. Very marked colon wall thickening (mean 15mm) with thumbprinting. Pericolic stranding. Accordion sign (trapping of +ve contrast between folds – also seen in ischaemia, cirrhosis, and infectious types of colitis). Ascites in up to 35% (unlike Crohn's disease). Often left-sided but maybe segmental.

Predominantly right-sided

1. **Crohn's disease** (skip lesions, mural thickening often >UC [mean 11mm vs 8mm] lymphadenopathy).
2. **Salmonella.**
3. **TB** (ileocaecal valve often involved. Distal colon can be involved, lymphadenopathy [low attenuation], sinuses, strictures. Ascites, peritoneal thickening may be [but not always] present. No fibrofatty infiltration [cf. Crohn's disease]).
4. **Yersinia.**
5. **Amoebiasis** (usually starts on the right but may be diffuse. Terminal ileum often spared. May produce toxic megacolon. Mass like amoebomas in 10%. Liver abscess).
6. **Neutropenic enterocolitis** (typhlitis). Immunosuppressive states (including AIDS). Marked thickening of right colon and terminal ileum. Pericolic stranding and fluid.
7. **Ischaemic colitis.** Hyopvolaemic states in young patients. Cocaine users.
8. **Omental infarction.** Well-circumscribed triangular or oval heterogeneous fatty mass with a whorled pattern of concentric linear fat stranding.

Predominantly left-sided

1. **Ulcerative colitis**.
2. **Shigellosis**.
3. **Gonorrhoea**.
4. **Lymphogranuloma venereum**.
5. **Ischaemic colitis**. Watershed areas in the sigmoid colon near the rectosigmoid junction and splenic flexure (especially the elderly). Rectum usually (but not always) spared.
6. **Radiation**.
7. **Diverticulitis**. May be right-sided. Differentiation from cancer not always possible. Features suggesting diverticulitis; >10cm involvement, pericolonic stranding, engorged mesenteric vessels, fluid in the mesentery. Features suggesting cancer; focal concentric mass, shouldering, pericolonic nodes.
8. **Epiploic appendagitis**. Often left-sided but can occur anywhere. Well-defined oval or round area of fat with an enhancing rim located immediately adjacent to the colon. High density central focus.

Further Reading

Thoeni RF, Cello JP. CT imaging of colitis. Radiology 2006;240(3):623–38.

6.25 PNEUMATOSIS INTESTINALIS (GAS IN THE BOWEL WALL)

Gas in the bowel wall. CT sensitivity much greater than plain films.

Benign causes

1. **Idiopathic** (up to 15% of cases and usually involves the colon) – pneumatosis cystoides intestinalis.
2. **Pulmonary** (asthma, emphysema, positive end-expiratory pressure [PEEP], cystic fibrosis).
3. **Intestinal** (pyloric stenosis, intestinal pseudo-obstruction, enteritis, bowel obstruction, adynamic ileus, inflammatory bowel disease, leukemia, collagen vascular disease [e.g. scleroderma]).
4. **Iatrogenic** (barium enema/CT colonography, jejunostomy tubes, postsurgical anastomosis, endoscopy).
5. **Medication** (corticosteroids, chemotherapeutic agents).
6. **Organ transplants** (and graft-versus-host disease).

Life-threatening causes

1. **Intestinal ischaemia.**
2. **Intestinal obstruction** (especially strangulation).
3. **Enteritis.**
4. **Toxic megacolon.**
5. **Trauma.**

Further Reading

Ho LM, Paulson EK, Thompson WM. Pneumatosis intestinalis in the adult: benign to life-threatening causes. Am J Roentgenol 2007;88:1604–13.

6.26 MEGACOLON IN AN ADULT

Colonic calibre greater than 5.5cm.

Non-toxic (without mucosal abnormalities)

1. **Distal obstruction** – e.g. carcinoma.
2. **Ileus** – paralytic or secondary to electrolyte imbalance.
3. **Pseudo-obstruction** – symptoms and signs of large bowel obstruction but with no organic lesion identifiable by barium enema or CT. A continuous, gas-filled colon with sharp, thin bowel wall, few fluid levels and gas or faeces in the rectum may differentiate from organic obstruction. Mortality is 25–30% and the risk of caecal necrosis and perforation is up to 15%.
4. **Purgative abuse**.

Toxic (with severe mucosal abnormalities)

Deep ulceration and inflammation produce a neuromuscular degeneration. Thick oedematous folds and extensive sloughing of the mucosa leaves mucosal islands. The underlying causes produce similar plain film changes. The presence of intramural gas indicates that perforation is imminent.

1. **Inflammatory**
   (a) Ulcerative colitis*.
   (b) Crohn's disease*.
   (c) Pseudomembranous colitis.
2. **Ischaemic colitis.**
3. **Dysentery**
   (a) Amoebiasis.
   (b) Salmonella.

Further Reading

Saunders MD. Acute colonic pseudo-obstruction. Best Pract Res Clin Gastroenterol 2007;21(4):671–87.

6.27 'THUMBPRINTING' IN THE COLON

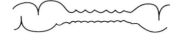

Colitides

1. **Ulcerative colitis*.**
2. **Crohn's disease*.**
3. **Ischaemic colitis** – commonest at the splenic flexure, but anywhere possible. Air insufflation may obliterate the 'thumbprinting'.
4. **Pseudomembranous colitis.**
5. **Amoebic colitis.**
6. **Schistosomiasis.**

Neoplastic

1. **Lymphoma*.**
2. **Metastases.**

Differential diagnosis

1. **Pneumatosis coli** – cysts may indent the mucosa, giving a similar appearance, but gas is seen in the wall.

6.28 APHTHOID ULCERS

Barium in a central ulcer surrounded by a halo of oedematous mucosa.

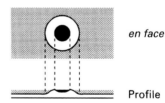

en face

Profile

In colon

1. **Crohn's disease*** – the earliest sign in the terminal ileum and colon. Observed in 50% of patients.
2. **Yersinia enterocolitis.**
3. **Amoebic colitis.**
4. **Ischaemic colitis.**
5. **Behçet's disease** – mostly resembles Crohn's disease, but can occasionally simulate an idiopathic ulcerative proctocolitis.

In small bowel

1. **Crohn's disease*.**
2. **Yersinia enterocolitis.**
3. **Polyarteritis nodosa.**

6.29 CT SIGNS OF INTESTINAL ISCHAEMIA

Approximately 40% arterial emboli, 50% arterial thrombus, 10% venous occlusion.

1. **Vascular occlusion** (CT around 60% sensitive).
2. **Dilatation** (occurs early).
3. **Hyperenhancement** (occurs early – may indicate reversibility).
4. **Reduced enhancement** (with or without target sign).
5. **Mural thickening** (more marked with venous infarction).
6. **Mesenteric hyperattenuation** (30–70%).
7. **Free fluid.**
8. **Pneumatosis.**
9. **Gas in portal venous system** (late sign).

Further Reading
Angelelli G. Acute bowel ischaemia: CT findings. Eur J Radiol 2004;50:37–47.

6.30 CROSS-SECTIONAL IMAGING SIGNS OF APPENDICITIS

1. **Diameter >6mm** (but uncompressed normal appendix can be 10mm diameter).
2. **Lack of luminal gas** (luminal gas does NOT exclude appendicitis).
3. **Mural thickening.**
4. **Periappendiceal inflammation** (absence does not exclude appendicitis).
5. **Caecal pole thickening** (arrow head sign).
6. **Periappendiceal abscess.**

Further Reading
Pinto Leite N, Pereira JM, Cunha R. CT evaluation of appendicitis and its complications: imaging techniques and key diagnostic findings. Am J Roentgenol 2005;185(2):406–17.

6.31 CAUSES OF INCREASED MESENTERIC ATTENUATION – 'MISTY MESENTRY'

Inflammatory

1. Pancreatitis.
2. Cholecystitis.
3. Diverticulitis.
4. TB.
5. Inflammatory bowel disease.
6. Appendicitis.

Haemorrhage

Oedema (heart failure, liver failure etc)

Neoplastic

1. Lymphoma.
2. Primary peritoneal malignancy.
3. Secondary malignancy.
4. Desmoid tumour.

Idiopathic

1. **Mesenteric panniculitis** (retractile/sclerosing mesenteritis)
   (a) Idiopathic condition characterized by fat necrosis, inflammation [notably lymphocytic] and variable fibrosis. Associated with idiopathic inflammatory disorders (retroperitoneal fibrosis, sclerosing cholangitis etc). Link with neoplasia controversial but reported association with malignancy in up to 50% of cases (particularly lymphoma).
   (b) CT features include increased mesenteric attenuation often with pseudo capsule (50–60%), surrounds but does not displace vessels (unlike liposarcoma) but may displace bowel loops. Discrete soft tissue nodules may be apparent in 80%. Lymph nodes greater than 1cm atypical (raises possibility of lymphoma). May progress to dense fibrosis (sclerosing mesenteritis).

Further Reading
Horton KM, Lawler LP, Fishman EK. CT findings in sclerosing mesenteritis (panniculitis): spectrum of disease. Radiographics 2003;23:1561–7.

6.32 WIDENING OF THE RETRORECTAL SPACE/PRESACRAL MASS

The post-rectal soft-tissue space at S3–S5 is greater than 1.5 cm.

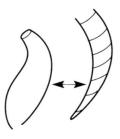

Normal variation

40% of cases and these are mostly large or obese individuals.

Inflammatory

1. **Ulcerative colitis*** – seen in 50% of these patients and the width increases as the disease progresses.
2. **Crohn's disease*** – the widening may diminish during the course of the disease.
3. **Radiotherapy**.
4. **Diverticulitis**.
5. **Abscess**.

Neoplastic

1. **Carcinoma of the rectum**.
2. **Metastases to the rectum** – especially from prostate, ovary and bladder.
3. **Sacral tumours** – metastases, plasmacytoma, chordoma.

Rectorectal development cysts

Epithelial lined developmental cysts. Associated with sacral anomalies. May communicate with rectum or anus. 50% asymptomatic. Complicated by infection, bleeding and malignant degeneration. Calcification rare.

1. **Epidermoid** (benign, unilocular).
2. **Dermoid**.
3. **Enteric cyst** (lined with intestinal mucosa)
   (a) Tailgut cyst (may be multiloculated).
   (b) Duplication cyst.

Others

1. **Anterior sacral meningocoele** – a sac containing CSF protrudes through a round or oval defect in the anterior wall of the sacrum. The diagnosis is confirmed by CT myelography or MRI.
2. **Pelvic lipomatosis.**
3. **Abscess.**
3. **Pseudomyxoma retroperitonei.**

Further Reading

Dahan H, Arrive L, Wendum D et al. Retrorectal developmental cysts in adults: clinical and radiologic-histopathologic review, differential diagnosis, and treatment. Radiographics 2001;21:575–84.

6.33 CT OF A RETROPERITONEAL CYSTIC MASS

Pancreas

1. **Pseudocyst** – can be mesenteric.
2. **Cystadenoma/carcinoma.**
3. **von Hippel–Lindau.**

Kidney – see 8.19
Para-aortic cystic nodes

1. **Testicular teratoma.**
2. **Carcinoma cervix.**

Retroperitoneal cystic tumour

1. **Lymphangioma** – can be mesenteric.
2. **Leiomyosarcoma** – can be mesenteric.
3. **Haemangiopericytoma.**
4. **Cystic teratoma** (fat and calcifications) – can be mesenteric.
5. **Mullerian cyst.**

NB. Any tumour with a fatty content can appear cystic due to density averaging, e.g. neurofibroma.

Others

1. **Haematoma** – late stage.
2. **Abscess.**
3. **Lymphocoele.**
4. **Meningocoele.**

Further Reading

Barwick TD, Malhotra A, Webb JA. Embryology of the adrenal glands and its relevance to diagnostic imaging. Clin Radiol 2005;60(9):953–9.

Nishino M, Hayakawa K, Minami M. Primary retroperitoneal neoplasms: CT and MR imaging findings with anatomic and pathologic diagnostic clues. Radiographics 2003;23(1):45–57.

6.34 NORMAL SIZE OF ABDOMINAL AND PELVIC LYMPH NODES

Normal size of pelvic and inguinal lymph nodes (short axis)

Site	Short axis size (mm)
Gastrohepatic	8
Porta hepatic	8
Porta caval	10
Coeliac axis to renal artery	10
Renal artery to aortic bifurcation	12

Site	Short axis size (mm)
Common iliac	9
External iliac	10
Internal iliac	7
Obturator	8
Inguinal	10

Further Reading

Royal College of Radiologists. Recommendations for cross-sectional imaging in cancer management. Royal College of Radiologists, London, 2006.

6.35 LOCALIZATION OF GASTROINTESTINAL BLEEDING

1. **Ulcers** – benign or malignant.
2. **Vascular lesions** – telangiectasia, haematoma, fistula, angiodysplasia.
3. **Tumours** – leiomyoma, adenoma.
4. **Inflammatory lesions** – gastritis, duodenitis.
5. **Varices** – oesophageal or stomach.
6. **Surgical anastomosis.**
7. **Meckel's diverticulum** (q.v.).
8. **Intussusception.**
9. **Metastatic disease.**
10. **Diverticula.**
11. **False positive**
    (a) Renal tract, liver, spleen, small bowel vascularity.
    (b) Uterus.
    (c) Accessory spleen.
    (d) Marrow uptake of colloid, especially if irregular.

Techniques

1. ^{99}mTc-labelled red blood cells. Labelling efficiency is important, as false positive scans can result from accumulations of free pertechnetate. Can detect a bleeding rate of more than 0.2ml/min
2. MDCT angiography – Pre-contrast, aorta triggered CT and delayed scans. Extravasation of IV contrast into the bowel lumen is diagnostic of GI bleeding. Can detect a bleeding rate of more than 0.3ml/min
3. Conventional angiography. Can detect a bleeding rate of more than 0.5ml/min

Further Reading

Holder LE. Radionuclide imaging in the evaluation of acute gastrointestinal bleeding. Radiographics 2000;20:1153–9.

Yoon M et al. Acute massive gastrointestinal bleeding. Gastrointest Bleed 2006;239:160–7.

6.36 CAUSES OF NON-MALIGNANT FDG UPTAKE IN ABDOMINAL PET CT

1. Attenuation correction artefacts.
2. Granulomatous disease (e.g. TB).
3. Abscesses.
4. Recent surgery (up to 6 weeks).
5. Foreign body.
6. Inflammation (diverticulitis, gastritis, pancreatitis).
7. Physiological uptake (liver, spleen, kidneys, bowel).
8. Urine.
9. Retroperitoneal fibrosis.
10. Adrenal adenoma (5%).
11. Portal vein thrombosis.
12. Uterine fibroid (18%).
13. Corpus luteum.
14. Paget's disease.
15. Bone marrow stimulation.
16. Brown fat (e.g. supra-adrenal).

6

6.37 ABDOMINAL MALIGNANCY WITH POOR FDG PET AVIDITY

1. Hepatoma (up to 50% show no uptake).
2. Lymphoma subtypes (e.g. MALT).
3. Necrotic and metastatic mucinous adenocarcinoma.
4. Renal cell carcinoma (around 60% sensitivity).
5. Early stage pancreatic cancer.
6. Prostate cancer.
7. Neuroendocrine tumours (e.g. carcinoid).

Further Reading

Blake M, Singh A, Getty B et al. Pearls and pitfalls in interpretation of abdominal and pelvic PET-CT. Radiographics 2006;26:1335–53.

Gallbladder, liver, spleen and pancreas

Stuart Taylor and Rebecca Greenhalgh

7.1 FILLING DEFECT IN THE GALLBLADDER

Multiple

1. **Calculi** – 30% are radio-opaque. Freely mobile.
2. **Cholesterosis ('strawberry' gallbladder)** – characteristically multiple fixed mural filling defects.

Single and small

1. **Calculus**.
2. **Adenomyomatosis** – three characteristic signs.
   (a) Fundal nodular filling defect.
   (b) Stricture – anywhere in the gallbladder. Sharply localized or a diffuse narrowing. More prominent following contraction after a fatty meal.
   (c) Rokitansky–Aschoff sinuses – may only be visible after gallbladder contraction.

Single and large

1. **Calculus**.
2. **Carcinoma** – difficult to diagnose as the radiological presentation is usually with a non-functioning gallbladder. Nearly always associated with gallstones and, therefore, if filling does occur it is indistinguishable from them. Cross-sectional imaging demonstrates a mass replacing the gallbladder (40–65%), focal or diffuse gallbladder wall thickening (20–30%) or an intraluminal polypoid mass (15–25%).

7.2 BILIARY TRACT DILATATION

CBD
>5mm at 50 years
>6mm at 60 years
>7mm at 70 years.
Intra hepatic ducts >2mm.

Benign

1. CBD stone.
2. Bile duct stricture.
3. Mirrizzi's syndrome.
4. Adenoma.
5. Iatrogenic.
6. Bile duct cysts.
7. Chronic pancreatitis.

Malignant

1. CBD cholangiocarcinoma.
2. Periampullary carcinoma.
3. Gallbladder carcinoma.
4. Porta hepatis lymphadenopathy.
5. Parenchymal metastases.
6. Pancreatic carcinoma.

7

Further Reading

Stroszczynski C, Hunerbein M. Malignant biliary obstruction: value of imaging findings. Abdom Imaging 2005;30(3):314–23.

Watanabe Y, Nagayama M, Okumura A. MR imaging of acute biliary disorders. Radiographics 2007;27(2):477–95.

7.3 GAS IN THE BILIARY TRACT

Irregularly branching gas shadows which do not reach to the liver edge, probably because of the direction of bile flow. The gallbladder may also be outlined.

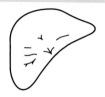

Within the bile ducts

Incompetence of the sphincter of Oddi
1. Following sphincterotomy.
2. Following passage of a gallstone.
3. Patulous sphincter in the elderly.

Postoperative
1. Cholecystoenterostomy.
2. Choledochoenterostomy.

Spontaneous biliary fistula
1. **Passage of a gallstone directly from an inflamed gallbladder into the bowel** – 90% of spontaneous fistulae. 57% erode into the duodenum and 18% into the colon. May result in a gallstone ileus.
2. **Duodenal ulcer perforating into the common bile duct** – 6% of spontaneous fistulae.
3. **Malignancy or trauma** – 4% of spontaneous fistulae.

Within the gallbladder

1. **All of the above.**
2. **Emphysematous cholecystitis** – due to gas-forming organisms and associated with diabetes in 20% of cases. There is intramural and intraluminal gas but, because there is usually cystic duct obstruction, gas is present in the bile ducts in only 20%. The erect film may show an air–bile interface.

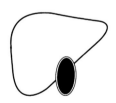

7.4 GAS IN THE PORTAL VEINS

Gas shadows which extend to within 2 cm of the liver capsule because of the direction of blood flow in the portal veins. Gas may also be present in the portal and mesenteric veins and the bowel wall.

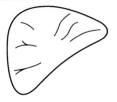

1. **Bowel infarction** – the majority of patients die soon after gas is seen in the portal veins.
2. **Sigmoid diverticulitis.**
3. **Haemorrhagic pancreatitis.**
4. **Pneumonia.**
5. **Air embolus during double contrast barium enema** – this has been observed during the examination of severely ulcerated colons and is not associated with a fatal outcome.
6. **Acute gastric dilatation** – in bed-ridden young people. May recover following decompression with a nasogastric tube.

7

7.5 SEGMENTAL ANATOMY OF THE LIVER

25% of colorectal carcinomas have liver secondaries at presentation. Of these, 10% have surgically resectable disease. Surgeons need to know the number, size, location and proximity to vessels.

The liver is divided into segments in the horizontal plane by the right and left main portal veins, and in the vertical plane by the right, middle and left hepatic veins.

> *Upper Segments*: above the level of the right and left portal veins.

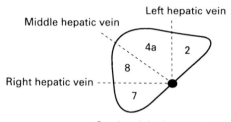

Caudate lobe is segment 1

> *Lower Segments*: below the level of the right and left portal veins.

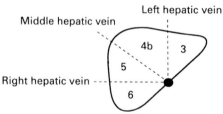

Further Reading

Foley WD. Liver: surgical planning. Eur Radiol 2005;15(Suppl 4):D89–95.
Nelson RC, Chezmer JL, Sugarbaker PH et al. Preoperative localisation of focal liver lesions to specific liver segments. Radiology 1990;176:86–94.

7.6 HEPATOMEGALY

Neoplastic

1. **Metastases.**
2. **Hepatoma.**
3. **Lymphoma*** – secondary involvement occurs in up to 50% of patients with systemic lymphoma, but is frequently occult. Primary hepatic lymphoma is very rare.

Raised venous pressure

1. **Congestive cardiac failure.**
2. **Constrictive pericarditis.**
3. **Tricuspid stenosis.**
4. **Budd–Chiari syndrome.**

Degenerative

1. **Cirrhosis** – especially alcoholic.
2. **Fatty infiltration.**

Myeloproliferative disorders

1. **Polycythaemia rubra vera.**
2. **Myelofibrosis.**

Infective

1. **Viral** – infectious and serum hepatitis; infectious mononucleosis.
2. **Bacterial** – abscess; brucellosis.
3. **Protozoal** – amoebic abscess, malaria, trypanosomiasis and kala-azar.
4. **Parasitic** – hydatid.

Storage disorders

1. **Amyloid.**
2. **Haemochromatosis.**
3. **Gaucher's disease.**
4. **Niemann–Pick disease.**

Congenital

1. **Riedel's lobe.**
2. **Polycystic disease*.**

7

7.7 HEPATIC CALCIFICATION

Multiple and small

1. **Healed granulomas** – tuberculosis, histoplasmosis and, less commonly, brucellosis and coccidioidomycosis. Usually <2cm. May be solitary. May be calcified granulomas in other organs.

Curvilinear

1. **Hydatid** – liver is the commonest site of hydatid disease. Most cysts are in the right lobe and are clinically silent but may cause pain, a palpable mass or a thrill. Calcification in 20–30% and, although calcification does not necessarily indicate death of the parasite, extensive calcification favours an inactive cyst. Calcification of daughter cysts produces several rings of calcification.
2. **Abscess** – especially amoebic abscess when the right lobe is most frequently affected.
3. **Calcified (porcelain) gallbladder** – strong association with gallbladder carcinoma.

Localized in mass

1. **Metastases** – calcification is uncommon but colloid carcinoma of the rectum, colon or stomach calcify most frequently. It may be amorphous, flaky, stippled or granular and solitary or multiple. Calcification may follow radiotherapy or chemotherapy.
2. **Adenoma** – rare. Calcifications are punctate, stippled or granular. Often placed eccentrically within a complex heterogeneous mass.

Sunray spiculation

1. **Haemangioma** – calcification in 10% (on AXR) to 20% (on CT). Phleboliths may also occur but are uncommon.
2. **Metastases** – infrequently in metastases from colloid carcinomas.
3. **Adenoma**.

Diffuse increased density

1. **Haemochromatosis***.

Further Reading
Paley MR, Ros PR. Hepatic calcification. Radiol Clin North Am 1998;36(2):391–8.

7.8 ULTRASOUND LIVER – GENERALIZED HYPOECHOIC

1. **Acute hepatitis** – mild hepatitis has normal echo pattern.
2. **Diffuse malignant infiltration**.

7.9 ULTRASOUND LIVER – GENERALIZED HYPERECHOIC

1. **Fatty infiltration**.
2. **Cirrhosis**.
3. **Hepatitis** – particularly chronic.
4. **Infiltration/deposition** – malignant, granulomata (e.g. TB, brucellosis, sarcoidosis), glycogen storage disease.

Further Reading

Karcaaltincaba M, Akhan O. Imaging of hepatic steatosis and fatty sparing. Eur J Radiol 2007;61(1):33–43
Vilgrain V. Ultrasound of diffuse liver disease and portal hypertension. Eur Radiol 2001;11:1563–77.

7.10 ULTRASOUND LIVER – FOCAL HYPERECHOIC

1. **Metastases** – gastrointestinal tract, ovary, pancreas, urogenital tract.
2. **Capillary haemangioma**.
3. **Adenoma** – particularly if associated haemorrhage.
4. **Focal nodular hyperplasia** – may be hyperechoic.
5. **Focal fatty infiltration**.
6. **Debris within lesion** – e.g. abscess, haematoma.
7. **Hepatocellular carcinoma** – can be hyperechoic or hypoechoic.

7.11 ULTRASOUND LIVER – FOCAL HYPOECHOIC

1. **Metastasis** – including cystic metastases (e.g. ovary, pancreas, stomach, colon).
2. **Lymphoma*.**
3. **Hepatocellular carcinoma** – can be hypoechoic or hyperechoic.
4. **Cysts** – benign, hydatid. Hydatid cysts can be classified according to their sonographic pattern. Type I, (commonest) uncomplicated unilocular cyst; Type II, a cyst with a split wall, i.e. a detached endocyst membrane; Type III, a cyst containing daughter cysts; Type IV, a cyst with a predominantly heterogeneous solid echo pattern with thick membranes and a few daughter cysts; Type V, a calcified cyst.
5. **Abscess** – ± hyperechoic wall due to fibrosis, ± surrounding hypoechoic rim due to oedema. Gas produces areas of very bright echoes.
6. **Haematoma** – acute stage.
7. **Cavernous haemangioma.**

Further Reading

Catalano O, Nunziata A, Lobianco R et al. Real-time harmonic contrast material-specific US of focal liver lesions. Radiographics 2005;25(2):333–49.

Harvey CJ, Albrecht T. Ultrasound of focal liver lesions. Eur Radiol 2001;11:1578–93.

Jang HJ, Kim TK, Wilson SR. Imaging of malignant liver masses: characterization and detection. Ultrasound Q 2006;22(1):19–29.

7.12 ULTRASOUND LIVER – PERIPORTAL HYPERECHOIC

1. **Air in biliary tree.**
2. **Schistosomiasis.**
3. **Cholecystitis.**
4. **Recurrent pyogenic cholangitis (oriental).**
5. **Peri-portal fibrosis.**

7.13 PERIPORTAL HYPOECHOGENICITY/ HYPOATTENUATION

Hepatic causes

1. Acute hepatitis.
2. Liver cirrhosis.
3. Abscess.
4. Tumour causing secondary lymphatic obstruction.
5. Orthotopic liver transplant rejection.
6. Trauma.

Extra-hepatic causes

1. Raised central venous pressure.
2. Hypoproteinaemia.
3. Bacteraemia.
4. Periportal lymphadenopathy.
5. Acute cholecystitis.
6. Acute pancreatitis.
7. Inflammatory bowel disease.

Further Reading
Karcaaltincaba M, Haliloglu M, Akpinar E et al. Multidetector CT and MRI findings in periportal space pathologies. Eur J Radiol 2007;61(1):3–10.

7.14 THICKENED GALLBLADDER WALL

>3mm – excluding the physiological, contracted (empty) gallbladder.

1. Cholecystitis.
2. Hepatitis.
3. Hypoalbuminaemia.
4. Cirrhosis.
5. Congestive heart failure.
6. Renal failure.

7.15 CT LIVER – FOCAL HYPODENSE LESION PRE-INTRAVENOUS CONTRAST MEDIUM

	Pre contrast	Arterial phase	Portal-venous phase	Delayed	Comments
Hepatocellular carcinoma	Low attenuation	Homogeneous enhancement	Washout of lesion	Isodense	± Irregular patchy enhancement
Adenoma	Low attenuation	Homogeneous enhancement 85%	Iso or hypodense	Iso or hypodense	Rapid washout often young woman
Haemangioma	Low attenuation may be heterogenous	Peripheral puddles	Partial fill in	Complete fill in	75% peripheral enhancement, 10% central enhancement, 74% progressively isodense on delayed scan, 24% partially isodense on delayed scan, 24% partially hypodense on delayed scan
Focal nodular hyperplasia	Iso/Low attenuation	Homogenous enhancement	Hypodense	Isodense	Often young female. Central scar. Most are hyperdense during arterial phase but rapidly (45s–1 min) becomes iso or hypodense, ± stellate central low density due to scar, but this is not specific and occurs in adenomas, haemangiomas and fibrolamellar hepatocellular carcinoma
Metastases – hypervascular	Low attenuation	Homogeneous enhancement	Hypodense		Melanoma, carcinoid, renal cell
Metastases	Low attenuation	Hypodense	Hypodense		Colorectal, lung
Cyst	Low attenuation	No enhancement			
Abscess	Low attenuation may have irregular margin	Transient regional increased enhancement	Ring enhancement		

Further Reading

Caseiro-Alves F, Brito J, Araujo AE et al. Liver haemangioma: common and uncommon findings and how to improve the differential diagnosis. Eur Radiol 2007;17:1544–54.

Grazioli L, Federle MP, Brancatelli G et al. Hepatic adenomas: imaging and pathologic findings. Radiographics 2001;21:877–94.

Kim HJ, Kim AY, Kim TK et al. Transient hepatic attenuation differences in focal hepatic lesions: dynamic CT features. AJR Am J Roentgenol 2005;1841:83–90.

Valls C, Iannacconne R, Alba E et al. Fat in the liver: diagnosis and characterization. Eur Radiol 2006;16:2292–308.

Winterer JT, Kotter E, Ghanem N et al. Detection and characterization of benign focal liver lesions with multislice CT. Eur Radiol 2006;16:2427–43.

7.16 CT LIVER – FOCAL HYPERENHANCING LESION

During the arterial phase

1. **Hepatocellular carcinoma.**
2. **Haemangioma.**
3. **Focal nodular hyperplasia.**
4. **Adenoma.**
5. **Metastases** – particularly carcinoid and pancreatic islet cell. Most metastases are hypovascular.

During the portal vein phase

1. **Haemangioma.**
2. **Hepatocellular carcinoma** – unusually. Most are iso- or low-attenuation during this phase.
3. **Venous collaterals** – from an obstructed SVC to the IVC via hepatic veins.

During the equilibrium phase

1. **Haemangioma** – because of progressive fill-in.
2. **Cholangiocarcinoma.**
3. **Solitary fibrous tumour.**
4. **Treated metastases.**

Further Reading

Hussain SM, Terkivatan T, Zondervan PE et al. Focal nodular hyperplasia: findings at state-of-the-art MR imaging, US, CT, and pathologic analysis. Radiographics 2004;24:3–17.

Kamel IR, Liapi E, Fishman EK. Liver and biliary system: evaluation by multidetector CT. Radiol Clin North Am 2005;43:977–97.

Kanematsu M, Kondo H, Goshima S et al. Imaging liver metastases: review and update. Eur J Radiol 2004;58:217–28.

7.17 CT LIVER – FOCAL HYPERDENSE LESION

Pre-intravenous contrast

1. **Calcification in:**
   (a) Metastasis – usually colorectal, but ovary, stomach, islet cell pancreas also possible.
   (b) Primary tumour – hepatoma, hepatoblastoma, haemangioendothelioma.
   (c) Infective lesion – hydatid, tuberculous granuloma.
2. **Acute haemorrhage** – post-traumatic or bleed into a vascular tumour, e.g. adenoma.

Post-intravenous contrast

1. **Hypervascular masses**
   (a) Metastases – carcinoid, renal cell carcinoma, islet cell pancreas and phaeochromocytoma.
   (b) Adenoma.
   (c) Focal nodular hyperplasia.
2. **Vascular abnormalities** – e.g. arterioportal shunts which may occur in hepatoma.

Further Reading

Kanematsu M, Kondo H, Goshima S et al. Imaging liver metastases: review and update. Eur J Radiol 2004;58:217–28.

7.18 CT LIVER – GENERALIZED LOW ATTENUATION PRE-INTRAVENOUS CONTRAST MEDIUM

Assess by comparing liver with spleen. Also intrahepatic vessels stand out as 'high' density against low density background of liver, but aorta shows normal soft-tissue density indicating the apparent high density of the intrahepatic vessels is not due to intravenous contrast.

1. **Fatty infiltration** – early cirrhosis, obesity, parenteral feeding, bypass surgery, malnourishment, cystic fibrosis, steroids, Cushing's, late pregnancy, carbon tetrachloride exposure, chemotherapy, high-dose tetracycline, and glycogen storage disease.
2. **Malignant infiltration**.
3. **Budd–Chiari**
   (a) Acute – big low-density liver with ascites. After intravenous contrast there is patchy enhancement of the hilum of the liver due to multiple collaterals, and non-visualization of the hepatic veins and/or IVC.

(b) Chronic – atrophied patchy low-density liver with sparing and hypertrophy of caudate lobe. Post-intravenous contrast scans show similar signs as the acute stage.

4. **Amyloid** – no change after intravenous contrast.

7.19 CT LIVER – GENERALIZED INCREASE IN ATTENUATION DENSITY PRE-INTRAVENOUS CONTRAST MEDIUM

Assess by comparing liver with spleen. Also intrahepatic vessels stand out as low-density against high-density background of liver.

1. **Haemochromatosis** – may be an associated hepatoma present.
2. **Haemosiderosis**.
3. **Iron overload** – e.g. from large number of blood transfusions.
4. **Glycogen storage disease** – liver may be increased or decreased in density.
5. **Amiodarone treatment** – contains iodine. Can also cause pulmonary interstitial and alveolar infiltrates.

7.20 MRI LIVER

	T_1W	T_2W	Gadolinium
Hepatocellular carcinoma	↓, iso or ↑ (due to fat degeneration)	↑	↑
Metastases	↓	↑	±↑
Haemangioma	↓	↑ ++ = to CSF at long TE	↑ (like CT)
Adenoma	↑ often	↑	↑
Focal nodular hyperplasia central scar	↓	↑+	↑ delayed
margins	isointense	↑	±↑
Regenerating nodule	↓, isointense	↓	
Haemochromatosis/ iron deposition	↓	↓++	

Further Reading

Bartolozzi C, Cioni D, Donati F et al. Focal liver lesions: MR imaging-pathologic correlation. Eur Radiol 2001;11:1374–88.

Elsayes KM, Narra VR, Yin Y et al. Focal hepatic lesions: diagnostic value of enhancement pattern approach with contrast-enhanced 3D gradient-echo MR imaging. Radiographics 2005;25:1299–320.

Martin DR, Semelka RC. Magnetic resonance imaging of the liver: review of techniques and approach to common diseases. Semin Ultrasound CT MR 2005;3:116–31.

Morana G, Salviato E, Guarise A. Contrast agents for hepatic MRI. Cancer Imaging. 2007;1(7 Spec No A):S24–7.

Namasivayam S, Martin DR, Saini S. Imaging of liver metastases: MRI. Cancer Imaging 2005;7:2–9.

7.21 LIVER SPECIFIC MRI CONTRAST MEDIA

	Superparamagnetic agents	Paramagnetic agents
	Reticuloendothelial system agents	Hepatocyte selective agents
Pharmacokinetics	Uptake by macrophages (Kuppfer cells)	Uptake by hepatocytes
Signal characteristics	Signal loss in T_2 weighted images	Signal rise in T_1 weighted images
Examples of compounds	SPIO particles (ferumoxides)	Mangafodipir trisodium
Scan timing	1–4 hours	3–10 min (parenchymal evaluation), 15–20 min (biliary evaluation)
Clinical applications	Typically, malignant liver lesions devoid of Kuppfer cells, such as metastases and HCC are hyperintense on T_2 against a background of normal dark liver parenchyma. Tumours with Kuppfer cells (FNH, adenoma and regenerative nodules) or a relevant blood pool (haemangiomas) show a decrease in signal intensity after SPIO administration.	Distinguishing metastases from hepatocellular lesions, metastases show ring-shaped peripheral enhancement esp. at 24 hours. Well differentiated HCCs, adenomas, FNH and regenerative nodules take up hepatocyte selective agents and has a limited ability to differentiate between them. MR cholangiopancreatography

Further Reading

Karabulut H et al. Contrast agents used in MR imaging of the liver. Diagn Interv Radiol 2006;12:22–30.

Namkung W et al. Superparamagnetic iron oxide (SPIO)-enhanced liver MRI with ferucarbotran: efficacy for characterization of focal liver lesions. J Magn Res Imag 2007;25:755.

Sunil N et al. MR contrast agents for liver imaging: what, when, how. Radiographics 2006;26:1621–36.

7.22 MRI LIVER – FOCAL HYPERINTENSE LESION ON T$_1$W

NB. Most lesions are hypointense on T$_1$W.

1. **Fat** – lipomas, angiomyolipomas, focal fatty deposits, surgical defect packed with omental fat, occasionally hepatomas undergo fatty degeneration.
2. **Blood** – in the acute stage due to methaemoglobin.
3. **Proteinaceous material** – occurs in dependent layer of fluid/fluid levels in abscesses and haematomas due to increased concentration of hydrated protein molecules.
4. **Melanoma metastases.**
5. **Chemical** – gadolinium, lipiodol (contains fat).
6. **'Relative'** – i.e. normal signal intensity liver surrounded by low signal intensity liver which may occur with iron deposition (haemochromatosis, i.v. ferrite particles), cirrhosis (unclear aetiology, but a regenerating nodule within a cirrhotic area may appear artifactually hyperintense), oedema.
7. **Artefact** – pulsation artefact from abdominal aorta can produce a periodic 'ghost' artefact along the phase-encoded direction which can be hypointense or hyperintense depending on the phase.

Further Reading

Elsayes KM, Narra VR, Yin Y et al. Focal hepatic lesions: diagnostic value of enhancement pattern approach with contrast-enhanced 3D gradient-echo MR imaging. Radiographics 2005;25:1299–320.

Martin DR, Semelka RC. Magnetic resonance imaging of the liver: review of techniques and approach to common diseases. Semin Ultrasound CT MR 2005;3:116–31.

7.23 MRI LIVER – RINGED HEPATIC LESIONS

One or several layers which may be a component of the lesion itself or a response of the liver to the presence of the adjacent lesion.

1. **Capsules of 1° liver tumours** – a low signal ring may be seen in 25–40% but does not differentiate between benign and malignant. A peritumoral halo of high signal on T_2W is seen in 30% of 1° tumours and more closely correlates with malignancy.
2. **Metastases** – halo of high signal on T_2W or with central liquefaction to give an even higher centre and a 'target' lesion. A peritumoral halo or a target on T_2W distinguishes metastasis from cavernous haemangioma.
3. **Subacute haematoma** – low-signal rim on T_1W and T_2W (because of iron) with an inner bright ring on T_1W (because of methaemoglobin).
4. **Hydatid cyst** – T_2W high-signal cyst contents with a low-signal capsule. The capsule is not well seen on T_1W.
5. **Amoebic abscess** – prior to treatment incomplete concentric rings of variable intensity, better seen on T_2W than T_1W. During antibiotic treatment, T_1W and T_2W images show the development of four concentric zones because of central liquefaction and resolution of hepatic oedema.

Further Reading
Elsayes KM, Narra VR, Yin Y et al. Focal hepatic lesions: diagnostic value of enhancement pattern approach with contrast-enhanced 3D gradient-echo MR imaging. Radiographics 2005;25:1299–320.

7.24 SPLENOMEGALY

Huge spleen
1. Chronic myeloid leukaemia.
2. Myelofibrosis.
3. Malaria.
4. Kala-azar.
5. Gaucher's disease.
6. Lymphoma*.

Moderately large spleen
1. All of the above.
2. Storage diseases.
3. Haemolytic anaemias.
4. Portal hypertension.
5. Leukaemias.

Slightly large spleen
1. All of the above.
2. Infections
   (a) Viral – infectious hepatitis, infectious mononucleosis.
   (b) Bacterial – septicaemia, brucellosis, typhoid and tuberculosis.
   (c) Rickettsial – typhus.
   (d) Fungal – histoplasmosis.
3. Sarcoidosis*.
4. Amyloidosis.
5. Rheumatoid arthritis (Felty's syndrome)*.
6. Systemic lupus erythematosus*.

7

7.25 SPLENIC CALCIFICATION

Curvilinear

1. **Splenic artery atherosclerosis** – including splenic artery aneurysm.
2. **Cyst** – hydatid or post-traumatic.

Multiple small nodular

1. **Phleboliths** – may have small central lucencies.
2. **Haemangioma** – phleboliths.
3. **Tuberculosis.**
4. **Histoplasmosis.**
5. **Brucellosis.**
6. **Sickle-cell anaemia*.**

Diffuse homogeneous or finely granular

1. **Sickle-cell anaemia*.**
2. *Pneumocystis carinii.*

Solitary greater than 1cm

1. **Healed infarct or haematoma.**
2. **Healed abscess.**
3. **Tuberculosis.**

7.26 SPLENIC LESION

Solid

1. **Lymphoma.**
2. **Metastases** – esp. melanoma, lung and breast.
3. **Langerhans cell histiocytosis.**
4. **Hamartoma.**
5. **Haemangioma** – rare, still remain the most common benign neoplasm of the spleen. Although the majority of patients are asymptomatic and are diagnosed incidentally, a 25% incidence of spontaneous rupture has been reported. Same US and CT characteristics as liver haemangioma.
6. **Sarcoid.**

Cystic

1. **False cyst (80%)** – usually past history of trauma.
2. **Congenital cyst.**
3. **Abscess** (pyogenic).
4. **TB.**
5. **Echinococcus infection.**

Further Reading

Abbott RM, Levy AD, Aguilera NS et al. From the archives of the AFIP: primary vascular neoplasms of the spleen: radiologic-pathologic correlation. Radiographics 2004;24:1137–63.

Bean MJ, Horton KM, Fishman EK. Concurrent focal hepatic and splenic lesions: a pictorial guide to differential diagnosis. J Comput Assist Tomogr 2004;28:605–12.

Elsayes KM, Narra VR, Mukundan G et al. MR imaging of the spleen: spectrum of abnormalities. Radiographics 2005;25(4):967–82.

7.27 PANCREATIC CALCIFICATION

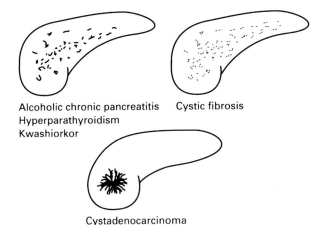

Alcoholic chronic pancreatitis
Hyperparathyroidism
Kwashiorkor

Cystic fibrosis

Cystadenocarcinoma

1. **Alcoholic pancreatitis** – calcification, which is almost exclusively due to intraductal calculi, is seen in 20–40% (compared with 2% of gallstone pancreatitis). Usually after 5–10 years of pain. Limited to head or tail in 25%. Rarely solitary. Calculi are numerous, irregular and generally small.

2. **Pseudocyst** – 12–20% exhibit calcification which is usually similar to that seen in chronic pancreatitis but may be curvilinear rim calcification.

3. **Carcinoma of the pancreas** – although for all practical purposes adenocarcinoma does not calcify there is an increased incidence of pancreatic cancer in chronic pancreatitis and the two will be found concurrently in about 2% of cases.

4. **Hyperparathyroidism*** – pancreatitis occurs as a complication of hyperparathyroidism in 10% of cases. 70% have nephrocalcinosis or urolithiasis and this should suggest the diagnosis.

5. **Cystic fibrosis*** – calcification occurs late in the disease when there is advanced pancreatic fibrosis associated with diabetes mellitus. Calcification is typically finely granular.
6. **Kwashiorkor** – pancreatic lithiasis is a frequent finding and appears before adulthood. Its pattern is similar to chronic alcoholic pancreatitis.
7. **Hereditary pancreatitis** – AD. 60% show calcification which is typically rounded and often larger than in other pancreatic diseases. 20% die from pancreatic malignancy. The diagnosis should be considered in young, non-alcoholic patients.
8. **Tumours** – calcification is observed in 10% of cystadenomas and cystadenocarcinomas. It is non-specific but occasionally 'sunburst'.
9. **Idiopathic.**

Further Reading

Lesniak RJ, Hohenwalter MD, Taylor AJ. Spectrum of causes of pancreatic calcifications. Am J Roentgenol 2002;178:79–86.
Paspulati RM. Multidetector CT of the pancreas. Radiol Clin North Am 2005;43:999–1020.

7.28 CYSTIC PANCREATIC LESION

1. **Pseudocyst** (85%).
2. **Intraductal papillary mucinous tumour.**
3. **Cystadenoma** (mucinous cystadenoma and cystadenocarcinoma) – majority of cases have a large central cyst surrounded by smaller cysts, usually in body or tail. Calcification may be more common in the malignant lesions. The thick walls may help to distinguish from pseudocysts. Usually in females aged over 60 years.
4. **True cyst** – associated with autosomal dominant polycystic kidney disease, Von Hippel–Lindau disease and cystic fibrosis.
5. **Cystic metastases** – esp. renal cell, melanoma and lung carcinoma.
6. **Pancreatic abscess.**

7.29 CT OF PANCREAS – SOLID MASS

1. **Adenocarcinoma** – 60% head, 10% body, 5% tail, 20% diffuse. 40% are isodense on pre-contrast scan, but most of these show reduced density on a post-contrast scan. Virtually never contain calcification. The presence of metastases (nodes, liver) or invasion around vascular structures (SMA, coeliac axis, portal and splenic vein) helps to distinguish this from focal pancreatitis.
2. **Focal pancreatitis** – usually in head of pancreas. Can contain calcification, but if not may be difficult to distinguish from carcinoma.
3. **Metastasis** – e.g. breast, lung, stomach, kidney, thyroid.
4. **Islet cell tumour** – equal incidence in head, body and tail. 80% are functioning and so will present at a relatively small size. 20% are non-functioning and so are larger and more frequently contain calcification at presentation. In general, functioning islet cell tumours, other than insulinomas, are often malignant, whereas 75% of non-functioning tumours are benign.
   - **(a)** Beta cell:
     - **(i)** Insulinoma – 90% benign, 10% multiple, 80% <2cm in diameter. Usually isodense with marked contrast enhancement. Can calcify.
   - **(b)** Non-beta cell:
     - **(i)** Gastrinoma – 60% malignant, 30% benign adenoma, 10% hyperplasia. 90% located in pancreas, 5% duodenum, occasionally stomach and splenic hilum. Shows marked contrast enhancement. Multiple adenomas seen as part of multiple endocrine adenopathy I syndrome (pituitary, parathyroid and pancreatic adenomas).
     - **(ii)** Glucagonoma – usually >4cm, since endocrine disturbance is often less marked.

Further Reading

Horton KM, Hruban RH, Yeo C et al. Multi-detector row CT of pancreatic islet cell tumors. Radiographics 2006;26:453–64.

Kawamoto S, Horton KM, Lawler LP et al. Intraductal papillary mucinous neoplasm of the pancreas: can benign lesions be differentiated from malignant lesions with multidetector CT? Radiographics 2005;256:1451–68.

Paspulati RM. Multidetector CT of the pancreas. Radiol Clin North Am 2005;43:999–1020.

Rha SE, Jung SE, Lee KH et al. CT and MR imaging findings of endocrine tumor of the pancreas according to WHO classification. Eur J Radiol 2007;62:371–7.

Schima W. MRI of the pancreas: tumours and tumour-simulating processes. Cancer Imaging 2006;6:199–203.

Scott J, Martin I, Redhead D et al. Mucinous cystic neoplasms of the pancreas: imaging features and diagnostic difficulties. Clin Radiol 2000;55:187–92.

8

Adrenals, urinary tract and testes

Sarfraz Nazir and Nigel Cowan

8.1 ADRENAL CALCIFICATION

1. **Cystic disease** – similar to that seen in the child. Bilateral in 15% of cases.
2. **Carcinoma** – irregular punctate calcifications seen in 30%. Average size of tumour is 14cm and there is frequently displacement of the ipsilateral kidney.
3. **Addison's disease** – now most commonly due to autoimmune disease or metastasis. In the past, when tuberculosis was a frequent cause, calcification was a common finding.
4. **Ganglioneuroma** – 40% occur over the age of 20 years. Slightly flocculent calcifications in a mass which is usually asymptomatic. If the tumour is large enough there will be displacement of the adjacent kidney and/or ureter.
5. **Inflammatory** – primary tuberculosis and histoplasmosis.
6. **Phaeochromocytoma** – calcification is rare but when present is usually an 'egg-shell' pattern.

Further Reading

Hindman N, Israel GM. Adrenal gland and adrenal mass calcification. Eur Radiol 2005;15(6):1163–7.

8.2 INCIDENTAL ADRENAL MASS (UNILATERAL)

Adrenal 'incidentalomas' are seen in 1% of all CT scans. The normal length of adrenal limbs is variable: can be up to 4cm. The width of a limb is normally less than 1cm. A mass less than 3cm in diameter is likely benign (87% cases) and a mass greater than 5cm in diameter is probably malignant. On unenhanced scans a mass <10 HU is likely a benign lipid-rich adenoma. For indeterminate lesions i.e. those >10 HU, a contrast enhanced scan with delayed imaging is required to assess degree of enhancement and washout values. Chemical shift MRI is also useful although ultimately biopsy may be required.

Functioning tumours

1. **Conn's adenoma** – accounts for 70% of Conn's syndrome. Usually small, 0.5–1.5cm. Homogeneous, relatively low density due to build up of cholesterol. 30% of Conn's syndrome due to hyperplasia which can occasionally be nodular and mimic an adenoma.
2. **Phaeochromocytoma** – usually large, >5cm, with marked contrast enhancement (beware hypertensive crisis with i.v. contrast medium). 10% malignant, 10% bilateral, 10% ectopic (of these 50% are located around the kidney, particularly renal hilum. If CT does not detect, MIBG isotope scan may be helpful). 10% are multiple and usually part of multiple endocrine neoplasia II (MEN II) syndrome, neurofibromatosis or von Hippel–Lindau.
3. **Cushing's adenoma** – accounts for 10% of Cushing's syndrome. Usually over 2cm in diameter. 40% show slight reduction in density. 80% of Cushing's syndrome due to excess ACTH from pituitary tumour or ectopic source (oat cell carcinoma, pancreatic islet cell, carcinoid, medullary carcinoma of thyroid, thymoma) which causes adrenal hyperplasia not visible on CT scan. Other 10% of Cushing's syndrome due to adrenal carcinoma. The possibilities for adrenal mass in Cushing's syndrome are:
   (a) Functioning adenoma/carcinoma.
   (b) Coincidental non-functioning adenoma.
   (c) Metastasis from oat cell primary.
   (d) Nodular hyperplasia, which occurs in 20% of Cushing's syndrome due to pituitary adenoma.
4. **Adrenal carcinoma** – 50% present as functioning tumours (Cushing's 35%, Cushing's with virilization 20%, virilization 20%, feminization 5%).

8

Malignant tumours

1. **Metastases** – may be bilateral, usually greater than 2–3cm, irregular outline with patchy contrast enhancement. Recent haemorrhage into a vascular metastasis (e.g. melanoma) can give a patchy high density on pre-contrast scan. In patients without a known extra-adrenal primary tumour the vast majority of adrenal masses are benign; even in the presence of a known primary malignant tumour many adrenal masses will still be benign (40% are metastases).
2. **Carcinoma** – Typical features are: (a) >5cm; (b) central areas of low attenuation due to tumour necrosis; (c) calcification; and (d) hepatic, nodal or venous spread.
3. **Lymphoma** – 25% also involve kidneys at autopsy. Lymphadenopathy will be seen elsewhere.
4. **Neuroblastoma** – greater than 5cm. Calcification in 90%. Extends across midline. Nodes commonly surround and displace the aorta and inferior vena cava.

Benign

1. **Non-functioning adenoma** – occurs in 5% at autopsy. Usually relatively small (50% less than 2cm), homogeneous and well-defined.
2. **Myelolipoma** – 0.2% at autopsy. Rare benign tumour composed of adipose and haematopoietic tissue. 85% are found in the adrenal but extra-adrenal tumours (liver, retroperitoneum, pelvis) have been reported. Low attenuation on CT and may enhance. Mean diameter of 10cm.
3. **Angiomyolipoma** – adrenal lesions are very rare in practice. Usually contain vascular tissue and fat density.
4. **Cyst** – well-defined, water density.
5. **Post-traumatic haemorrhage** – homogeneous, hyperdense. Occurs in 25% of severe trauma, 20% bilateral, 85% on right. Adrenal haemorrhage can also occur in vascular metastases, anticoagulant treatment, and severe stress (e.g. surgery, sepsis, burns, hypotension).
6. **Granulomatous disease** (TB, histoplasmosis). Present as diffuse enlargement or as discrete mass. Can have a central cystic component, with/without calcification.

Further Reading

Korobkin M, Francis IR, Kloos RT et al. The incidental adrenal mass. Radiol Clin North Am 1996;34(5):1037–54.

Mayo-Smith W, Boland GW, Noto RB et al. State-of-the-art adrenal imaging. Radiographics 2001;21:995–1012.

Park BK, Kim CK, Lee JH. Comparison of delayed enhanced CT and chemical shift MR for evaluating hyperattenuating incidental adrenal masses. Radiology 2007;243(3):760–5.

Pender SM, Boland GW, Lee MJ. The incidental nonhyperfunctioning
   adrenal mass: an imaging algorithm for characterization. Clin Radiol
   1998;53:796–804.

8.3 BILATERAL ADRENAL MASSES

1. **Metastases** – bilateral in 15%. Common at autopsy. Most common
   primary sites are lung or breast; also melanoma, renal cell
   carcinoma, GI tract, thyroid, contralateral adrenal gland. Usually
   does not affect adrenal function; may cause adrenal insufficiency if
   extensive (replacing >80% of adrenal gland).
2. **Phaeochromocytoma** – bilateral in 10%.
3. **Hyperplasia** – adrenogenital syndromes result in symmetrically
   enlarged and thickened adrenal glands. Adrenocortical hyperplasia
   can cause bilateral adrenal enlargement but usually these are not
   visible on CT.
4. **Spontaneous adrenal haemorrhage.**
5. **Lymphoma** – primary adrenal lymphoma is rare. Usually presents
   with bilateral adrenal masses, often with adrenal hypofunction.
   Usually diffuse large B-cell lymphomas. Adrenal involvement occurs
   at autopsy in up to 25% with disseminated lymphoma, usually with
   no associated adrenal insufficiency.
6. **Granulomatous disease** – Histoplasmosis/TB. Can be acute or
   chronic. Patients with adrenal masses and adrenal failure caused by
   chronic disseminated histoplasmosis may have symptoms and CT
   findings that are indistinguishable from those of malignancy.

Further Reading
Gibb WRG, Ramsay AD, McNeil NI et al. Bilateral adrenal masses. Br Med J (Clin
   Res Ed) 1985;291(6489):203–4.

8.4 ADRENAL PSEUDOTUMOURS

Soft tissue density in the location of the adrenal glands on plain films of the abdomen or on CT. This almost always occurs on the left side. Right-sided lesions are usually liver, gallbladder or renal masses.

The right adrenal lies behind inferior vena cava and above right kidney, i.e. not on same slice as the kidney. The left adrenal lies in front of upper pole of left kidney, i.e. on same slice as the kidney – do not mistake upper pole of left kidney for an adrenal mass.

Imaging structures mimicking adrenal mass

1. **Exophytic upper pole renal mass** – requires sagittal or coronal reconstructions and thin-section CT.
2. **Gastric diverticulum** – give oral contrast.
3. **Splenic lobulation/accessory spleen** – give intravenous contrast, should enhance to the same level as the body of the spleen.
4. **Prominent lobation of the hepatic lobe, or hepatic tumour.**
5. **Varices** – give intravenous contrast.
6. **Large mass in tail of pancreas** – give intravenous contrast, pancreatic mass usually displaces splenic vein posteriorly, whereas adrenal mass displaces it anteriorly.
7. **Fluid filled colon** – give intraluminal contrast and thin-section CT. Intraluminal gas is diagnostic.

Further Reading
Gokan T, Ohgiya Y, Nobusawa H et al. Commonly encountered adrenal pseudotumours on CT. Br J Radiol 2005;78:170–4.

8.5 META-IODO-BENZYL-GUANIDINE (MIBG) IMAGING

The scintigraphic distribution of I-131 MIBG occurs in organs with adrenergic innervation or those that process catecholamines for excretion.

Normal uptake

1. Myocardium.
2. Liver and spleen.
3. Bladder.
4. Adrenal glands – more marked with ^{123}I MIBG.
5. Salivary glands.
6. Nasopharynx.
7. Thyroid.
8. Colon.

Abnormal uptake

1. Phaeochromocytoma.
2. Neuroblastoma.
3. Carcinoid tumour.
4. Paraganglioma.
5. Medullary thyroid carcinoma.
6. Ganglioneuroma.

Further Reading

McEwan AH, Shapiro B, Sisson JC et al. Radioiodobenzylguanidine for the scintigraphic localization and therapy of adrenergic tumours. Semin Nucl Med 1985;15:132–53.

Standalick RC. The biodistribution of metaiodobenzylguanidine. Semin Nucl Med 1992;22:46–7.

8.6 CONGENITAL RENAL ANOMALIES

These may be anomalies of position, of form or of number.

Anomalies of position

All malpositioned kidneys are malrotated. Most commonly malrotation occurs around the vertical axis with collecting structures positioned ventrally.

1. **Pelvic kidney** – ectopic kidney due to failure of renal ascent. There is non-rotation with anteriorly positioned renal pelvis in most cases. Blood supply is from the iliac artery or the aorta. Most ectopic kidneys are asymptomatic notwithstanding the fact pelvic kidneys are more susceptible to trauma and infection and may complicate natural childbirth later in life.
2. **Ectopic kidney** – in the case of intrathoracic kidney, usually an acquired duplication through the foramen of Bochdalek. Can also be pre-sacral or at the lower lumbar level.

Anomalies of form

1. **Horseshoe kidney** – two kidneys joined by parenchymal/fibrous isthmus. Most common fusion anomaly with incidence of 1 in 400 births. Fusion of right and left kidney at lower pole in 90%. Abnormal axis of each kidney (bilateral malrotation). Renal pelves and ureters situated anteriorly and renal long axis medially oriented. Associated with other anomalies in 50% (e.g. vesicoureteral reflux, ureteral duplication, genital anomalies, Turner's syndrome).

2. **Pancake/discoid kidney** – bilateral fused pelvic kidneys, usually near the aortic bifurcation.
3. **Crossed renal ectopia** – kidney is located on opposite side of midline from its ureteral orifice. Usually L>R. The lower kidney is usually ectopic. In 90% there is fusion of both kidneys (=crossed fused ectopia). May be associated with anorectal anomalies and renal dysplasia. Slightly increased incidence of calculi.
4. **Renal hypoplasia** – incomplete development results in a smaller (<50% of normal size) kidney with fewer calyces and papillae. Normal function.

Anomalies of number

1. **Unilateral renal agenesis** – 1:1000 live births. Increased incidence of extrarenal abnormalities (meningomyelocoele, ventricular septal defect, intestinal tract strictures, imperforate anus, unicornuate uterus skeletal abnormalities). Hyperplastic normal solitary kidney – up to twice normal size.
2. **Bilateral renal agenesis** – Potter syndrome. 1:10000 live births. Invariably fatal in first few days of life due to pulmonary hypoplasia secondary to the associated oligohydramnios.
3. **Supernumerary kidney** – very rare. Most commonly on left side caudal to normal kidney.

Further Reading

Cohen HL, Kravets F, Zucconi W et al. Congenital abnormalities of the genitourinary system. Semin Roentgenol 2004;39(2):282–303.

Philip J, Kenney PJ, Spirt BA et al. Genitourinary anomalies: radiologic-anatomic correlations. Radiographics 1984;4:233–60.

8.7 LOCALIZED BULGE OF THE RENAL OUTLINE

RENAL CYST
US confirms typical
echo-free cyst

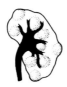

**MULTIPLE RENAL
CYSTS**
e.g. adult type
polycystic disease.
Spider leg deformity
of calyces

TUMOUR
Replacement of much
or all of normal renal
tissue

DROMEDARY HUMP
Left sided variant

**PROMINENT SEPTUM
OF BERTIN**
Increased activity on
Tc-DMSA scanning

HILAR LIP
Hyperplasia of
parenchyma adjacent
to the renal hilum.
Normal on Tc-DMSA scan

8

**PSEUDOTUMOUR IN
REFLUX
NEPHROPATHY**
Hypertrophy of
unscarred renal
parenchyma

**DUPLEX KIDNEY WITH
HYDRONEPHROTIC
UPPER MOIETY**
Drooping flower
appearance

**DILATATION OF A
SINGLE CALYX**
Most commonly due
to extrinsic
compression by an
intrarenal artery
(Fraley syndrome)

Redrawn from Taylor C.M. & Chapman S. (1989) *Handbook of Renal Investigations in Children*. London: Wright. By kind permission of the publisher.

1. **Cyst** – well-defined nephrographic defect with a thin wall on the outer margin. Beak sign. Displacement and distortion of smooth-walled calyces without obliteration.
2. **Tumour** – mostly renal cell carcinoma in adults and Wilms' tumour in children. See 8.22.

3. **Fetal lobation** – the lobule directly overlies a normal calyx. Normal interpapillary line. See 8.10.

4. **Dromedary hump** – on the midportion of the lateral border of the left kidney. Occurs secondary to prolonged pressure by spleen during fetal development. The arc of the interpapillary line parallels the renal contour.

5. **Splenic impression** – on the left side only. This produces an apparent bulge inferiorly.

6. **Enlarged septum of Bertin** – overgrowth of renal cortex from two adjacent renal lobules. Usually between upper and interpolar portion. Excretory urography shows a pseudomass with calyceal splaying and associated short calyx ± attempted duplication. Tc-DMSA accumulates normally or in excess. On US echogenicity is usually similar to normal renal cortex but may be of increased echogenicity. CT – enhances similar to cortex.

7. **Localized compensatory hypertrophy** – e.g. adjacent to an area of pyelonephritic scarring.

8. **Acute focal nephritis (lobar nephronia)** – usually an ill-defined hypoechoic mass on US, but may be hyperechoic. CT shows an ill-defined, low attenuation, wedge-shaped mass with reduced contrast enhancement.

9. **Abscess** – loss of renal outline and psoas margin on the control film. Scoliosis concave to the involved side. Initially there is no nephrographic defect, but following central necrosis there will be a central defect surrounded by a thick irregular wall. Adjacent calyces are displaced or effaced.

10. **Non-functioning moiety of a duplex** – usually a hydronephrotic upper moiety. Delayed films may show contrast medium in the upper moiety calyces. Lower moiety calyces display the 'drooping lily' appearance.

Further Reading

Felson B, Moskowitz M. Renal pseudotumours. The regenerated nodule and other lumps, bumps and dromedary humps. Am J Roentgenol 1969;107:720–9.

Kawashima A, Goldman SM, Sandler CM. The indeterminate renal mass. Radiol Clin North Am 1996;34(5):997–1015.

Levitin A, Becker JA. Tumorlike conditions of the kidney. Semin Roentgenol 1995;30(2):185–99.

8.8 PSEUDOKIDNEY SIGN

Refers to a sonographic mass of reniform appearance with a central hyperechoic region surrounded by a hyperechoic region.

1. **Intussusception** – the most common cause by far.
2. **Necrotizing enterocolitis.**
3. **Midgut volvulus.**
4. **Sigmoid volvulus.**
5. **Crohn's disease.**

False positives

1. **Faeces in colon.**
2. **Psoas muscle.**
3. **Perforated Meckel's diverticulum with malrotation.**
4. **Haematoma.**

Further Reading
Anderson DR. The pseudokidney sign. Radiology 1999;211:395–7.

8.9 NON-VISUALIZATION OF ONE KIDNEY DURING EXCRETION UROGRAPHY

Absence of kidney

1. **Agenesis.**
2. **Postnephrectomy.**
3. **Ectopic kidney.**

Loss of perfusion

1. **Chronic infarction.**
2. **Unilateral renal vein occlusion** – see 8.29.

Trauma

1. **Main renal artery occlusion/thrombosis.**

Urinary obstruction

1. **Chronic obstructive uropathy.**

Replaced renal parenchyma

1. **Multicystic kidney.**

2. **Tumour** – an avascular tumour completely replacing the kidney or preventing normal function of residual renal tissue by occluding the renal vein or pelvis.
3. **Infection** – Pyonephrosis, xanthogranulomatous pyelonephritis or tuberculosis.

8.10 UNILATERAL SCARRED KIDNEY

NORMAL
Cortex parallel to
interpapillary line

FETAL LOBULATION
Normal size.
Cortical depressions
between papillae

DUPLEX KIDNEY
Renal size usually
larger than normal

SPLEEN IMPRESSION
Right kidney may
show hepatic
impression

OVERLYING BOWEL
Spurious
loss of cortex

REFLUX
NEPHROPATHY
Focal scars over
dilated calyces. Most
prominent at upper
and lower poles. May
be bilateral

LOBAR INFARCTION
Broad depression
over a normal calyx

Redrawn from Taylor C.M. & Chapman S. (1989) *Handbook of Renal Investigations in Children*. London: Wright. By kind permission of the publisher.

1. **Reflux nephropathy** – a focal scar over a dilated calyx. Usually multifocal and may be bilateral. Scarring is most prominent in the upper and lower poles. Minimal scarring, especially at a pole, may produce decreased cortical thickness with a normal papilla and is then indistinguishable from lobar infarction.
2. **Tuberculosis** – calcification differentiates it from the other members of this section.
3. **Lobar infarction** – a broad contour depression over a normal calyx. Normal interpapillary line.
4. **Renal dysplasia** – a forme fruste multicystic kidney. Dilated calyces. Indistinguishable from chronic pyelonephritis. Arteriography outlines a small threadlike renal artery.

Differential diagnosis

1. Persistent fetal lobulation – lobules overlie calyces with interlobular septa between the calyces. Normal size kidney.

Further Reading

Davidson AJ et al. Renal parenchymal disease. In: Davidson AJ (ed) Radiology of the Kidney and Genitourinary Tract, 3rd edn. WB Saunders, Philadelphia, p73–358.

8.11 UNILATERAL SMALL SMOOTH KIDNEY

8

In all these conditions chronic unilateral disease is associated with compensatory hypertrophy of the contralateral kidney.

Prerenal = vascular

Usually with a small volume collecting system. This is a sign of diminished urinary volume and, together with global cortical thinning, delayed opacification of the calyces, increased density of the opacified collecting system and delayed wash-out following oral fluids or diuretics, indicates ischaemia.

1. **Ischaemia due to renal artery stenosis** – ureteric notching is due to enlarged collateral vessels and differentiates this from the other causes in this group. See 8.28.
2. **Radiation nephritis** – at least 23 Gy over 5 weeks. The collecting system may be normal or small. Depending on the size of the radiation field both, one or just part of one kidney may be affected. There may be other sequelae of radiotherapy, e.g. scoliosis following radiotherapy in childhood.
3. **End result of renal infarction** – due to previous severe trauma involving the renal artery or renal vein thrombosis. The collecting system does not usually opacify during excretion urography.

Renal = parenchymal

1. **Congenital hypoplasia** – five or less calyces. The pelvicalyceal system is otherwise normal.
2. **Multicystic dysplastic kidney (adult).**

Post-renal = collecting system

Usually with a dilated collecting system.

1. **Post-obstructive atrophy** – ± thinning of the renal cortex and if there is impaired renal function this will be revealed by poor contrast medium density in the collecting system.

Further Reading

Davidson AJ et al. Renal parenchymal disease. In: Davidson AJ (ed) Radiology of the Kidney and Genitourinary Tract, 3rd edn. WB Saunders, Philadelphia, p73–358.

8.12 BILATERAL SMALL SMOOTH KIDNEYS

Prerenal = vascular

1. **Arterial hypotension** – distinguished by the time relationship to the contrast medium injection and its transient nature.
2. **Generalized arteriosclerosis** – normal calyces.

Renal = parenchymal

1. **Chronic glomerulonephritis** – normal calyces. Reduced nephrogram density and poor calyceal opacification.
2. **Hereditary nephropathies** – e.g. Alport syndrome

Post-renal = collecting system

1. **Chronic papillary necrosis** (see 8.26) – with other signs of necrotic papillae.

Cause of unilateral small kidney

– but occurring bilaterally see 8.11.

Further Reading

Davidson AJ et al. Renal parenchymal disease. In: Davidson AJ (ed) Radiology of the Kidney and Genitourinary Tract, 3rd edn. WB Saunders, Philadelphia, p73–358.

8.13 UNILATERAL LARGE SMOOTH KIDNEY

Prerenal = vascular

1. **Renal vein thrombosis** – see 8.29.
2. **Acute arterial infarction.**

Renal = parenchymal

1. **Autosomal dominant polycystic kidney disease*** – asymmetrical bilateral enlargement, but 8% of cases are unilateral. Lobulated rather than completely smooth.
2. **Duplex kidney** – female:male, 2:1. Equal incidence on both sides and 20% are bilateral. Incomplete more common than complete. Only 50% are bigger than the contralateral kidney; 40% are the same size; 10% are smaller.
3. **Crossed fused ectopia** – see 8.6.
4. **Multicystic kidney.**
6. **Acute pyelonephritis** – impaired excretion of contrast medium ± dense nephrogram. Attenuated calyces but may have non-obstructive pelvicalyceal or ureteric dilatation. Completely reversible within a few weeks of clinical recovery.
7. **Trauma** – haematoma or urinoma.
8. **Tumour** – see 8.22.
9. **Compensatory hypertrophy.**

Post-renal = collecting system

1. **Obstructed kidney** – dilated calyces.
2. **Pyonephrosis.**

Further Reading

Davidson AJ et al. Renal parenchymal disease. In: Davidson AJ (ed) Radiology of the Kidney and Genitourinary Tract, 3rd edn. WB Saunders, Philadelphia, p73–358.

Pickhardt PJ, Lonergan GJ, Davis CJ Jr et al. Infiltrative renal lesions: radiologic-pathologic correlation. Radiographics 2000;20:215–43.

8

8.14 BILATERAL LARGE SMOOTH KIDNEYS

It is often difficult to distinguish, radiologically, the members of this group from one another. The appearance of the nephrogram may be helpful – see 8.25. Associated clinical and radiological abnormalities elsewhere are often more useful, e.g. in sickle-cell anaemia, Goodpasture's disease and acromegaly.

Developmental
1. **Polycystic disease*** – infantile form has smooth outlines.
2. **Bilateral renal duplication.**

Proliferative and necrotizing disorders
1. **Acute glomerulonephritis.**
2. **Polyarteritis nodosa.**
3. **Wegener's granulomatosis.**
4. **Goodpasture's disease.**
5. **Systemic lupus erythematosus*.**

Deposition of abnormal proteins
1. **Amyloid** – renal involvement in 80% of secondary and 35% of primary amyloid. Chronic deposition results in small kidneys.
2. **Multiple myeloma*.**

Interstitial fluid accumulation
1. **Acute tubular necrosis.**
2. **Acute cortical necrosis** – may show an opacified medulla and outer rim with non-opacified cortex. Cortical calcification is a late finding.
3. **Acute renal infarction.**
4. **Renal vein thrombosis** (see 8.29).

Neoplastic infiltration
1. **Leukaemia and lymphoma.**

Inflammatory cell infiltration
1. **Acute interstitial nephritis.**

Miscellaneous
1. **Acute renal papillary necrosis** (see 8.26).
2. **Acute urate nephropathy.**
3. **Sickle-cell anaemia*.**

4. **Bilateral hydronephrosis.**
5. **Acromegaly* and gigantism** – as part of the generalized visceromegaly.

Further Reading
Davidson AJ et al. Renal parenchymal disease. In: Davidson AJ (ed) Radiology of the Kidney and Genitourinary Tract, 3rd edn. WB Saunders, Philadelphia, p73–358.

8.15   RENAL CALCIFICATION

Calculi (see 8.16)
Nephrocalcinosis (see 8.17)
Dystrophic calcification due to localized disease

Usually one kidney or part of one kidney.

1. **Infections**
   (a) Tuberculosis – variable appearance of nodular, curvilinear or amorphous calcification. Typically multifocal with calcification elsewhere in the urinary tract.
   (b) Hydatid – the cyst is usually polar and calcification is curvilinear or heterogeneous. 50% of echinococcal cysts calcify.
   (c) Xanthogranulomatous pyelonephritis – large obstructive calculus in 80% of cases.
   (d) Abscess – tuberculous abscess frequently calcifies. Pyogenic abscesses rarely calcify.
2. **Tumours**
   (a) Carcinoma – in 6% of carcinomas. Usually amorphous or irregular, but occasionally curvilinear.
   (b) Wilms tumour.
   (c) Transitional cell carcinoma – very rare.
   (d) Metastasis.
3. **Cysts** – usually related to previous infection of haemorrhage.
   (a) Simple renal cyst – calcifies in up to 3%.
   (b) Multicystic dysplastic kidney.
   (c) Autosomal polycystic kidney disease.
4. **Vascular**
   (a) Subcapsular/perirenal haematoma.
   (b) Aneurysm – of the renal artery. Curvilinear.

Further Reading
Daniel WW, Hartman GW, Witten DM et al. Calcified renal masses. Radiology 1972;103:503–8.

8.16 RENAL CALCULI

Nephrolithiasis is the most common cause of calcification within the kidney. 12% of the population develop a renal stone by the age of 70.

Opaque

Calcium phosphate/calcium oxalate, calcium oxalate, calcium phosphate/magnesium ammonium phosphate and calcium phosphate. Calcium oxalate stones are more opaque than triple phosphate stones.

Poorly opaque

Cystine (in cystinuria).

Non-opaque

Uric acid, xanthine, matrix (mucoprotein) and stones related to treatment with indinavir.

Calcium-containing

1. **With normocalcaemia** – obstruction, urinary tract infection, prolonged bed rest, 'horseshoe' kidney, vesical diverticulum, renal tubular acidosis, medullary sponge kidney and idiopathic hypercalciuria.
2. **With hypercalcaemia** – hyperparathyroidism, milk-alkali syndrome, excess vitamin D, idiopathic hypercalcaemia of infancy and sarcoidosis.

Pure calcium oxalate due to hyperoxaluria

1. **Primary hyperoxaluria** – rare. AR. 65% present below 5 years of age. Radiologically – nephrocalcinosis (generally diffuse and homogeneous but may be patchy), recurrent nephrolithiasis, dense vascular calcification, osteopenia or renal osteodystrophy and abnormal metaphyses (dense and/or lucent bands).
2. **Enteric hyperoxaluria** – due to a disturbance of bile acid metabolism. Mainly in patients with small bowel disease, either Crohn's disease or surgical resection.

Uric acid

1. **With hyperuricaemia** – gout, myeloproliferative disorders and during the treatment of tumours with antimitotic agents.
2. **With normouricaemia** – idiopathic or associated with acid, concentrated urine (in hot climate and in ileostomy patients).

Xanthine

Due to a failure of normal oxidation of purines.

Matrix

Rare. In poorly functioning, infected urinary tracts.

Indinavir

Protease inhibitor used in the treatment of HIV. Rare cause of non-opaque calculi.

Helical unenhanced CT is the most accurate technique for detecting urinary tract calculi (97% sensitive, 96% specific). All stone compositions are readily detectable except stones related to indinavir.

Further Reading

Banner MP, Pollack HM. Urolithiasis in the lower urinary tract. Semin Roentgenol 1982;17(2):140–8.

Blake SP, McNicholas MM, Raptopoulos V. Nonopaque crystal deposition causing ureteric obstruction in patients with HIV undergoing indinavir therapy. Am J Roentgenol 1999;171(3):717–20.

Sandhu C, Anson KM, Patel U. Urinary tract stones – Part I: role of radiological imaging in diagnosis and treatment planning. Clin Radiol 2003;58 (6):415–21.

Sandhu C, Anson KM, Patel U. Urinary tract stones – Part II: current state of treatment. Clin Radiol 2003;58(6):422–23.

Singh EO, Malek RS. Calculus disease in the upper urinary tract. Semin Roentgenol 1982;17(2):113–32.

8

8.17   NEPHROCALCINOSIS

Parenchymal calcification associated with a diffuse renal lesion (i.e. dystrophic calcification) or metabolic abnormality, e.g. hypercalcaemia (metabolic or metastatic calcification). May be medullary (95%) or cortical (5%).

Medullary (pyramidal)

The first three causes account for 70% of cases.

1. **Medullary sponge kidney** – a variable portion of one or both kidneys contains numerous small medullary cysts which communicate with tubules and therefore opacify during excretion urography. The cysts contain small calculi, giving a 'bunch of grapes' appearance. Big kidneys. ± Multiple cysts or large medullary

cystic cavities which may be >2cm in diameter. (Although not strictly a cause of nephrocalcinosis, because it comprises calculi in ectatic ducts, it is included here because of the plain film findings which simulate nephrocalcinosis.)

2. **Hyperparathyroidism*.**
3. **Renal tubular acidosis** – may be associated with osteomalacia or rickets. Calcification tends to be more severe than that due to other causes. It is the commonest cause in children. Almost always a distal tubular defect.
4. **Renal papillary necrosis** – calcification of necrotic papillae. See 8.26.
5. **Causes of hypercalcaemia or hypercalciuria**
   (a) Milk-alkali syndrome.
   (b) Idiopathic hypercalciuria.
   (c) Sarcoidosis*.
   (d) Hypervitaminosis D.
6. **Preterm infants** – in up to two-thirds. Risk factors include extreme prematurity, severe respiratory disease, gentamicin use and high urinary oxalate and urate excretion. 50% resolve spontaneously.
7. **Primary hyperoxaluria** – rare. AR. 65% present below 5 years of age (younger than the other causes). Radiologically – nephrocalcinosis (generally diffuse and homogeneous but may be patchy), recurrent nephrolithiasis, dense vascular calcification, osteopenia or renal osteodystrophy and abnormal metaphyses (dense and/or lucent bands).

Cortical

1. **Acute cortical necrosis** – classically 'tramline' calcification.
2. **Chronic glomerulonephritis** – rarely.
3. **Chronic transplant rejection.**
4. **Alports syndrome.**

Further Reading

Kellett MJ. Calculus disease and urothelial lesions. In: Grainger & Allison's Diagnostic Radiology: A Textbook of Medical Imaging. Churchill Livingstone, New York, 2002, p1582–5.

Lalli AF. Renal parenchyma calcifications. Semin Roentgenol 1982;17(2):101–12.

Narendra A, White MP, Rolton HA et al. Nephrocalcinosis in preterm babies. Arch Dis Child Fetal Neonatal Ed 2001;85:F207–213.

Wrong OM, Feest TG. Nephrocalcinosis. Adv Med 1976;12: 394–406.

8.18 CORTICAL DEFECTS IN RADIONUCLIDE RENAL IMAGES

1. **Scars** – note that apparent scars present during infection may resolve later. Oblique views are required.
2. **Hydronephrosis.**
3. **Trauma** – subcapsular or intrarenal.
4. **Renal cysts.**
5. **Carcinoma.**
6. **Infarct or ischaemia.**
7. **Abscesses.**
8. **Metastases.**
9. **Wilms' tumour.**

Further Reading
Fogelman I, Maisey M. An Atlas of Clinical Nuclear Medicine. Martin Dunitz, London, 1988, p217–373.

8.19 RENAL CYSTIC DISEASE

Renal dysplasia
1. **Multicystic kidney.**
2. **Focal and segmental cystic dysplasia.**
3. **Multiple cysts associated with lower urinary tract obstruction** – usually posterior urethral valves in males.

Polycystic disease*
1. **Autosomal recessive polycystic kidney disease.**
2. **Autosomal dominant polycystic kidney disease.**

Cortical cysts
1. **Simple cyst** – unilocular. Increase in size and number with age.
2. **Multilocular cystic nephroma.**
3. **Syndromes associated with cysts** – Zellweger's syndrome, tuberous sclerosis, Turner's syndrome, von Hippel–Lindau disease, trisomy 13 and 18.
4. **End-stage renal disease and haemodialysis** – in 8–13% of patients in renal failure not on dialysis; 10–20% of patients after 1–3 years of dialysis; >90% of patients after 5–10 years of dialysis. Diagnosis based on finding at least 3–5 cysts in each kidney. Cysts are of variable size and occur in cortex and medulla. Increased incidence of renal cell carcinoma, particularly when on dialysis.

Medullary cysts

1. **Calyceal cysts (diverticulum)** – small, usually solitary cyst communicating via an isthmus with the fornix of a calyx.
2. **Medullary sponge kidney** – bilateral in 60–80%. Multiple, small, mainly pyramidal cysts which opacify during excretion urography and contain calculi.
3. **Papillary necrosis** – see 8.26.
4. **Juvenile nephronophthisis** (medullary cystic disease) – usually presents with polyuria and progressive renal failure. Positive family history. Normal or small kidneys. US shows a few medullary or corticomedullary cysts, loss of corticomedullary differentiation and increased parenchymal echogenicity.

Miscellaneous intrarenal cysts

1. **Inflammatory**
   (a) Tuberculosis.
   (b) Calculus disease.
   (c) Hydatid.
2. **Neoplastic** – cystic degeneration of a carcinoma.
3. **Traumatic** – intrarenal haematoma.

Extraparenchymal renal cysts

1. **Parapelvic cyst** – located in or near the hilum, but does not communicate with the renal pelvis and therefore does not opacify during urography. Simple or multilocular; single or multiple, unilateral or bilateral. It compresses the renal pelvis and may cause hydronephrosis.
2. **Perinephric cyst** – beneath the capsule or between the capsule and perinephric fat. Secondary to trauma, obstruction or replacement of haematoma. It may compress the kidney, pelvis or ureter, leading to hydronephrosis or causing displacement of the kidney.

Further Reading

Choyke PL. Inherited cystic diseases of the kidney. Radiol Clin North Am 1996;34(5):925–46.

Choyke PL. Acquired cystic kidney disease. Eur Radiol 2000;10:1716–21.

Levine E. Acquired cystic kidney disease. Radiol Clin North Am 1996; 34(5):947–64.

Pedrosa I, Saiz A, Arrazola L et al. Hydatid disease: radiologic and pathologic features and complications. Radiographics 2000;20:795–817.

Saunders AJ, Denton E, Stephens S et al. Cystic kidney disease presenting in infancy. Clin Radiol 1999;54:370–6.

Tattersall DJ, Moore NR. Von Hippel–Lindau disease: MRI of abdominal manifestations. Clin Radiol 2002;57:85–92.

8.20 CT FINDINGS IN RENAL CYSTIC DISEASE

See also 8.19.

1. **Simple** – thin-walled, no enhancement. Occasionally haemorrhage can occur within one, producing a round hyperdense lesion.
2. **Malignant** – 5% of renal cell carcinomas are cystic. Suspect if thick walls or separations but this may just indicate previous infection/ haemorrhage in cyst.
3. **Polycystic** – associated with hepatic cysts in approximately 60% of cases. Haemorrhage into cysts relatively common, so may be of varying density. Associated with increased incidence of renal cell carcinoma.
4. **Haemodialysis-related cysts** – cysts develop in approximately 50% of long-term haemodialysis patients, but can involute after a successful renal transplant. 7% incidence of associated renal cell carcinoma.
5. **von Hippel–Lindau** – associated pancreatic, hepatic cysts and renal cell carcinoma and phaeochromocytoma.
6. **Hydatid** – affected in 10% of cases. ± Curvilinear calcification in wall.
7. **Multicystic** – usually detected in infancy.
8. **Cystic hamartoma** – usually large with thick capsule and septations.

Further Reading

Cho C, Friedland GW, Swenson RS. Acquired renal cystic disease and renal neoplasms in haemodialysis patients. Urol Radiol 1984;6:153–7.
Jennings CM, Gaines PA. The abdominal manifestation of von Hippel–Lindau disease and a radiological screening protocol for an affected family. Clin Radiol 1988;39:363–7.

8.21 FAT-CONTAINING RENAL MASS

1. **Angiomyolipoma** – 80% of cases are sporadic and 20% are associated with tuberous sclerosis. 80% of sporadic cases are on the R side. Angiomyolipomas are seen in up to 80% of patients with tuberous sclerosis where they are commonly large, bilateral and multifocal. May be the only evidence of tuberous sclerosis. Also seen in neurofibromatosis and von Hippel–Lindau.
   Ultrasound, CT and MRI: fat densities within the tumours. NB. Fat may occasionally be identified within Wilms' tumour.
2. **Renal cell carcinoma** (RCC) – invasion of perirenal fat or intratumoral metaplasia into fatty marrow (in one-third of RCCs if <3cm).
3. **Lipoma** – no different on CT to angiomyolipoma. Diagnosis only confirmed at pathologic inspection.

4. **Liposarcoma** – large, bulky and peripheral. Usually capsular, extends into perirenal space and hypovascular at angiography.
5. **Wilms tumour.**
6. **Oncocytoma** – entrapment of perirenal or sinus fat or production of fatty marrow in association with osseous metaplasia.
7. **Xanthogranulomatous pyelonephritis.**
8. **Teratoma** – very rare. Contains varying amounts of fat and calcification.

Further Reading

Choi DJ, Wallace C, Fraire AE et al. Intrarenal teratoma. Radiographics 2005;25:481–5.

Helenon O, Merran S, Paraf F et al. Unusual fat-containing tumors of the kidney – a diagnostic dilemma. Radiographics 1997;1:129–144.

8.22 RENAL NEOPLASMS IN AN ADULT

Malignant

1. **Renal cell carcinoma** – 90% of adult malignant tumours. Bilateral in 10% and an increased incidence of bilaterality in polycystic kidneys and von Hippel–Lindau disease. A mass lesion (showing irregular or amorphous calcification in 10% of cases). Calyces are obliterated, distorted and/or displaced. Half-shadow filling defect in a calyx or pelvis. Arteriography shows a typical pathological circulation in the majority.
2. **Transitional cell carcinoma** – usually papilliferous. May obstruct or obliterate a calyx or obstruct a whole kidney. Seeding may produce a second lesion further down the urinary tract. Bilateral tumours are rare. Calcification in 2%.
3. **Squamous cell carcinoma** – ulcerated plaque or stricture. 50% are associated with calculi. There is usually a large parenchymal mass before there is any sizeable intrapelvic mass. No calcification. Avascular at arteriography.
4. **Leukaemia/lymphoma** – bilateral large smooth kidneys. Thickened parenchyma with compression of the pelvicalyceal systems.
5. **Metastases** – not uncommon. Usually multiple. Bronchus, breast and stomach.

Benign

1. **Hamartoma** – usually solitary but often multiple and bilateral in tuberous sclerosis. Diagnostic appearance on the plain film of radiolucent fat (but only observed in 9%). Other signs are of any mass lesion, and angiography does not differentiate from renal cell carcinoma.

2. **Adenoma** – usually small and frequently multiple. Majority are found at autopsy. Hypovascular at arteriography.
3. **Others** – myoma, lipoma, haemangioma and fibroma are all rare.

Further Reading

Helenon O, Correas JM, Balleyguier C et al. Ultrasound of renal tumours. Eur Radiol 2001;11:1890–901.

Meilstrup JW, Mosher TJ, Dhadha RS et al. Other renal tumours. Semin Roentgenol 1995;30(2):168–84.

Patel U. Small and indeterminate renal masses: characterisation and management. CME J Radiol 1999;1:47–55.

Ramchandani P, Pollack HM. Tumors of the urothelium. Semin Roentgenol 1995;30(2):149–67.

Zhang J, Lefkowitz RA, Ishill NM et al. Solid renal cortical tumors: differentiation with CT. 2007;244(2):494–504.

8.23 CT OF FOCAL HYPODENSE RENAL LESIONS

Tumours

1. **Malignant**
   (a) Renal cell carcinoma – usually inhomogeneous and irregular if large.
   (b) Metastases.
   (c) Lymphoma – usually late-stage non-Hodgkin's lymphoma; only 5% at initial staging. 70% multiple and bilateral. Usually rounded in appearance.
   (d) Transitional cell carcinoma – can infiltrate and mimic renal cell carcinoma.
   (e) Wilms' tumour.
2. **Benign**
   (a) Oncocytoma – adenoma arising from proximal tubular cells. Round, well-defined, homogeneous (usually high density pre-contrast, low density post-contrast), ± central stellate low-density scar if tumour bigger than 3cm.
   (b) Angiomyolipoma – well-defined containing fat densities. Association with tuberous sclerosis.

Infection

1. **Abscess** – thick irregular walls ± perirenal fascial thickening, but this can occur in malignancy.
2. **Xanthogranulomatous pyelonephritis** – obstructing calculus seen in 80% cases leading to chronic sepsis, perinephric fluid collections and fistula formation.

3. **Acute focal bacterial nephritis** – wedge-shaped low density $\pm$ radiating striations after intravenous contrast.

Vascular

1. **Infarcts** – well-defined, peripheral, wedge-shaped.

Cyst – see 8.19 and 8.20

Further Reading

Ishikawa I, Saito Y, Onouchi Z et al. Delayed contrast enhancement in acute focal bacterial nephritis: CT features. J Comput Assist Tomogr 1985;9(5):894–7.

Neirius D, Braedel HU, Schindler E et al. Computed tomographic and angiographic findings in renal oncocytoma. Br J Radiol 1988;61:1019–25.

Rabushka LS, Fishman EK, Goldman SM et al. Pictorial review: computed tomography of renal inflammatory disease. Urology 1994;44:473–80.

Sheth S, Scatarige JC, Horton KM et al. Current concepts in the diagnosis and management of renal cell carcinoma: role of multidetector CT and three-dimensional CT. Radiographics 2001;21:S237–54.

Urban BA, Fishman EK. Renal lymphoma: CT patterns with emphasis on helical CT. Radiographics 2000;20:197–212.

Yuh BI, Cohan RH. Different phases of renal enhancement: role in detecting and characterizing renal masses during helical CT. Am J Roentgenol 1999;173:747–55.

8.24 RENAL SINUS MASS

Neoplastic

1. **Transitional cell carcinoma** – intraluminal filling defect on excretory urography, centred in the renal pelvis which secondarily invades the renal sinus and the renal parenchyma.
2. **Squamous cell carcinoma** – strongly associated with renal calculi.
3. **Metastasis to sinus lymph nodes.**
4. **Mesenchymal tumour** – e.g. lipoma, fibroma, haemangioma.
5. **Retroperitoneal tumours that extend into the renal sinus** – any retroperitoneal tumour but lymphoma most commonly.
6. **Renal parenchymal tumours that project into the renal sinus** – renal cell carcinoma, multilocular cystic nephroma.

Non-neoplastic lesions

1. **Sinus lipomatosis** – echogenic central sinus complex on ultrasound. CT and MRI directly reveal fatty nature.

2. **Peripelvic cyst** – multiple, small, benign, extraparenchymal cysts, probably lymphatic in origin, which appear to arise in the sinus itself. Distinguished from hydronephrosis by contrast-enhanced CT.
3. **Parapelvic cyst** – single, larger cyst protruding into the sinus, most likely originating from the adjacent parenchyma. Large cysts may cause haematuria, hypertension or hydronephrosis by local compression.
4. **Vascular** – renal artery aneurysm, arteriovenous communication or renal vein varix can manifest as parapelvic masses or peripelvic lesions. Colour-Doppler or contrast-enhanced CT used for diagnosis.
5. **Inflammatory** – usually extension into the sinus from chronic or severe pyelonephritis.
6. **Haematoma** – as a complication of anticoagulant therapy or less commonly secondary to trauma.
7. **Urinoma** – usually associated with ureteral obstruction secondary to stone disease or trauma.

Further Reading
Rha SE, Byun JY, Jung SE et al. The renal sinus: pathologic spectrum and multimodality imaging approach. Radiographics 2004;24(Suppl 1):S117–31.

8.25 NEPHROGRAPHIC PATTERNS

8

Global absence of nephrogram
Complete renal ischaemia secondary to occlusion of main renal artery.

1. **Injury to vascular pedicle** during blunt abdominal trauma.
2. **Thromboembolic disease.**
3. **Renal artery dissection.**

Segmental absence of nephrogram
1. **Neoplasm.**
2. **Cyst.**
3. **Abscess.**
4. **Focal renal infarction** – arterial embolus or thrombosis/renal vein thrombosis/sepsis/vasculitis

Immediate faint persistent nephrogram
1. **Proliferative/necrotizing disorders** – e.g. acute glomerulonephritis. See 8.14.
2. **Renal vein thrombosis.**
3. **Chronic severe ischaemia.**

Immediate distinct persistent nephrogram

1. **Acute tubular necrosis** – in 60% of cases.
2. **Other causes of acute renal failure.**
3. **Acute-on-chronic renal failure.**
4. **Acute hypotension** – uncommonly.

Increasingly dense nephrogram

Increasingly faint nephrogram becoming increasingly dense over hours to days.

1. **Acute obstruction** – including urate nephropathy.
2. **Acute hypotension.**
3. **Acute tubular necrosis** – in 30% of cases.
4. **Acute pyelonephritis.**
5. **Multiple myeloma.**
6. **Renal vein thrombosis.**
7. **Acute glomerulonephritis.**
8. **Amyloid.**
9. **Acute papillary necrosis** – and rarely chronic papillary necrosis.

Rim nephrogram

Rim of cortex receiving collateral blood flow from capsular, peripelvic, and periureteric vessels. This is the most specific indicator of renovascular compromise.

1. **Severe hydronephrosis** – scalloped nephrogram with a negative pyelogram.
2. **Acute complete arterial occlusion** – smooth nephrogram from cortical perfusion by capsular arteries.

Striated nephrogram

Streaky linear bands of alternating hyper- and hypoattenuation parallel to the axis of tubules and collecting ducts during the excretory phase.

1. **Acute ureteric obstruction.**
2. **Infantile polycystic disease** – contrast medium in dilated tubules.
3. **Medullary sponge kidney** – in the medulla only. Parallel or fan-shaped streaks radiating from the papilla to the periphery of the kidney.
4. **Acute pyelonephritis.**

Further Reading

Newhouse JH, Pfister RC. The nephrogram. Radiol Clin North Am 1979;17:213–26.

Saunders HS, Dyer RB, Shifrin RY et al. The CT nephrogram: implications for evaluation of urinary tract disease. Radiographics 1995;15:1069–85.

8.26 RENAL PAPILLARY NECROSIS

Ischaemic necrobiosis of medulla secondary to interstitial nephritis (interstitial oedema) or intrinsic vascular obstruction.

1. Normal – small kidneys with smooth outlines.
2. Bilateral in 85% with multiple papillae affected – usually a systemic cause.
3. Unilateral – usually obstruction, renal vein thrombosis or acute bacterial nephritis.
4. Papillae may show:
   (a) Enlargement (early).
   (b) Partial sloughing – a fissure forms and may communicate with a central irregular cavity.
   (c) Total sloughing – the sloughed papillary tissue may: (i) fragment and be passed in the urine; (ii) cause ureteric obstruction; (iii) remain free in a calyx; or (iv) remain in the pelvis and form a ball calculus.
   (d) Necrosis-in-situ – the papilla is shrunken and necrotic but has not separated.
5. Calyces will appear dilated following total sloughing of a papilla.
6. Calcification and occasionally ossification of a shrunken, necrotic papilla. If marginal, it appears as a calculus with a radiolucent centre.

    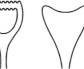

| Normal | Swollen | Partial papillary necrosis | Total papillary necrosis | Necrosis-in-situ |

8

A useful mnemonic is ADIPOSE:

A   Analgesics – phenacetin and aspirin.
D   Diabetes.
I   Infants in shock.
P   Pyelonephritis.
O   Obstruction.
S   Sickle-cell disease.
E   Ethanol.

However, diabetes, analgesics and sickle-cell anaemia are the most important, with diabetes (50%) the most frequent cause.

Further Reading

Jung DC, Kim SH, Jung SI et al. Renal papillary necrosis: review and comparison of findings at multi-detector row CT and intravenous urography. Radiographics 2006;26(6):1827–36.

8.27 RENAL-INDUCED HYPERTENSION

Renal artery stenosis – see 8.28
Chronic bilateral parenchymal disease

1. **Chronic glomerulonephritis.**
2. **Reflux nephropathy.**
3. **Adult polycystic disease*.**
4. **Diabetic glomerulosclerosis.**
5. **Connective tissue disorders** – systemic lupus erythematosus, scleroderma and polyarthritis nodosa.
6. **Radiotherapy.**
7. **Hydronephrosis.**
8. **Analgesic nephropathy.**
9. **Renal vein thrombosis.**

Unilateral parenchymal disease

Much less common as a cause of hypertension.

1. **Reflux nephropathy.**
2. **Hydronephrosis.**
3. **Tumours** – hypertension is more common with Wilms' tumour than with renal cell carcinoma. The rare juxtaglomerular cell tumour secretes renin.
4. **Tuberculosis.**
5. **Xanthogranulomatous pyelonephritis.**
6. **Radiotherapy.**
7. **Renal vein thrombosis.**

8.28 RENAL ARTERY STENOSIS

Aetiology

1. **Arteriosclerosis** – 66% of renovascular causes. Stenosis of the proximal 2cm of the renal artery; less frequently the distal artery or early branches at bifurcations. More common in males.
2. **Fibromuscular dysplasia** – 33% of renovascular causes. Stenoses ± dilatations which may give the characteristic 'string of beads' appearance. Mainly females less than 40 years. Bilateral in 60% of cases.
3. **Thrombosis/embolism.**
4. **Arteritis** – polyarteritis nodosa, thromboangiitis obliterans. Takayasu's disease, syphilis, congenital rubella or idiopathic.
5. **Neurofibromatosis*** – coarctation of the aorta. ± Stenoses of other arteries. ± Intrarenal arterial abnormalities.
6. **Trauma.**
7. **Aneurysm** – of the aorta or the renal artery.
8. **Arteriovenous fistula** – traumatic, congenital or a stump fistula following nephrectomy.
9. **Extrinsic compression** – neoplasm, aneurysm or lymph nodes.

Signs of unilateral renal artery stenosis on CT

1. **Direct visualization of the stenotic segment.**
2. **Post-stenotic dilatation.**
3. **Nephrogram asymmetry.**
4. **Reduction in kidney size and cortical thinning.**
5. **Differential urine concentration on delayed CT.**

Signs of unilateral renal artery stenosis on IVU

1. **Unilateral delayed nephrogram.**
2. **Small, smooth kidney.**
3. **Unilateral delay of 1 minute or more in the appearance of opacified calyces.**
4. **Increased density of opacified calyces.**
5. **Ureteric notching by collateral vessels.**

Signs of unilateral renal artery stenosis on ACE inhibitor renal scintigraphy

1. **Low probability** suggested by a normal study.
2. **Intermediate probability** when: (a) small kidney contributing <30% of total renal function; (b) time to maximum activity (T_{max}) =2 minutes, and shows no change following administration of ACE inhibitor; and (c) bilateral symmetrical cortical retention of tracer.

3. **High probability** when unilateral parenchymal retention, indicated by: (a) a change in the 20-minute/peak uptake ratio = 0.15, delayed excretion of tracer into the renal pelvis >2 minutes, or increase in the T_{max} of = 2 minutes or 40% after administration of ACE inhibitor.
4. **Decreased sensitivity** when bilateral renal artery stenosis, impaired renal function, urinary obstruction or long-term ACE therapy.

Signs of unilateral renal artery stenosis on Doppler sonography

1. **Peak velocity in the renal artery** >100cm/s.
2. **Renal artery velocity** >3.5 × aortic velocity.
3. **Tardus-parvus waveform** – slope of the systolic upstroke <3 m/s^2 and acceleration time (time from onset of systole to peak systole) >0.07 s.
4. **Turbulent flow in the post-stenotic renal artery.**

Further Reading

Joesphs SC. Techniques in interventional radiology: renal CT angiography. Tech Vasc Interv Radiol 2006;9(4):167–71.

Kawashima A, Sandler CM, Ernst RD et al. CT evaluation of renovascular disease. Radiographics 2000;20:1321–40.

Rankin S, Saunders AJ, Cook GJ et al. Renovascular disease. Clin Radiol 2000;55:1–12.

Soulez G, Oliva VL, Turpin S et al. Imaging of renovascular hypertension: respective values of renal scintigraphy, renal Doppler US, and MR angiography. Radiographics 2000;20:1355–68.

Sung CJ, Chung JW, Kim SH et al. Urine attenuation ratio: a new CT indicator of renal artery stenosis. Am J Radiol 2006;187:532–540.

8.29 RENAL VEIN THROMBOSIS

Unilateral or bilateral. The ultrasound findings (after Cremin et al 1991) are:

1st week
1. Globular renal enlargement.
2. Increase in echogenicity which may be more prominent in the cortex.
3. Loss of corticomedullary differentiation.
4. Echogenic streaks in the direction of the interlobular vessels.
5. Loss of definition of normal renal sinus echoes.

2nd week
1. Diffuse renal enlargement is more obvious.
2. Diffuse 'snow storm' appearance of increased echogenicity.
3. Loss of corticomedullary differentiation.
4. Mixed hyperechoic areas (haemorrhage) and hypoechoic areas (oedema and/or resolving haemorrhage).
5. Thrombus in main renal vein or IVC.

Late
1. Kidney returns to normal size or becomes small and atrophic.
2. Calcification may occur in kidney or IVC.

Conventional radiography findings are:

Sudden occlusion
1. Large non-functioning kidney which, over a period of several months, becomes small and atrophic.
2. Retrograde pyelography reveals thickened parenchyma (due to oedema) with elongation and compression of the major calyces.
3. Arteriography shows stretching and separation of arterial branches with decreased flow and a poor persistent nephrogram. No opacification of the renal vein.

Gradual occlusion
1. Large kidney.
2. Nephrogram may be normal, poor persistent or increasingly dense.
3. Thickened parenchyma with elongation of major calyces.
4. Ureteric notching due to venous collaterals.

Children
1. **Dehydration and shock** – especially in infants delivered of diabetic mothers.
2. **Nephrotic syndrome**.
3. **Cyanotic heart disease**.

Adults

1. Extension of renal cell carcinoma into the renal vein.
2. Local compression by tumour or retroperitoneal nodes.
3. Extension of thrombus from the IVC.
4. Trauma.
5. Sickle cell disease.
6. Secondary to renal disease – especially amyloid and chronic glomerulonephritis with nephrotic syndrome.

A useful mnemonic is MEAN TEST:

M   Membranous glomerulonephritis.
E   Extension from IVC.
A   Amyloidosis.
N   Neoplasm. Nephrotic syndrome.
T   Trauma.
E   Enterocolitis (resultant dehydration).
S   Sickle-cell disease/SLE
T   Thrombophleblitis.

Further Reading
Argyropoulou MI, Giapros VI, Papadopoulou F et al. Renal venous thrombosis in an infant with predisposing thrombotic factors: color Doppler ultrasound and MR evaluation. Eur Radiol 2003;13(8):2027–30.
Cremin BJ, Davey H, Oleszczuk-Raszke K. Neonatal renal venous thrombosis: sequential ultrasonic appearances. Clin Radiol 1991;44:52–5.

8.30 NON-OPACIFICATION OF A CALYX ON CT OR EXCRETORY UROGRAPHY

1. **Technical factors** – incomplete filling during excretory urography.
2. **Tumour** – most commonly a renal cell carcinoma (adult) or Wilms' tumour (child).
3. **Obstructed infundibulum** – due to tumour, calculus or tuberculosis.
4. **Duplex kidney** – with a non-functioning upper or lower moiety. Signs suggesting a non-functioning upper moiety are:
   (a) Fewer calyces than the contralateral kidney. This sign is only reliable in unilateral duplication. (Calyceal distribution is symmetrical in 80% of normal individuals.)
   (b) A shortened upper calyx which does not reach into the upper pole.
   (c) The upper calyx of the lower moiety may be deformed by a dilated upper pole pelvis.
   (d) The kidney may be displaced downward by a dilated upper moiety pelvis. The appearances mimic a space-occupying lesion in the upper pole.

(e) The upper pole may be rotated laterally and downward by a dilated upper moiety pelvis and the lower pole calyces adopt a 'drooping lily' appearance.

(f) Lateral displacement of the entire kidney by a dilated upper moiety ureter.

(g) The lower moiety ureter may be displaced or compressed by the upper pole ureter, resulting in a series of scalloped curves.

(h) The lower moiety renal pelvis may be displaced laterally and its ureter then takes a direct oblique course to the lumbosacral junction.

5. **Infection** – abscess or tuberculosis.

6. **Partial nephrectomy** – with a surgical defect in the twelfth rib.

Further Reading
Fernbach SK, Feinstein KA, Spencer K et al. Ureteral duplication and its complications. Radiographics 1997;17:109–27.

8.31 RADIOLUCENT FILLING DEFECT IN THE RENAL PELVIS OR A CALYX

Technical factors

1. **Incomplete filling during excretion urography.**
2. **Overlying gas shadows.**

Extrinsic with a smooth margin

1. **Cyst** – see 8.19.
2. **Vascular impression** – an intrarenal artery producing linear transverse or oblique compression lines and most commonly indenting an upper pole calyx, especially on the right side.
3. **Renal sinus lipomatosis** – most commonly in older patients with a wasting disease of the kidney. Fat in the renal hilum produces a relative lucency and narrows and elongates the major calyces.
4. **Collateral vessels** – most commonly ureteric artery collaterals in renal artery stenosis. Multiple small irregularities in the pelvic wall.

Inseparable from the wall and with smooth margins

1. **Blood clot** – due to trauma, tumour or bleeding diathesis. May be adherent to the wall or free in the lumen. Change in size or shape over several days.
2. **Papilloma** – solitary or multiple.
3. **Pyeloureteritis cystica** – due to chronic infection. Multiple well-defined submucosal cysts project into the lumen of the pelvis and/or ureter.

Arising from the wall with an irregular margin

1. **Transitional cell carcinoma.**
2. **Squamous cell carcinoma** – see 8.22.
3. **Renal cell carcinoma.**
4. **Squamous metaplasia (cholesteatoma)** – occurs rarely in association with chronic irritation from a calculus. Indistinguishable from tumour and may be premalignant.

In the lumen

1. **Blood clot.**
2. **Lucent calculus** – see 8.16.
3. **Sloughed papilla.**
4. **Air** – see 8.43.

Further Reading

Brown RC, Jones MC, Boldus R et al. Lesions causing radiolucent defects in the renal pelvis. Am J Roentgenol 1973;119:770–8.

8.32 SPONTANEOUS URINARY CONTRAST EXTRAVASATION

Pyelorenal backflow

Seen on excretory urography. Also known as spontaneous pyelorenal backflow. Described as being 'spontaneous' but is more commonly due to sudden increased pressure in the collecting system e.g. stone or tumour. Complications are rare and treatment is conservative.

1. **Pyelosinus backflow** – contrast extravasation from fornix rupture.
2. **Pyelotubular 'backflow'** – opacification of terminal portions of collecting ducts so not really 'backflow'. May be physiological. Fan like streaks from calyx toward periphery.
3. **Pyelointerstitial backflow** – contrast flows from pyramids into subcapsular tubules. More amorphous than pyelotubular.
4. **Pyelolymphatic backflow** – dilated lymphatics. Visualization of small lymphatics draining medially.
5. **Pyelovenous backflow** – forniceal rupture into arcuate or interloper veins. Very rare.

The first two are the most common.

Further Reading

Cooke GM, Batiks JP. Spontaneous extravasation of contrast medium during intravenous urography. Report of fourteen cases and a review of the literature. Clin Radiol 1974;25(1):87–93.

8.33 DILATED CALYX

With a narrow infundibulum

1. **Stricture** – tumour, calculus or tuberculosis.
2. **Extrinsic impression by an artery** – most commonly a right upper pole calyx (Fraley syndrome).
3. **Hydrocalycosis** – may be a congenital anomaly. Can only be safely diagnosed in childhood when calculus, tumour and tuberculosis are uncommon.

With a wide infundibulum

1. **Post-obstructive atrophy** – generally all the calyces are affected and associated with parenchymal thinning.
2. **Megacalyces** – dilated calyces ± a slightly dilated pelvis. ± Stones. Increased number of calyces: 20–25 (normal 8–12). Because of the large volume collecting system full visualization during urography is delayed. Normal cortical thickness and good renal function differentiate it from post-obstructive atrophy.
3. **Polycalycosis** – rare. ± Ureteric abnormalities.

Further Reading
Gabutti L, Alerci M, Marone C. Spiral CT angiography for discriminating between megacalyces and intermittent hydronephrosis. Nephrol Dial Transplant 1997;12(7):1487–9.
Sethi R, Yang DC, Mittal P et al. Congenital megacalyces. Studies with different imaging modalities. Clin Nucl Med 1997;22(9):653–5.

8.34 DILATED URETER

Obstruction

Within the lumen
1. **Calculus** – see 8.16.
2. **Blood clot.**
3. **Sloughed papilla.**

In the wall
1. **Oedema or stricture due to calculus**.
2. **Tumour** – carcinoma or papilloma.
3. **Tuberculous stricture** – a particular hazard during the early weeks of treatment.
4. **Schistosomiasis** – especially the distal ureter. ± Calcification in the ureter or bladder.
5. **Post-surgical trauma** – e.g. a misplaced ligature.

6. **Ureterocoele.**
7. **Megaureter** – symmetrical tapered narrowing above the ureterovesical junction.

Outside the wall
1. **Retroperitoneal fibrosis** (q.v.).
2. **Carcinoma of cervix, bladder or prostate.**
3. **Retrocaval ureter** – right side only. Distal ureter lies medial to the dilated proximal portion.
4. **Aortic aneurysm.**

Vesicoureteric reflux
No obstruction or reflux

1. **Postpartum** – more common on the right side.
2. **Following relief of obstruction** – most commonly calculus or prostatectomy.
3. **Urinary tract infection** – due to the effect of P fimbriated *E. coli* on the urothelium.
4. **Primary non-obstructive megaureter** – children > adults. The juxtavesical segment of ureter is of normal calibre but fails to transmit an effective peristaltic wave due to faulty development of muscle layers.

Further Reading
Mostbeck GH, Zontsich T, Turetschek K. Ultrasound of the kidney: obstruction and medical diseases. Eur Radiol 2001;11:1878–89.

8.35 STRICTURE OF THE URETER

Wide differential. CT urography ± retrograde pyelography is used to determine if there is a true stricture or a mass and how long the narrowing is.

Congenital

1. **Ectopic ureterocoele.**
2. **Primary megaureter.**
3. **Congenital stenosis.**

Inflammatory

1. **Ureterolithiasis.**
2. **TB** – corkscrew appearance.
3. **Schistosomiasis.**

4. **Inflammatory bowel disease** – Crohn's disease, diverticulitis.
5. **Endometriosis** – ureteral involvement is rare and indicates widespread disease. Abrupt, smooth stricture.
6. **Retroperitoneal fibrosis** – any cause.

Neoplastic

1. **Transitional cell carcinoma.**
2. **Metastases** – cervix, endometrium, ovary, rectum, prostate, breast, lymphoma.

Infection

1. **Abscess** – tubo-ovarian, appendiceal, perisigmoidal.

Vascular

1. **Aortic or iliac artery aneurysm** – perianeurysmal fibrosis.

Trauma

1. **Iatrogenic** – hysterectomy, endoscopic stone extraction.
2. **Radiation.**

A useful mnemonic is SMARTIE:

S   Schistosomiasis.
M   Metastases.
A   Abscess.
R   Radiation / Retroperitoneal fibrosis.
T   TB / TCC / Trauma.
I   Inflammation – from calculus and other inflammatory conditions.
E   Endometriosis.

8.36 FILLING DEFECT WITHIN THE URETER

Solitary

Within the lumen
1. Calculus.
2. Blood clot.
3. Sloughed papilla.
4. Benign fibroepithelial polyp.

In the wall
1. Urothelial neoplasm.
2. Metastasis.
3. Tuberculosis.
4. Endometriosis.

MULTIPLE

Within the lumen
1. Calculi.
2. Blood clots.
3. Sloughed papillae.
4. Multiple fibroepithelial polyps.
5. Air bubbles.
6. Fungus ball.

In the wall
1. **Ureteritis cystica** – asymptomatic multiple, small (2–4 mm) cysts usually related to infection or calculi. Usually upper ureter.
2. **Allergic mucosal bullae.**
3. **Pseudodiverticulosis** – associated with malignancy and 50% eventually develop uroepithelial malignancy.
4. **Vascular impressions** (collateral veins in IVC obstruction).
5. **Multiple papillomas.**
6. **Multiple metastases** – melanoma.
7. **Suburothelial haemorrhage** – usually associated with a coagulopathy. Less discrete than ureteritis cystica.

8.37 RETROPERITONEAL FIBROSIS

1. Dense retroperitoneal, periaortic fibrous tissue mass which typically begins around the aortic bifurcation and extends superiorly to the renal hila. Rarely extends below the pelvic rim.
2. Envelops the aorta and IVC, lymphatics and ureter(s) en route.
3. Demonstrable by CT (= muscle), US (hypoechoic) or MRI (low signal on T_1W, high signal on T_2W in the active stage, low signal on T_2W in the chronic stage). Contrast enhancement in the early, active stage.
4. Ureteric obstruction is of variable severity. 75% bilateral.
5. Tapering ureteral lumen or complete obstruction – usually at L4–5 level and never extreme lower end.
6. Medial deviation of the ureters – more significant if there is a right-angled step in the course of the ureter rather than a gentle drift. The position of the ureters is frequently normal.
7. Easy retrograde catheterization of ureter(s).
8. Clinically – back pain, high ESR and elevated creatinine.

Aetiology

1. **Idiopathic** – >50% all cases. May be due to an immune reaction to artheromatous material in the aorta. In 10% cases, associated with fibrosis in other organ systems (e.g. mediastinal fibrosis, sclerosing cholangitis, orbital pseudotumour).
2. **Retroperitoneal malignancy** – lymphoma and metastases from colon and breast especially. The tumour initiates a fibrotic reaction around itself.
3. **Aortic aneurysm** ⎫ fibrosis occurs secondary
4. **Trauma** ⎬ to blood in the
5. **Surgery** ⎭ retroperitoneal tissues.
6. **Inflammatory conditions** – Crohn's disease, diverticular disease, actinomycosis, pancreatitis and extravasation of urine from the pelvicalyceal system.
7. **Connective tissue diseases** – ankylosing spondylitis, systemic lupus erythematosus, Wegener's granulomatosis and polyarteritis nodosa.
8. **Drugs** – methysergide, methyldopa, beta-blockers amongst others.
9. **Radiation therapy.**

Further Reading
Brooks AP. Computed tomography of idiopathic retroperitoneal fibrosis ('periaortitis'): variants, variations, patterns and pitfalls. Clin Radiol 1990;42:75–9.
Geoghegan T, Byrne AT, Benfayed W et al. Imaging and intervention of retroperitoneal fibrosis. Australas Radiol 2007;1:26–34.
Vivas I, Nicolas AI, Velazquez P. Retroperitoneal fibrosis: typical and atypical manifestations. Br J Radiol 2000;73:214–22.

8.38 DEVIATED URETERS

Medial deviation

1. **Normal variant** – 15% of individuals. Commoner in blacks, in whom bilateral displacement is also commoner.
2. **Retroperitoneal fibrosis** – see 8.37.
3. **Retrocaval ureter** – the right ureter passes behind the IVC at the level of L4. The distal ureter lies medial to the dilated proximal portion.
4. **Pelvic lipomatosis** – other signs suggesting the diagnosis are:
   (a) Elevation and elongation of the bladder.
   (b) Elongation of the rectum and sigmoid with widening of the rectorectal space.
   (c) Increased lucency of the pelvic wall.
5. **Following abdominoperineal resection** – the ureters are medially placed inferiorly.
6. **Iliac lymphadenopathy.**
7. **Aneurysmal dilatation of the iliac vessels.**

Lateral deviation

Much commoner than medial deviation.

1. **Hypertrophy of psoas muscle.**
2. **Paracaval/para-aortic lymphadenopathy.**
3. **Pelvic mass** (fibroids, ovarian tumour).
4. **Aneurysmal aortic dilatation.**
5. **Neurogenic tumours.**
6. **Fluid collection** (abscess, urinoma, lymphocoele, haematoma)

8.39 VESICOURETERIC REFLUX

Congenital (= primary reflux)

Renal scarring with UTI in 50%.

1. **Congenital reflux** – due to incompetence of vesicoureteric junction secondary to abnormal tunnelling of distal ureter through bladder. 10% of normal Caucasian babies and 30% of children with a first episode of ITI. Renal scars in up to 50%. Usually disappears in 80% but can cause end-stage renal disease in 10% adults.

Acquired (= secondary reflux)

1. **Hutch diverticulum.**
2. **Cystitis** – in 50%.

3. **Neurogenic bladder.**
4. **Urethral obstruction** – posterior urethral valves. Mainly on L side (reflux in 33%).
5. **Duplication with ureterocoele.**
6. **Prune-belly syndrome** – almost exclusively males. High mortality. Bilateral hydronephrosis and hydroureters with a distended bladder are associated with undescended testes, hypoplasia of the anterior abdominal wall and urethral obstruction.

Further Reading

Buckley O, Geoghegan T, O'Brien J et al. Vesicoureteric reflux in the adult. Br J Radiol 2007;80(954):392–400.

Fernbach SK, Feinstein KA, Schmidt MB. Pediatric voiding cystourethrography: a pictorial guide. Radiographics 2000;20(1):155–71.

8.40 FILLING DEFECT IN THE BLADDER

Within the lumen

1. **Calculus.**
2. **Instrumentation** – urethral or suprapubic catheter.
3. **Blood clot.**
4. **Enlarged prostate.**
5. **Ureterocoele.**

In the wall

1. **Primary neoplasm** – especially transitional cell carcinoma in an adult and rhabdomyosarcoma in a child.
2. **Polyps.**
3. **Metastases.**
4. **Schistosomiasis.**
5. **Malakoplakia** – uncommon chronic inflammatory response to gram negative infection. Yellow-brown submucosal histiocytic granuloma causing multiple mural filling defects on IVU.
6. **Endometriosis.**

8.41 BLADDER WALL THICKENING

Normal bladder wall thickness is defined as <5mm in non-distended bladders, <3mm in well-distended bladders.

Neoplastic

1. Transitional cell carcinoma.
2. Lymphoma.
3. Metastases.
4. Neurofibromatosis.

Inflammatory

1. Any cause of cystitis – e.g. radiation, infection.
2. TB.
3. Schistosomiasis.
4. Malakoplakia.
5. Inflammatory bowel disease, appendicitis, focal diverticulitis.

Muscular hypertrophy

1. Neurogenic bladder.
2. Bladder outlet obstruction – BPH, urethral stricture, posterior urethral valves.

Trauma

1. Haemorrhage/haematoma – bleeding diatheses, iatrogenic.

Underdistended bladder

Further Reading
Wong-You-Cheong JJ, Woodward PJ, Manning MA et al. Inflammatory and non-neoplastic bladder masses: radiologic-pathologic correlation. Radiographics 2006;26(6):1847–68.

8.42 BLADDER CALCIFICATION

In the lumen
1. **Calculus.**
2. **Foreign body** – encrustation of the balloon of a Foley catheter.

In the wall
1. **Transitional and squamous cell carcinoma** – radiographic incidence about 0.5%. Usually surface calcification which may be linear, curvilinear or stippled. Punctate calcification of a villous tumour may suggest chronicity. No extravesical calcification.
2. **Schistosomiasis** – an infrequent cause in the Western hemisphere but the commonest cause of mural calcification worldwide. Thin curvilinear calcification outlines a bladder of normal size and shape. Calcification spreads proximally to involve the distal ureters in 15%.
3. **Tuberculosis** – rare and usually accompanied by calcification elsewhere in the urogenital tract. Unlike schistosomiasis, the disease begins in the kidney and spreads distally. Contracted bladder.
4. **Cyclophosphamide-induced cystitis.**
5. **Radiation.**

A useful mnemonic is STRICT:

S   Schistosomiasis.
T   Transitional cell carcinoma.
R   Radiation.
I   Interstitial cystitis.
C   Cyclophosphamide/Calculus
T   Tuberculosis.

Further Reading
Dyer RB, Chen MY, Zagoria RJ. Abnormal calcifications in the urinary tract. Radiographics 1998;18(6):1405–24.
Pollack HM, Banner MP, Martinez LO et al. Diagnostic considerations in urinary bladder wall calcification. Am J Roentgenol 1986;136:791–7.

8.43 BLADDER FISTULA

Congenital
1. **Ectopia vesicae.**
2. **Imperforate anus** – high type.
3. **Patent urachus.**

Inflammatory
1. **Diverticular disease** – most common cause.
2. **Crohn's disease*.**
3. **Appendix abscess** – and other pelvic sepsis.

Neoplastic
1. **Carcinoma of the colon, bladder or reproductive organs.**
2. **Radiotherapy.**

Trauma
1. **Accidental.**
2. **Iatrogenic** – particularly in obstetrics and gynaecology.

Further Reading
Yu NC, Raman SS, Patel M et al. Fistulas of the genitourinary tract: a radiologic review. Radiographics 2004;24(5):1331–52.

8.44 GAS IN THE URINARY SYSTEM

Gas shadows which conform to the position and shape of the bladder, ureters or pelvicalyceal systems.

Gas inside the bladder
1. **Vesicointestinal fistula** – diverticular disease, carcinoma of the colon or rectum and Crohn's disease.
2. **Cystitis** – due to gas-forming organisms and fermentation, especially in diabetics. Usually *Escherichia coli*. Clostridial infections are rare and usually secondary to septicaemia.
3. **Following instrumentation.**
4. **Penetrating wounds.**

Gas in the bladder wall

1. **Emphysematous cystitis** – usually in diabetics.

Gas in the ureters and pelvicalyceal systems

1. **Any cause of gas in the bladder.**
2. **Ureteric diversion** – into the colon or bladder.
3. **Fistula** – Crohn's disease or perforated duodenal ulcer.
4. **Infection** – usually in diabetics. Gas may also be present in the renal parenchyma and retroperitoneal tissues.

Further Reading

Roy C, Pfleger DD, Tuchmann CM et al. Emphysematous pyelitis. Findings in five patients. Radiology 2001;218:647–50.

8.45 CALCIFICATIONS OF THE MALE GENITAL TRACT

1. **Diabetes mellitus** – the cause in the vast majority of cases.
2. **Chronic infection** – tuberculosis, schistosomiasis, chronic urinary tract infection and syphilis.
3. **Ejaculatory duct calculi** – rare.
4. **Idiopathic.**

Prostate

1. **Calcified corpora amylacea** – dense accumulations of calcified proteinaceous material which may obstruct the lumens of the prostatic ducts, and may underlie some cases of BPH.
2. **Chronic prostatitis.**
3. **Tuberculosis.**

Further Reading

King JC, Rosenbaum HD. Calcification of the vasa deferentia in non-diabetes. Radiology 1971;100:603–6.

8.46 ULTRASOUND OF INTRATESTICULAR ABNORMALITIES

Neoplastic

Colour Doppler does not accurately differentiate neoplasm from acute inflammation or benign from malignant tumours.

1. **Germ cell tumours** – 95% of primary testicular tumours. 40% are of mixed histology. 8% are bilateral.

   (a) *Seminoma* – most common testicular tumour in the adult. 40–50% of testicular germ cell tumours. 25% have metastases at presentation. Most common tumour in the undescended testis. A solid, homogeneous, hypoechoic, round or oval mass which is sharply delineated from normal testicular tissue.

   (b) *Embryonal carcinoma* – 20–25% of germ cell tumours. More aggressive than seminoma and more heterogeneous because of necrosis, haemorrhage, cysts and calcification.

   (c) *Choriocarcinoma* – rare.

   (d) *Teratoma* – 5–10% and most common in infants and children. Heterogeneous echo texture because of the different tissue elements present.

2. **Non-Germ cell tumours** – usually benign. May secrete oestrogens (Sertoli cell) or testosterone (Leydig cell). Non-specific appearance but usually solid hypoechoic mass ± cystic areas.

3. **Metastases** – kidney, prostate, bronchus, pancreas. More common than germ cell tumours in the over 50-year age group. Patients with leukaemia or lymphoma may relapse in the testis and present as focal or diffuse decreased echogenicity in an enlarged testis.

Vascular

1. **Testicular torsion**

   (a) *Acute* – presentation within 24 hours. Enlarged hypoechoic or heterogeneous testis ± hydrocoele and enlargement of the epididymis. Colour Doppler: absent testicular flow; normal peritesticular flow.

   (b) *Subacute or missed* – presentation at 1–10 days. Colour Doppler: absent testicular flow; increased peritesticular flow.

   (c) *Spontaneous detorsion* – colour Doppler: normal or increased testicular flow; increased peritesticular flow.

Inflammatory

1. **Orchitis** – generalized testicular swelling and hypoechogenicity, initially; progresses to patch focal low reflectivity. Hypoechoic areas are hypervascular. There may be swelling of the epididymis,

hydrocoele and scrotal wall oedema. Complications occur in 50% – abscess formation, necrosis, haematoma and testicular atrophy.
2. **Abscess** – complicating epididymo-orchitis, often in a diabetic patient or those with mumps. Hypoechoic or mixed echogenic mass.

Idiopathic non-neoplastic cysts

1. **Tunica albuginea cyst** – 2–5mm; typically in the upper anterior or lateral part of the testis; unilocular or multilocular.
2. **Simple cyst** – >40 years of age; 2–20mm; usually solitary and most are located near the mediastinum.

Further Reading

Atchley JT, Dewbury KC. Ultrasound appearances of testicular epidermoid cysts. Clin Radiol 2000;55:493–502.

Cook JL, Dewbury K. The changes seen on high-resolution ultrasound in orchitis. Clin Radiol 2000;55:13–18.

Dogra VS, Gottlieb RH, Rubens DJ et al. Benign intratesticular cystic lesions: US features. Radiographics 2001;21:S273–81.

Howlett DC, Marchbank ND, Sallomi DF. Ultrasound of the testis. Clin Radiol 2000;55:595–601.

Sidhu PS. Clinical and imaging features of testicular torsion: role of ultrasound. Clin Radiol 1999;54:343–52.

Siegel MJ. The acute scrotum. Radiol Clin North Am 1997;35(4):959–76.

Strauss S, Gottlieb P, Kessler A et al. Non-neoplastic intratesticular lesions mimicking tumour on ultrasound. Eur Radiol 2000;10:1628–35.

8

8.47 ULTRASOUND OF EXTRATESTICULAR ABNORMALITIES

Inflammatory

1. **Epididymitis** – enlarged, hypoechoic, hypervascular epididymis with a hydrocoele and skin thickening. Normal testis in the absence of orchitis but frequently coexists with orchitis.

Idiopathic

1. **Hydrocoele** – fluid collection anterolaterally in the scrotum.
    (a) Congenital – due to persistence of the processus vaginalis.
    (b) Infantile – accumulation of fluid along the processus vaginalis but with no communication with the abdominal cavity.
    (c) Secondary to trauma, infection, torsion or neoplasm.

Neoplastic

1. **Adenomatoid tumour of the epididymis** – a benign tumour which accounts for 30% of extratesticular tumours. Other tumours are varied and uncommon.

Vascular

1. **Varicocoele** – dilated pampiniform plexus of veins posterior to the testis. In 15% of adult males and virtually always on the left side. Important to exclude a compressive retroperitoneal aetiology if the varicocoele is right-sided or does not decompress in the erect position or with a Valsalva manoeuvre.

Further Reading
Woodward PJ, Schwab CM, Sesterhenn IA. Extratesticular scrotal masses: radiologic-pathologic correlation. Radiographics 2003;23(1):215–40.

Soft tissues

Stephen Davies

9.1 GYNAECOMASTIA

Physiological

1. **Neonatal** – due to high placental oestrogens.
2. **Pubertal** – due to an excess of oestradiol over testosterone.
3. **Senile** – due to falling androgen and rising oestrogen levels with age.

Pathological

1. **Carcinoma of the bronchus, gastric carcinoma, renal carcinoma, hepatoma** ⎫ secreting human chorionic
2. **Teratoma of the testis** ⎭ gonadotrophin
3. **Cirrhosis** – due to increased conversion of androgens to oestrogens.
4. **Hypogonadism** – e.g. Klinefelter's syndrome and testicular trauma.
5. **Hypopituitarism** – including acromegaly.
6. **Androgen insensitivity syndrome**.
7. **Adrenal tumours** ⎫ secreting
8. **Leydig cell tumours** ⎭ oestrogens.

Pharmacological

1. **Oestrogens or drugs with oestrogen like activity** – treatment of carcinoma of the prostate; digitalis.
2. **Enhanced oestrogen synthesis** – gonadotrophins, phenytoin.
3. **Anti-androgens** – spironolactone, metronidazole, alkylating agents, ketoconazole.
4. **Idiopathic** – phenothiazines, tricyclic antidepressants, ACE inhibitors, omeprazole.

9.2 LINEAR AND CURVILINEAR CALCIFICATION IN SOFT TISSUES

Arterial

1. **Atheroma/aneurysm.**
2. **Diabetes.**
3. **Hyperparathyroidism*** – more common in secondary than primary.

Nerve

1. **Leprosy.**
2. **Neurofibromatosis*.**

Ligament

1. **Tendonitis** – supraspinatus.
2. **Ankylosing spondylitis*.**
3. **Fluorosis.**
4. **Diabetes.**
5. **Alkaptonuria.**

Bismuth injection

In the buttocks. ± Neuropathic joints.

Parasites

1. Cysticerci — oval with lucent centre. Often arranged in the direction of muscle fibres.

2. Guinea worm — irregular coiled appearance.

3. Loa loa — thread-like coil. Particularly in the web spaces of the hand.

4. Armillifer — 'comma'-shaped. Only in trunk muscles.

See also 9.4.

Further Reading
Rahalkar MD, Shetty DD, Kelkar AB et al. The many faces of cysticercosis. Clin Radiol 2000;55:668–74.

9.3 'SHEETS' OF CALCIFICATION/ OSSIFICATION IN SOFT TISSUES

1. **Dermatomyositis.**
2. **Polymyositis.**
3. **Systemic lupus erythematosus.**

9.4 SOFT TISSUE CALCIFICATION

Connective tissue disorder

1. **Scleroderma.***
2. **Dermatomyositis.**
3. **Polymyositis.**
4. **Mixed connective tissue disease.**
5. **Bursitis** – can be dense and lobulated.
6. **Ehlers–Danlos syndrome.**

Metabolic

1. **Hyperparathyroidism*** – more common in secondary hyperparathyroidism. Vascular calcification is common.
2. **Treatment with 1-α-OHD$_3$** – particularly shoulder, hip and metacarpophalangeal joints.
3. **Sarcoidosis*** – rare. Hypercalcaemia. Affects hands and feet.
3. **Gout*** – calcified tophi. Punched-out erosions.
4. **Calcium hydroxyapatite deposition disease.**
5. **Calcium pyrophosphate deposition disease*.**
6. **Tumoral calcinosis** – age 20–30 years. Adjacent to a major joint. Firm, non-tender, moveable mass which is well-defined, lobulated and calcified on x-ray. Osseous involvement is rare. Usually hyperphosphataemia. ± Calcium fluid level.
7. **Hypervitaminosis D.**

Traumatic

1. **Myositis ossificans** – outer part is more densely calcified than the centre.
2. **Haematoma.**
3. **Calcifying myonecrosis.**
4. **Burns.**

9

Neoplastic

1. **Benign**
   (a) Parosteal lipoma – lucent. ± Pressure erosion of adjacent bone.
   (b) Haemangioma – Suspect if phleboliths present in an unusual site. ± Soft-tissue mass with adjacent bone destruction.
   (c) Synovial osteochondromatosis – age 20–50 years. Most commonly affects a large joint. Multiple calcified loose bodies. ± Secondary degenerative changes or pressure erosion of bone.

2. **Malignant**
   (a) Parosteal osteosarcoma – age 20–40 years. Lobulated calcification around a metaphysis. Inner part is more densely calcified than the periphery. Early – a thin lucent line may separate it from underlying bone.
   (b) Extraskeletal osteosarcoma*.
   (c) Synovial sarcoma – age 20–50 years. Soft-tissue mass with amorphous calcification, irregular bone destruction and osteoporosis.

Further Reading

Olsen KM, Chew FS. Tumoural calcinosis: pearls, polemics and alternative possibilities. Radiographics 2006;26:871–85.

9.5 SOFT-TISSUE OSSIFICATION

Traumatic

1. **Myositis ossificans.**
2. **Burns.**
3. **Neurogenic** – paraplegia and post-comatose states.

Neoplastic

1. **Synovial sarcoma.**
2. **Parosteal osteosarcoma.**
3. **Liposarcoma.**

Idiopathic

1. **Fibrodysplasia ossificans progressiva.**

Breast disease and mammography

Aisling Butler

10.1　INTRODUCTION

The accuracy of mammography for detection of breast cancer is dependant on image quality. Modern mammography demands meticulously high standards in all its aspects. These include x-ray equipment, radiographic technique, film–screen combinations, processing, viewing conditions and interpretation. Shortcomings in any of these factors will lead to serious errors. Other factors that lead to difficulty include dense parenchymal background that may obscure malignancy. The DMIST study has shown that digital mammography is comparable to conventional mammography in detection of breast cancer but has significantly higher accuracy in those under the age of 50, those with heterogeneously dense or extremely dense breasts, and pre- or perimenopausal women. Digital mammography has also been shown to be better at detecting microcalcification.

The concept of 'triple assessment' in breast diagnosis is accepted as the gold standard and incorporates clinical breast examination, imaging in the form of mammography ± ultrasound and pathological analysis where appropriate, with core breast biopsy or fine needle aspiration and cytology. The radiologist plays a key and integral role in this process. This approach is unique to breast disease and is strictly regulated by local multidisciplinary teams ensuring high standards of care.

Further Reading

Bassett LW. Imaging of breast masses. Radiol Clin North Am 2000;38(4):669–91.

Orel SG, Schnall MD. MR imaging of the breast for detection, diagnosis and staging of breast cancer. Radiology 2001;220:13–30.

Pisano ED, Gatsonis C, Hendrick E et al. Digital Mammographic Imaging Screening Trial (DMIST) Investigators Group. Diagnostic Performance of digital versus film mammography for breast-cancer screening. N Engl J Med 2005;353(17):1773–83.

Tabar L, Vitak B, Chen HH et al. The Swedish two county trial twenty years later. Updated mortality results and new insights from long term follow-up. Radiol Clin North Am 2000;38(4):625–51.

10.2 THE NORMAL BREAST

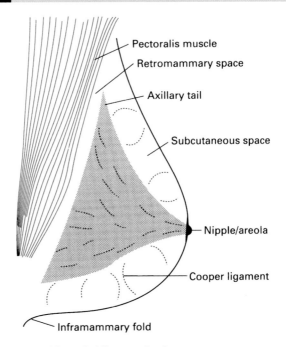

Pectoralis muscle

Retromammary space

Axillary tail

Subcutaneous space

Nipple/areola

Cooper ligament

Inframammary fold

Normal lateral oblique projection

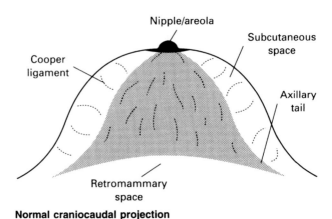

Nipple/areola

Subcutaneous space

Cooper ligament

Axillary tail

Retromammary space

Normal craniocaudal projection

10.3 BENIGN v. MALIGNANT

1. Opacity	Smooth margin	Ill-defined margin – stellate, spiculated, comet tail.
	Low density	High density
	Homogeneous	Inhomogeneous
	Thin 'halo'	Wide 'halo'
2. Calcification		see 10.4
3. Surrounding parenchyma	Normal	Disrupted
4. Nipple/areola	± Retracted	± Retracted
5. Skin	Normal	Thickened
6. Cooper ligaments	Normal	Thickened, increased number
7. Ducts	Normal	Focal dilatation
8. Subcutaneous/ retromammary space	Normal	Obliterated

NB. The above distinguishing features are not invariable and may be found in 'classic cases' only.

10

10.4 CALCIFICATION

1. Microcalcification is defined as individual calcific opacities measuring < 0.5mm in diameter.
2. Macrocalcification – opacities > 0.5mm in diameter.
3. Microcalcification is not specific to carcinoma.
4. Microcalcification is seen in 30–40% of carcinomas on mammography.
5. Macrocalcification may be found in carcinoma.

Definitely benign (see figure, p. 241)

1. Arterial – tortuous, tramline.
2. Smooth, widely separated, some with radiolucent centre.
3. Linear thick, rod-like, widespread, some with radiolucent centre.
4. 'Egg-shell' curvilinear – margin of cyst, fat necrosis.
5. 'Pop-corn' in fibroadenoma.
6. Large individual calcific opacity > 2mm, e.g. involutional fibroadenoma.
7. 'Floating' calcification – seen as calcific/fluid level on lateral oblique projection in 'milk of calcium' cysts.

Probably benign

1. Widespread – all one/both breasts.
2. Macrocalcification of one size.
3. Symmetrical distribution.
4. Widely separated opacities.
5. Superficial distribution.
6. Normal parenchyma.

Possibly malignant

Biopsy indicated – see microcalcification figure.

1. Microcalcification – particularly segmental, cluster distribution (> 5 particles in $1.0cm^3$ space; of these 30% will be malignant).
2. Mixture of sizes and shapes – linear, branching, punctate.
3. Associated suspicious soft-tissue opacity.
4. Microcalcification eccentrically located in soft-tissue mass.
5. Deterioration on serial mammography.

Examples of definitely benign calcification:

1. Arterial

2. Smooth ± lucent centre
widely separated

3. Linear, thick, rod-like
± lucent centres

4 'Egg-shell'

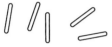

5. 'Pop-corn'

6. Large calcific opacity

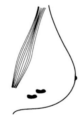

7. Floating calcification

Microcalcification; mixture of sizes,
shapes, cluster, haphazard arrangement,
linear branching patterns

10

Further Reading
Hogge JP, Robinson RE, Magnant CM et al. The mammographic spectrum of fat
    necrosis of the breast. Radiographics 1995;15:1347–56.
Monsees BS. Evaluation of breast microcalcifications. Radiol Clin North Am
    1995;33(6):1109–21.
Sickles E. Breast calcification: mammographic evaluation. Radiology
    1986;160:289–93.

10.5 DISAPPEARANCE OF CALCIFICATION

1. Surgery.
2. Radiotherapy.
3. Chemotherapy.
4. Spontaneous.

10.6 BENIGN LESIONS WITH TYPICAL APPEARANCES

1. **Lipoma** – large, rounded, radiolucent, well-defined with compression of adjacent parenchyma.
2. **Fibroadenoma** – rounded, lobulated, well-defined homogeneously dense soft-tissue opacity with eccentrically sited 'pop-corn' calcification.
3. **Intramammary lymph node** – well-defined, usually approximately 1.0 cm in diameter soft-tissue opacity, often with an eccentric radiolucency situated most often in the upper outer quadrant of the breast.
4. **Lipid cyst** – well-defined, multiple, lucent, 'egg-shell' calcification.
5. **Hamartoma/fibroadenolipoma.** 'Breast within a breast' appearance on a mammogram.

10.7 SINGLE WELL-DEFINED SOFT-TISSUE OPACITY

Benign

1. Cyst.
2. Fibroadenoma.
3. **Intramammary lymph node**.
   Intramammary lymph nodes occur in up to 40% of breasts, causes include breast cancer, lymphoma, melanoma, regional inflammation/dermatitis, fungal infection, tuberculosis/granulomatous disease, foreign body reactions, e.g. gold injections for rheumatoid arthritis, silicone adenopathy, HIV and sinus histiocytosis.
4. **Skin lesion**.
5. **Papilloma**.
6. **Nipple not in profile**.
7. **Hamartoma**.
8. **Galactocoele**.

Malignant

1. **Cystosarcoma phylloides** – usually large, may be benign but have malignant potential (5–10%), calcification rare, median age 45–49, rare <30 or >60. High tendency to recur, both in the benign and malignant. Malignant lesions metastasise to lung and bone and may invade chest wall.
2. **Carcinoma** – a small group of carcinomas look 'benign' on mammography, medullary, encephaloid, mucoid, papillary.

NB. Any well-defined opacity >1.0cm in diameter should be subjected to ultrasound; if solid, biopsy should be performed.

10

10.8 MULTIPLE WELL-DEFINED SOFT-TISSUE OPACITIES

1. **Cysts**.
2. **Fibroadenomas** – 10–20% are multiple.
3. **Skin lesions** – e.g. neurofibromas.
4. **Silicone injections** – usually dense.
5. **Intramammary lymph nodes**.
6. **Metastases** – Melanoma most common, lymphoma second most common non-mammary breast tumour, then lung, ovarian, soft tissue sarcomas, GI/GU malignancy, carcinoid and sporadically thyroid, osteosarcoma, cervical vaginal and endometrial. Mean survival after diagnosis of metastasis within the breast is <1 year.

10.9 LARGE (>5 cm) WELL-DEFINED OPACITY

1. Giant cyst.
2. Giant fibroadenoma.
3. Lipoma.
4. Sebaceous cyst.
5. Cystosarcoma phylloides.

10.10 BENIGN CONDITIONS THAT MIMIC MALIGNANCY

1. **Microcalcification**
   (a) Sclerosing adenosis – one/both breasts, widely separated opacities.
2. **Suspicious soft-tissue opacity**
   (a) Fibroadenoma – when one margin ill-defined.
   (b) Fat necrosis – ill-defined, sometimes with radiolucent centre.
   (c) Post-biopsy scar.
   (d) Radial scar. 22% of excised radial scars show invasive cancer or DCIS not diagnosed at core biopsy and therefore excision generally recommended. Carries a 2× risk of developing a subsequent breast cancer in either breast and this increases to 4–5× risk if associated atypical ductal hyperplasia.
   (e) Plasma cell mastitis.
   (f) Haematoma.
   (g) Summation of normal tissues.
   (h) Irregular skin lesion, e.g. wart.

10.11 CARCINOMA

Primary features

1. **Opacity** – ill-defined, spiculated outline, comet tail. Usually dense.
2. **Microcalcification** – mixture of sizes, shapes; linear, branching, punctate cluster arrangement. Eccentric to and/or outside soft-tissue opacity.

Secondary features

1. **Distortion** – adjacent tissues, obliteration subcutaneous, retromammary spaces.
2. **Skin, nipple retraction**.
3. **Oedema** – all or part of breast.
4. **Halo** – wide around primary opacity.
5. **Duct dilatation**.
6. **Venous engorgement**.

NB Approximately 10% of palpable carcinomas in premenopausal women are not diagnosable on mammography, but this is likely to decrease with digital mammography.

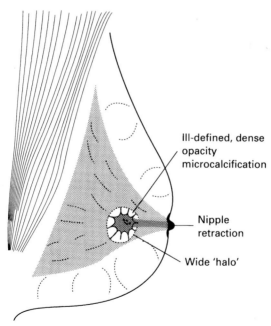

Ill-defined, dense opacity microcalcification

Nipple retraction

Wide 'halo'

Typical carcinoma

10

Risk factors for breast cancer

1. **Gender,** 100× more common in women.
2. **Age,** majority of cases occur after age of 50.
3. **Family history and genetic factors** (see below).
4. **Personal history of breast cancer,** 3–4× risk of developing a new cancer in the other breast or another part of the same breast.
5. **Previous chest irradiation.** Women who received mantle radiotherapy for Hodgkin's and non-Hodgkin's lymphoma have significantly higher risk and should undergo annual MRI screening.
6. **Early menarche, late menopause, nulliparity** and having first child after the age of 30 associated with slightly raised risk.
7. **Alcohol, obesity and physical inactivity.**

Family and genetic factors

1. **First-degree relative** (mother, sister, daughter) approx doubles risk, two first-degree relatives increase risk 5-fold, however 70–80% of women who develop breast cancer do not have a family history.
2. **Genetic factors** – 5–10% of all breast cancers, of which BRCA1 mutation accounts for 20–40%, Ch 17, autosomal dominant, lifetime risk of breast cancer is 50–85%. BRCA2 mutation accounts for 10–30%, Ch 13, autosomal dominant, lifetime risk of breast cancer is 50–85%. P53 mutation accounts for <1%. Li Fraumeni syndrome. Rare cause of breast cancer but individuals have a greater than 90% lifetime risk of developing breast cancer and at a young age. PTEN mutations account for <1%, Cowden syndrome, 25–50% lifetime risk of breast cancer. 30–70% are due to other gene mutations.

NB NICE guidance recommends offering annual mammographic screening for those at documented raised or higher risk from 40–49 years and that this should be digital in preference to conventional mammography when available. MRI surveillance annually in BRCA1 and BRCA2 mutation carriers from 30–39 and from 20 years or older with the P53 mutation.

10.12 OEDEMATOUS BREAST

Signs on mammography
1. Diffuse increased density.
2. Skin thickening (>1.5mm).
3. Coarse reticular pattern.
4. Prominent Cooper ligaments.

Causes
1. Inflammatory carcinoma.
2. Radiotherapy.
3. Lymphatic obstruction.
4. Venous obstruction.
5. Recent surgery.
6. Breast abscess.

10

10.13 ULTRASOUND IN BREAST DISEASE

Uses and indications

1. Assessing a palpable abnormality
   (a) In combination with mammography 97% sensitivity, 98.6% NPV.
   (b) Direct correlation of imaging and clinical findings.
   (c) Nodularity, a common cause of concern.
   (d) Initial modality in those <35.
2. Assessing a mammographic abnormality.
3. Assessment of nipple discharge, diagnosis of papilloma, DCIS may be diagnosed with US.
4. Biopsy guidance.
5. Guide aspiration of cysts/breast abscesses and insertion of drainage catheters.
6. Lesion localization for surgery, skin marking and wire localization of impalpable tumours.
7. Assessment of axillary adenopathy in proven cancers may preclude sentinel node imaging and avoid unnecessary second surgery for nodal clearance.
8. Distinguishing local recurrence from surgical scar.
9. Targetted/second-look US for MRI detected abnormality.
10. Vacuum-assisted biopsy devices are being used in many institutions for the removal of benign lesions such as fibroadenomas.

Typical appearances of carcinoma

1. **Poorly reflective mass.**
2. **Ill-defined mass.**
3. **Heterogeneous internal echo pattern.**
4. **Absent 'far wall' echoes.**
5. **Posterior acoustic shadowing.**

Typical appearances of simple cysts

1. **Round, oval in shape.**
2. **Well-defined.**
3. **Anechoic (echo-free).**
4. **Posterior wall enhancement.**
5. **Posterior acoustic enhancement.**

10.14 APPEARANCES AND FEATURES OF FIBROADENOMAS

1. Most common benign breast tumour and most common solid mass <35 years. 10–20% multiple and bilateral in 4%.
2. Palpable in up to 70%.
3. On US generally oval, but may be round, homogenous echotexture hypo/isoechoic. 2–4% contain small cystic foci. Posterior enhancement variable and can have posterior acoustic shadowing when hyalinized or contain calcium.
3. Tend to regress with age, undergo myxoid degeneration giving pathognomic 'popcorn' calcification on mammography.
4. Juvenile FA occur most commonly between 10–20 years, but majority of teenage fibroadenomas are of adult type. Juvenile FAs usually solitary.
5. Giant FA are >5 cm, may grow to 15cm, more common in African-American women.
6. Fibroadenomas are well described on treatment with ciclosporin A following renal transplantation and may be single, multiple or Giant in type.

10.15 GYNAECOMASTIA

1. 85% of all breast masses in males.
2. Bilateral in 63%.
3. Trimodal distribution – neonatal, pubertal and senescence.
4. Differential includes pseudogynaecomastia (fat rather than glandular tissue), diabetic mastopathy, male breast cancer.

10

Causes

1. **Drugs** – alcohol, amiodarone, alkylating agents, amphetamines, anabolic steroids, captopril, cimetidine, cocaine, diazepam, digoxin, haloperidol, heroin, izoniazid, marijuana, metronidazole, nifedipine, omeprazole, phenytoin, spironolactone, tricyclic antidepressants, thiazides, verapamil.
2. **Systemic causes** – chronic renal failure, cirrhosis, HIV, hypo and hyperthyroidism, refeeding gynaecomastia following nutritional deprivation.
3. **Tumours** – Germ cell, Leydig, Sertoli tumours; adrenal, liver, lung and renal (secondary to ectopic human chorionic gonadotrophin secretion)

10.16 MRI IN BREAST DISEASE

Performed using a dedicated phased array breast coil, ideally =1.5T. Performed in prone position with both breasts imaged simultaneously. Dynamic post-contrast imaging with subtraction of pre-contrast images. Scheduling examination 7–10 days after onset of last menstruation decreases background parenchymal enhancement. MRI is sensitive but not highly specific and may pick up lesions/areas of enhancement requiring further evaluation. MR biopsy is not widely available, targetted US often used to evaluate MR findings.

Indications

1. Evaluate local extent of cancer in those anticipating breast conservation when tumour size uncertain on conventional imaging.
2. Lobular carcinoma – typically mammographically occult and may be multifocal/bilateral.
3. Metastatic axillary adenopathy of unknown primary, may find occult breast cancer.
4. High risk screening, those with history of mantle radiotherapy or genetic mutation.
5. Evaluation of implant integrity.
6. Monitor response to neoadjuvant chemotherapy.
7. Problem solving tool. Possible suspicious finding on conventional imaging, should not be used to preclude biopsy.

Further Reading

Baker JA, Soo MS, Rosen EL. Artifacts and pitfalls in sonographic imaging of the breast. Am J Roentgenol 2001;176:1261–6.

Lister D, Evans AJ, Burrell HC et al. The accuracy of breast ultrasound in the evaluation of clinically benign, discrete symptomatic breast lumps. Clin Radiol 1998;53:490–2.

Smith DN. Breast ultrasound. Radiol Clin North Am 2001;39(3):485–97.

Berg WA et al. Diagnostic imaging: breast. Amirsys, Salt Lake City, 2006.

National Institute for Health and Clinical Excellence. CG41 Familial breast cancer – full guideline (October 2006). NICE, London, 2006

Leach MO, Boggis CR, Dixon AK et al. MARIBS study group. Screening with magnetic resonance imaging and mammography of a UK population at high familial risk of breast cancer: a prospective multicentre cohort study (MARIBS). Lancet 2005;365(9473):1769–78.

11

Face and neck

Neil Stoodley

11.1 ORBITAL MASS LESIONS

Many lesions are inflammatory and/or vascular. Therefore enhancement following contrast is common and not a useful discriminatory feature. Classification by site: globe or relationship to muscle cone

Lesions involving the globe

1. **Retinoblastoma** – usually presents with white pupil; 20–40% bilateral, 10% have family history; four main subgroups:
   (a) Sporadic.
   (b) Inherited: autosomal dominant.
   (c) Chromosomal: associated with partial deletion of chromosome 13.
   (d) 'Trilateral' retinoblastoma: bilateral retinoblastoma with pineal tumour.

90% show (various patterns of) calcification.

2. **Melanoma** – increased incidence from middle age; avidly enhances; may be high signal on pre-contrast T_1 if melanotic.
3. **Retinal detachment with choroidal effusion**.

Intraconal lesions

1. **Optic nerve glioma** – painless visual loss; in NF1 other soft tissue neurofibromas may be evident or hamartomatous lesions in brain.
2. **Optic nerve meningioma**.
3. **Haemangioma (usually cavernous) or AVM (rarer)**.
4. **Orbital pseudotumour** – inflammatory mass can involve nerve and/ or muscle.

5. Metastases.
6. Lymphoma.
7. Haematoma.
8. Isolated neurofibroma.

Conal lesions

1. **Orbital pseudotumour.**
2. **Thyroid eye disease** – enlargement of muscles; swelling of intraorbital fat.
3. **Rhabdomyosarcoma** – 10% arise in orbit, 50% less than 7 years of age; rapid onset proptosis with deviation of globe; although arises in muscle most of tumour usually extraconal; differentiation between orbital and extra-orbital (parameningeal) origin important as treatment differs.

Extraconal lesions

1. **Orbital cellulitis and abscess** – coronal sections with contrast most sensitive esp. for small subperiosteal collections; secondary to paranasal sinus infection.
2. **Lymphoma.**
3. **Metastases.**
4. **Dermoid** – commonest at external angle.
5. **Lymphangioma/lymphaemangioma.**
6. **Direct extension of lacrimal gland tumour.**
7. **Langerhans cell histiocytosis.**
8. **Direct extension of ethmoidal or maxillary antrum tumour.**
9. **Paranasal sinus mucocoele.**

Further Reading

Kantarci M, Karasen RM, Alper F et al. Remarkable anatomic variations in paranasal sinus region and their clinical importance. Eur J Radiol 2004; 50(3):296–302.

11.2 OPTIC NERVE GLIOMA V OPTIC NERVE SHEATH MENINGIOMA. CLINICAL AND RADIOLOGICAL DIFFERENTIATION

Glioma	Meningioma
50% less than 5 years of age	Usually middle-aged women
± Bilateral	Usually unilateral
Slowly progressive, painless loss of vision; central scotoma. Childhood tumours may remain quiescent for years, particularly in the presence of NF. Adult tumours are aggressive.	Slowly progressive, painless loss of vision; proptosis
Neurofibromatosis* NF1 in 25%; 15% of NF1 have optic nerve glioma; bilateral disease strongly suggests neurofibromatosis.	Neurofibromatosis (1 or 2) in 4–6%; bilateral disease may occur with or without NF.
No orbital hyperostosis	Hyperostosis
Widened optic canal in 90% but intracranial extension is unusual	Widened optical canal in 10%
Kinking and buckling of the optic nerve is common. Smooth outline	Straight optic nerve, but tumour may be eccentric
Well-defined margins	More infiltrative Localized or fusiform thickening
Calcification rare without prior radiotherapy	Calcification (linear, plaque-like or granular) are more common
Isointense to brain on T_1W MRI; Hyperintense on T_2W MRI	Similar signal to optic nerve on most unenhanced MR pulse sequences
Variable contrast enhancement with mottled lucencies due to mucinous degeneration	Diffuse homogeneous enhancement ± serrated margins
	Negative image of optic nerve within the tumour (tram-track sign)

Further Reading

Hollander MD, FitzPatrick M, O'Connor SG et al. Optic gliomas. Radiol Clin North Am 1999;37(1):59–71.

Mafee MF, Goodwin J, Dorodi S. Optic nerve sheath meningiomas. Radiol Clin North Am 1999;37(1):37–58.

11

11.3 ENLARGED ORBIT

1. **Neurofibromatosis**: dysplasia of sphenoid wing.
2. **Congenital glaucoma** (buphthalmos).
3. **Long-standing space occupying lesion.**

11.4 BARE ORBIT

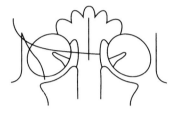

1. **Neurofibromatosis.**
2. **Lytic metastasis.**
3. **Meningioma.**

11.5 ENLARGED OPTIC FORAMEN

Normal range = 4.4–6 mm; 7+mm, or greater than 1 mm difference with asymptomatic side = abnormal.

Concentric enlargement

1. **Optic nerve glioma** – 25% associated with neurofibromatosis.
2. **Neurofibroma.**
3. **Extension of orbital tumour.**
4. **Vascular**: ophthalmic artery aneurysm, AVM.
5. **Granuloma**: sarcoidosis or pseudotumour.

Focal defect

1. **Adjacent tumour.**
2. **Adjacent mucocoele.**
3. **Raised intracranial pressure** (can cause thinning of orbital roof).

11.6 ENLARGED SUPERIOR ORBITAL FISSURE

1. **Normal variant.**
2. **Neurofibromatosis.**
3. **Extension of intracranial lesion:**
   (a) Meningioma.
   (b) Infraclinoid aneurysm (usually associated with erosion of inferior aspect of anterior clinoid).
   (c) Parasellar chordoma.
4. **Sphenoid wing lytic metastasis.**
5. **Extension of orbital lesion:**
   (a) AVM.
   (b) Haemangioma.
   (c) Orbital meningioma.
   (d) Lymphoma.

11.7 INTRAORBITAL CALCIFICATION

Within the globe

1. **Cataract.**
2. **Retinoblastoma.**
3. **Previous trauma.**
4. **Previous infection.**

Outside the globe

1. **Phleboliths** – usually associated with AVM.
2. **Orbital meningioma.**
3. **Neurofibroma.**
4. **Intraorbital dermoid.**
5. **Carcinoma of the lacrimal gland.**

11

11.8 ORBITAL HYPEROSTOSIS

1. **Meningioma.**
2. **Sclerotic metastases.**
3. **Fibrous dysplasia.**
4. **Paget's disease.**
5. **Osteopetrosis.**
6. **Chronic osteomyelitis.**
7. **Lacrimal gland tumour.**
8. **Langerhans cell histiocytosis.**
9. **Post radiotherapy.**

Further Reading

Chung EM, Smirniotopoulos JG, Specht CS et al. From the archives of the AFIP: Pediatric orbit tumors and tumorlike lesions: nonosseous lesions of the extraocular orbit. Radiographics 2007;27(6):1777–99.

Chung EM, Specht CS, Schroeder JW. From the archives of the AFIP: Pediatric orbit tumors and tumorlike lesions: neuroepithelial lesions of the ocular globe and optic nerve. Radiographics 2007;27(4):1159–86.

11.9 SMALL OR ABSENT SINUSES

Congenital

1. **Normal variant** (5% of population).
2. **Congenital hypothyroidism.**
3. **Down's syndrome** (frontal sinuses absent in 90%).
4. **Kartagener's syndrome.**

Acquired

Secondary to overgrowth of bony wall

1. **Paget's disease.**
2. **Fibrous dysplasia.**
3. **Haemolytic anaemias.**
4. **Post operative.**

11.10 OPAQUE MAXILLARY ANTRUM

Traumatic
1. Fracture.
2. Overlying soft tissue swelling.
3. Post-operative.
4. Epistaxis.
5. Barotrauma.

Inflammatory
1. Sinusitis.
2. Allergy.
3. Mucocoele.

Neoplastic
1. **Carcinoma**; usually associated with bony destruction and soft tissue mass.
2. **Lymphoma.**

Other
1. Fibrous dysplasia.
2. **Cysts**: dentigerous or mucous retention cysts.
3. Wegener's granulomatosis.
4. Anatomical.
5. **Radiographic**: over tilted view.

11.11 MASS IN MAXILLARY ANTRUM

1. **Cyst**
   (a) Mucous retention cyst; often arises from floor.
   (b) Dentigerous cyst: expands up into floor of antrum; displaced tooth may be seen in antrum.
2. **Trauma**: herniation of orbital muscle through fracture.
3. **Neoplastic**
   (a) Polyp.
   (b) Carcinoma.
4. **Wegener's granulomatosis**: usually presents in 40–50-year-olds; mucosal thickening progresses to formation of soft tissue mass with extensive bony destruction.

11

11.12 CYSTIC LESIONS IN THE MANDIBLE/MAXILLA

Dental

1. **Periodontal/periapical/radicular cyst**: develops in carious tooth; well defined lucency with thin sclerotic margin at tooth apex.
2. **Dentigerous cyst**: adjacent to crown of unerupted tooth; well defined uni- or multilocular; multiple cysts in Gorlin's syndrome.

Non-dental

1. **Developmental cysts.**
2. **Hyperparathyroidism**: brown tumours.
3. **Ameloblastoma**: commonest in mandible (80%), usually near angle; slow growing painless mass; well defined uni- or multilocular expansile mass. May extend through cortex.
4. **Langerhans cell histiocytosis.**
5. **Aneurysmal bone cyst.**
6. **Giant cell tumour.**
7. **Haemangioma.**
8. **Metastases.**
9. **Fibrous dysplasia.**
10. **Bone cyst**: may be post traumatic; unilocular asymptomatic cyst; indistinct borders.

Further Reading

Kaneda T, Minami M, Kurabayashi T. Benign odontogenic tumors of the mandible and maxilla. Neuroimaging Clin N Am 2003;13(3):495–507.

Weber AL, Bui C, Kaneda T. Malignant tumors of the mandible and maxilla. Neuroimaging Clin N Am 2003;13(3):509–24.

11.13 'FLOATING' TEETH

1. **Severe periodontal disease.**
2. **Langerhans cell histiocytosis.**
3. **Hyperparathyroidism.**
4. **Metastases.**
5. **Myeloma.**

11.14 LOSS OF LAMINA DURA OF TEETH

Generalized

1. **Osteoporosis.**
2. **Hyperparathyroidism.**
3. **Cushing's syndrome.**
4. **Osteomalacia.**
5. **Paget's disease.**
6. **Scleroderma**: thickened periodontal membrane.

Focal

1. **Local infection.**
2. **Leukaemia.**
3. **Metastasis.**
4. **Myeloma.**
5. **Langerhans cell histiocytosis.**
6. **Burkitt's lymphoma.**

11.15 NASOPHARYNGEAL MASS

1. **Adenoidal hypertrophy.**
2. **Trauma**: haematoma.
3. **Infection**: abscess confined above C2 level by strong attachment of pre-vertebral fascia.
4. **Benign neoplasm**
   (a) Angiofibroma.
   (b) Antro-choanal polyp.
5. **Malignant neoplasm**
   (a) Nasopharyngeal carcinoma.
   (b) Lymphoma.
   (c) Rhabdomyosarcoma.
   (d) Plasmacytoma.
   (e) Direct extension of paranasal sinus tumour.
6. **Encephalocoele**: midline defect on skull base with herniation of meninges and brain.

11

Further Reading

Weber AL, al-Arayedh S, Rashid A Nasopharynx: clinical, pathologic and radiologic assessment. Neuroimaging Clin N Am 2003;13(3):465–83.

11.16 PRE-VERTEBRAL SOFT-TISSUE MASS IN AN ADULT ON LATERAL CERVICAL X-RAY

1. **Trauma.**
2. **Abscess.**
3. **Post-cricoid carcinoma.**
4. **Lymphoma.**
5. **Chordoma.**
6. **Pharyngeal pouch:** air/fluid level.
7. **Retropharyngeal goitre.**

Further Reading
Turkington JR, Paterson A, Sweeney LE et al. Neck masses in children. Br J Radiol 2005;78(925):75–78.

Connor SE, Flis C, Langdon JD. Vascular masses of the head and neck. Clin Radiol 2005;60(8):856–68.

11.17 PHOTOPENIC AREAS IN RADIONUCLIDE THYROID IMAGING

Localized

1. **Colloid cyst.**
2. **Adenoma:** non-functioning.
3. **Carcinoma:** medullary may be bilateral.
4. **Multinodular goitre.**
5. **Local thyroiditis:** may show increased uptake.
   (a) Acute.
   (b) De Quervain's.
   (c) Hashimoto's.
   (d) Riedel's.
6. **Vascular.**
7. **Abscess.**
8. **Artefact.**

Generalized

1. **Concurrent medication.**
2. **Hypothyroidism.**
3. **Ectopic hormone production.**
4. **De Quervain's thyroiditis.**
5. **Ectopic thyroid.**

12

Skull and brain

Neil Stoodley

12.1 ACUTE ARTERIAL INFARCT: CT

1. Initial appearances often normal in first few hours. Larger infarcts more conspicuous.
2. Initial signs:
   (a) Low density with reduced grey/white differentiation (cell and tissue swelling): wedge shaped involving grey and white matter; 'insular ribbon sign' (loss of g/w differentiation in perisylvian region; loss of normal anatomical differentiation of basal ganglia).
   (b) Mass effect: local (sulcal effacement).
   (c) Hyperdense vessels due to thrombus (luminal/mural); usually middle cerebral or basilar arteries (mural calcification may mimic hyperdense artery sign).
3. Later signs:
   (a) More extensive area of low attenuation or progressive decreased attenuation.
   (b) Generalized mass effect (ventricular or basal cistern effacement $\pm$ midline shift [subfalcine herniation] or other herniation syndromes: uncal, transtentorial).
   (c) Secondary haemorrhagic transformation (usually occurs after a few days unless anticoagulated; reperfusion injury) if haemorrhage from outset consider embolus or venous stroke.
4. Contrast enhancement usually unhelpful and often confusing; simply reflects breakdown of blood–brain barrier. Any enhancement pattern possible.
5. CT perfusion study may demonstrate decreased perfusion in wider area of brain (ischaemic penumbra) suggesting further tissue at risk.
6. CT angiography can demonstrate dissection/stenosis/occlusion (embolic or thrombotic).

12.2 ACUTE ARTERIAL INFARCT: MRI

1. More sensitive than CT but signs similar (reduced attenuation on CT = increased T_2 signal on MRI). Wedge shaped; grey and white matter involvement; often initially cortical change). Signal change usually (but not always) evident within 3–6 hours (within minutes on diffusion weighted imaging [DWI]). Increased T_2 signal due to cytotoxic oedema (cell swelling; restricted diffusion).
2. Acute infarcts show increased DWI signal and low ADC (apparent diffusion coefficient). Low ADC signal 'pseudonormalizes' i.e. becomes bright at around 7–10 days post-infarct.
3. Mass effect: local and/or general as on CT.
4. Absent flow voids in affected major vessels; increased signal on T_2 and FLAIR; most often seen in MCA (check carotid canal at skull base) or basilar.
5. Contrast enhancement may be confusing as on CT; prolonged transit time of contrast through distal or collateral vessels may be seen on post-gadolinium T_1 sequences.
6. Perfusion weighted imaging may show poor perfusion in wider territory than changes on standard sequences: diffusion/perfusion mismatch may demonstrate ischaemic penumbra representing potentially salvageable brain tissue.
7. MR angiography may show vessel stenosis/occlusion in extra- or intracranial vessels.

12.3 VENOUS INFARCTS

1. Usually secondary to venous sinus thrombosis:
   (a) CT: hyperdense and expanded sinus precontrast; peripheral enhancement around luminal thrombus postcontrast (delta sign).
   (b) MR: absence of normal flow void: acute thrombus high signal on T_1 (methaemoglobin); variable signal on T_2; (beware normal variation in venous sinus anatomy with areas of hypoplasia).
   (c) Check for evidence of underlying cause on scans (mastoid infection, paranasal sinus infection etc).
2. If an area of infarction seen which is not in arterial distribution consider sinus thrombosis.
3. Venous infarction often haemorrhagic (but this is not a contraindication to anticoagulation; aim of anticoagulation is to stop propagation of thrombus).
4. Beware symmetrical low attenuation in deep grey matter structures (especially thalami); suggests involvement of deep cerebral veins which may not otherwise be seen on scans.

12.4 INDICATIONS FOR CT AND MR IMAGING IN ACUTE STROKE

Indications for CT in suspected stroke

1. Early diagnosis if possible.
2. Differentiation between ischaemic and haemorrhagic stroke (overt haemorrhage a contraindication to thrombolysis).
3. Exclusion of stroke mimics: tumour, other space occupying lesions e.g. extra-axial haematoma.

Indications for MRI in suspected stroke

1. If CT normal but clinical suspicion high, MRI more sensitive for early detection.
2. Assessment of diffusion/perfusion mismatch and suitability for thrombolysis.
3. Detection of stroke in distribution not well seen on CT (vertebro-basilar circulation in posterior fossa especially).
4. Detection of underlying cause such as arterial dissection or thrombosis (absent flow voids on standard sequences; narrowing/occlusion on MR angiography).
5. Assessment of intra- and extracranial vessels by MR angiography.
6. Exclusion of venous sinus thrombosis.

12.5 DIFFERENTIATION BETWEEN INFARCT AND TUMOUR

1. **Clinical history**: abrupt v gradual onset and development of symptoms.
2. **Distribution**: tumours not confined to vascular territory.
3. **Shape**: infarcts usually wedge shaped with base at periphery; tumours *tend* to be spherical/ovoid.
4. **Tissue involvement**: infarcts involve grey and white matter; most metastases or higher grade gliomas involve white matter primarily; lower grade primary tumours may involve grey matter.
5. **Advanced imaging techniques** such as DWI or MR spectroscopy may be useful in cases which remain unclear on standard sequences.

12

12.6 APPEARANCES OF BLOOD ON SCANS

CT

Blood changes appearance with time as haemoglobin breaks down but rate of change variable depending on factors such as:

(a) Where blood is (intraparenchymal v extra-axial).
(b) Haemoglobin level at time of haemorrhage (acute blood may not be bright if patient severely anaemic).
(c) Volume of haematoma.
(d) Normal clotting function.
(e) Haematoma is discrete collection of blood and not mixed with other fluids such as CSF.

In general:

1. **Acute** = higher attenuation than underlying brain (soon after episode of bleeding for up to 7–10 days).
2. **Subacute** = similar attenuation to underlying brain (transition usually occurs between 1–2 weeks).
3. **Chronic** = lower attenuation than underlying brain (suggests at least 2–3 weeks old but could be older).

MR

Similar change in appearances with time but due to different magnetic properties of blood breakdown products. Typical age ranges given below but these not absolute and again depend on discrete collection of blood and not mixture of different fluids.

1. Oxyhaemoglobin: iso/hypointense T_1; hyperintense T_2 (less than 24 hours approx).
2. Deoxyhaemoglobin: iso/hypointense T_1; hypointense T_2 (1–3 days approx).
3. Intracellular methaemoglobin: hyperintense T_1; hypointense T_2 (3–7 days approx).
4. Extracellular methaemoglobin: hyperintense T_1; hyperintense T_2 (1–2+ weeks approx).
5. Haemosiderin: isointense/hypointense T_1; hypointense T_2.

Further Reading

Srinivasan A, Goyal M, Al Azri F et al. State of the art imaging of acute stroke. Radiographics 2006;26(Suppl 1):S75–95.

Muir KW, Buchan A, von Kummer R et al. Imaging of acute stroke. Lancet Neurol 2006;5(9):755–68.

12.7 SUBARACHNOID HAEMORRHAGE

Causes

1. **Ruptured intracranial aneurysm** (75%): potentially devastating condition with 50% immediate mortality and high long-term morbidity.
2. **Bleeding from vascular malformation** (cerebral or spinal) (5%).
3. **Trauma**: tends to have peripheral distribution in sulci rather than concentrated in basal cisterns.
4. **Extension from parenchymal haematoma** (often hypertensive bleed) (5%).
5. **Perimesencephalic haemorrhage**: low pressure probable venous haemorrhage; few symptoms and signs and good prognosis.
6. **Miscellaneous**: anticoagulants, vasculopathy.

Diagnosis and investigation

1. **CT**: most sensitive in first few days (98% on day 1, 50% positive by 7 days). Check review areas on scans: anterior interhemispheric fissure, Sylvian fissure, posterior horns of lateral ventricles, third ventricle, basal cisterns, foramen magnum. CT angiography may be performed.
2. **Lumbar puncture**: negative CT scan does not exclude SAH, especially if scan performed days after ictus, therefore LP mandatory if CT negative.
3. **Late MRI more sensitive than CT** (proton density, gradient echo T_2 and FLAIR sequences most sensitive.
4. **Catheter angiography** now used less often in initial work-up as CT angiography often used at time of diagnosis of aneurysmal SAH and for planning therapy (neurointerventional v surgical).

Complications

1. **High mortality and morbidity.**
2. **Hydrocephalus** (communicating, obstructive or combination).
3. **Vasospasm leading to ischaemia** (often reversible).
4. **Infarction.**

12

Further Reading

van Gijn J, Kerr RS, Rinkel GJ. Subarachnoid haemorrhage. Lancet 2007;369 (9558):306–18.

U-King-Im JM, Koo B, Trivedi RA et al. Current diagnostic approaches to subarachnoid hemorrhage. Eur Radiol 2005;15(6):1135–47.

12.8 INTRACRANIAL ANEURYSMS

Presentation

1. **Sudden onset** of severe headache ± neurological signs ± reduced level of consciousness with scan findings of:
   (a) Subarachnoid haemorrhage.
   (b) Parenchymal haemorrhage (usually with associated subarachnoid haemorrhage).
   (c) Intraventricular haemorrhage (most often secondary to bleeding in the general subarachnoid space, occasionally primary).
2. **Mass effect**
   (a) Cranial nerve palsies (esp. III palsy with posterior communication artery aneurysm).
   (b) Horner's syndrome.
   (c) Brain stem dysfunction.
   (d) Hydrocephalus.
3. **Thromboembolic events**
4. **Incidental finding** on scan performed for another reason.

Incidence in general population ~2–3%. Overall risk of rupture = 0.5–1.5% per annum: variable according to size and position of aneurysm, sex, smoking etc.

Diagnosis

1. **CT and CTA**: extra-axial mass in subarachnoid space; enhances if patent; may be thrombosed and/or have calcification (especially giant aneurysms). CTA demonstrates site and morphology of aneurysm and may allow planning of treatment (neurointervention v surgery) without need for catheter angiography.
2. **MR and MRA**: patent aneurysm will show flow void; giant or partially thrombosed aneurysms can show complex flow patterns with heterogeneous signals on standard sequences. Not reliable for treatment planning.
3. **Catheter angiography**: invasive with 0.1–0.5% inherent stroke risk. Still considered gold standard but may soon be superseded by CTA.

12.9 VASCULAR MALFORMATIONS

Two main types: those with arteriovenous shunts and those without shunts.

Malformations with AV shunts:

1. **Arteriovenous malformations** – present in young–middle-age adults with one or combination of haemorrhage (40%), seizures (30%), neurological deficit or headache (20%). Annual cumulative rupture risk ~3% per year. Consist of one or more arterial pedicles draining directly to enlarged draining veins through nidus. Multiple lesions in various syndromes e.g. Osler–Weber–Rendu and Wyburn–Mason.
   (a) *CT*: hyperdense enlarged serpiginous vessels; often speckled calcification; enhance strongly.
   (b) *MR*: serpiginous flow voids; may be evidence of local atrophy and gliosis or previous haemorrhage.
   (c) *Catheter angiography*: gold standard for assessment of morphology and nidal architecture including presence of associated arterial or venous aneurysms, varices and stenoses.
2. **Dural arteriovenous fistulas** – acquired lesions presenting in older population (50–70 years) compared to AVMs (20–40 years). Occur following damage to venous structures (post-thrombosis, surgery, trauma). Symptoms and signs secondary to arterialization of venous system: bruit, venous hypertension, pulsatile tinnitus (if primary involvement is sinuses); haemorrhage, focal neurology, seizures (if primary or major secondary involvement of cortical veins). Caroticocavernous fistula may give rise to proptosis and chemosis.
   (a) *CT*: often normal unless complications e.g. haemorrhage; enlargement of cavernous sinus and superior ophthalmic veins if carotico-cavernous fistula.
   (b) *MR*: standard sequences often normal unless complication; dynamic subtraction angiography demonstrates lesions well.
   (c) *Catheter angiography*: still gold standard for diagnosis and demonstration of morphology on which classification and treatment planning based.

Malformations without AV shunts

1. **Cavernous angioma** (cavernoma) – sinusoidal spaces lined with endothelium; occur anywhere in CNS, commonest pons. Present with small haemorrhages (not associated with large haemorrhages) or seizures; often incidental findings. Multiple cavernomas may be familial.
   (a) *CT*: iso/hyperdense lesion, often calcification.
   (b) *MR*: characteristic appearance is heterogeneous signal centre with low T_2 signal (haemosiderin) rim. Gradient echo most sensitive sequence for detection.

12

2. **Developmental venous anomaly** (venous angioma) – probably due to persistent embryonic veins which drain normal brain. Not thought to have increased haemorrhage risk.
   (a) *CT*: enhanced scans may show linear vein draining to ependymal lining of ventricle or cortex with umbrella shaped leash of vessels draining toward anomalous vein.
   (b) *MR*: as above but larger lesions may be visible on non-enhanced scans as flow void.

12.10 CNS INFECTION

Meningitis

Diagnosis made by lumbar puncture not imaging. Indications for neuroimaging in possible meningitis are to assess complications: ischaemia/infarction, hydrocephalus, venous thrombosis, subdural empyema, ventriculitis and cerebral abscess.

1. **Bacterial meningitis** – CT usually normal. May see generalized brain swelling and/or focal or generalized ischaemia. Scanning only post-contrast may mask pathology. If contrast to be used, pre- and post-contrast scans should be obtained. Lack of enhancement does not exclude meningitis. Hydrocephalus may be communicating and/or obstructive.
2. **Subdural effusion or empyema** – low attenuation extra-axial collection which may or may not show rim enhancement. May be very subtle, especially if parafalcine. Parafalcine empyemas rapidly lead to sinus thrombosis. If frontal look at frontal sinuses carefully.
3. **Cerebritis** – diffuse area of parenchymal low attenuation which may develop into abscess.
4. **Abscess** – thin-walled rim enhancing lesion; may be very little systemic evidence of cerebral abscess.
5. **Viral meningitis** – neuroimaging usually entirely normal in viral meningitis.

Encephalitis and encephalitis like disorders

Usually viral or post-viral. Herpes simplex (HSV) is the commonest causative organism in developed world. May cause rapidly progressive necrotizing encephalitis affecting whole brain in neonates and infants but with predilection for limbic system in older children and adults.

1. **CT**: less sensitive than MRI, often normal in early HSV encephalitis; low attenuation in medial temporal lobes later usually unilateral; may be haemorrhagic.

2. **MRI**: increased T_2 signal in medial temporal lobes, insula, cingulate gyrus; usually bilateral but asymmetrical. Atrophy, gliosis and encephalomalacia long-term.

Slow viruses

1. **Subacute sclerosing panencephalitis** (SSPE): progressive increased T_2 signal and atrophy several years after primary measles infection.
2. **Rasmussen's encephalitis**: progressive neurological deficits and intractable seizures in children; increased T_2 signal and atrophy in one cerebral hemisphere.

Prion diseases

1. **Sporadic Creutzfeldt–Jakob disease** (CJD): rapidly progressive dementing illness associated with myoclonus, ataxia, pyramidal and extra-pyramidal signs, cortical blindness.
   MRI: increased T_2 and FLAIR signal in caudate and putamen (corpus striatum); less often signal change in thalamus, globus pallidus and periacqueductal grey.
2. **Variant CJD**: sensory disturbances, depression, abnormal eye movements and involuntary movements.
   MRI: increased T_2 and FLAIR signal in pulvinar nuclei of thalamus (hockey stick sign).

12.11 HIV AND THE BRAIN

HIV is a neurotropic virus that can affect the brain directly or can predispose to opportunistic infection (commonest toxoplasma, Cryptococcus, progressive multifocal leukoencephalopathy). Increased incidence of intracerebral lymphoma.

Infections

Viral
1. **HIV**: progressive dementia and atrophy due to subacute encephalitis.
   (a) CT: diffuse white matter low attenuation.
   (b) MRI: diffuse/patchy white matter high T_2 signal, may involve basal ganglia. Mass effect and contrast enhancement usually absent.
3. **Cytomegalovirus**: typically signal abnormalities seen in periventricular distribution.

12

4. **Progressive multifocal leukencephalopathy** (PML); papovavirus infection.
   (a) MRI: multifocal/confluent, asymmetrical increased T_2 signal in white matter; mass effect minimal if at all, grey matter spared, no atrophy.

Fungal
1. **Cryptococcus**: meningitis spread along perivascular spaces.
   (a) MRI: multiple focal areas of increased T_2 signal in basal ganglia and brain stem.
2. **Aspergillus and Candida** are rare in HIV; commoner in other immunocompromised groups e.g. bone marrow transplants.

Protozoal
1. **Toxoplasma**: multiple small nodules or ring enhancing lesions in basal ganglia, thalami and grey-white junction. May mimic lymphoma but multiple lesions more suggestive of toxo.

Bacterial
Typical pyogenic infections.

1. **TB**: tuberculous meningitis with leptomeningeal thickening, hydrocephalus, perforating vessel infarcts, cerebritis and abscess.

Tumour

1. **Lymphoma**: periventricular location with subependymal spread suggestive of lymphoma instead of toxoplasmosis. Lymphoma in HIV can cavitate prior to treatment and be ring enhancing (cf. immunocompetent).

12.12 CONGENITAL CNS INFECTIONS

1. **CMV**: damages germinal matrix causing periventricular calcification. Earlier infection leads to more extensive damage.
2. **Toxoplasmosis**: focal areas of calcification more widespread than with CMV and involve basal ganglia, periventricular regions and cortex.
3. **Rubella**: microcephaly, parenchymal calcification and atrophy.
4. **HIV**: diffuse cerebral atrophy; may cause calcification of basal ganglia after first year.

12.13 HEAD INJURY

Primary effects

1. **Fracture**: impact head injury; commonest = linear; complex fractures (diastatic, stellate, depressed) tend to occur with mechanisms involving greater degrees of force; skull base fractures may be occult (look for secondary clues such as fluid in sphenoid sinus or mastoid air cells; pneumocephalus); facial nerve palsy or ossicular disruption in temporal fractures.
2. **Extradural haemorrhage**: usually arterial bleed (middle meningeal); biconvex lentiform haematoma (limited by coronal and lambdoid sutures as inner layer of dura bound to sutures but may cross sagittal suture); mixed attenuation haematoma may mean ongoing bleeding.
3. **Subdural haemorrhage**: usually venous low pressure bleed; crescentic biconcave collection over cerebral hemisphere (can cross coronal and lambdoid but not usually sagittal sutures).
4. **Subarachnoid haemorrhage**: post-traumatic SAH usually low volume scattered bleeds; peripheral distribution.
5. **Contusions**: larger mixed attenuation (CT) or signal (MR) intra-axial lesions; tend to occur in inferior frontal and anterior temporal lobes (impact against bony anterior walls of anterior and middle cranial fossae); usually surrounding oedema adding to mass effect.
6. **Diffuse axonal injury**: smaller lesions than contusions; shearing injury secondary to rotational or acceleration/deceleration forces; tend to be widespread occurring at grey-white junction, corpus callosum, internal capsule and brain stem.
   - (a) CT: may be normal even with extensive DAI; scattered low attenuation lesions at grey-white junction (high attenuation if haemorrhagic).
   - (b) MRI: much more sensitive than CT (by at least factor of 10); gradient echo T_2 most sensitive sequence.

Secondary effects

1. **Cerebral oedema and ischaemia**: may lead to cerebral herniation syndromes.
2. **Subfalcine**: midline shift which can give rise to ischaemia in distribution of anterior cerebral artery; contralateral hydrocephalus with obstruction at foramen of Munro.
3. **Uncal**: medial aspect of medial temporal lobe presses on 3rd nerve (fixed dilated pupil).
4. **Transtentorial**: descending transtentorial herniation causes brain stem distortion and ischaemia in distribution of posterior cerebral artery.
5. **Coning**.
6. **Embolic complications if arterial damage** (dissection).

12

Delayed effects

1. **Atrophy**: focal (following contusion etc); generalized (following DAI or large extra-axial haematomas which required surgical evacuation).
2. **CSF leak**: secondary to fractures of frontal sinus, anterior cranial fossa, sphenoid sinus, temporal bone.
3. **Arteriovenous fistula**: direct carotico-cavernous fistula.
4. **Pseudoaneurysm**: following arterial wall tear.
5. **Leptomeningeal cyst**: dura trapped within fracture line, CSF pulsation prevents fracture healing leading to 'growing fracture'.

Further Reading

Davis PC; Expert Panel on Neurologic Imaging. Head trauma. Am J Neuroradiol 2007;28(8):1619–21.
Gallagher CN, Hutchinson PJ, Pickard JD. Neuroimaging in trauma. Curr Opin Neurol 2007;20(4):403–9.
Jaspan T, Griffiths PD, McConachie NS et al. Neuroimaging for non-accidental head injury: a proposed protocol. Clin Radiol 2003;58(1):44–53.
Stoodley N. Neuroimaging in non-accidental head injury: if, when, why and how. Clin Radiol 2005;60(1):22–30.

12.14 HYDROCEPHALUS

Large ventricles not always due to increased CSF volume: cerebral atrophic processes can lead to relative enlargement of ventricles; ventricles may be congenitally large (probably secondary to reduced white matter volume).

Hydrocephalus more likely if:

1. Commensurate enlargement of temporal horns.
2. Ventricles disproportionately enlarged compared to sulci.
3. Effacement of third ventricular recesses.
4. Evidence of CSF transudation (periventricular).

Increased CSF volume may be due to:

1. Over-production.
2. Obstruction of flow (non-communicating/obstructive).
3. Reduced CSF resorption (communicating).

CSF overproduction

1. **Choroid plexus tumours** (papilloma, carcinoma).

Non-communicating/obstructive

Pattern of ventricular enlargement depends on level of obstruction: intraventricular, foramen of Munro, third ventricle, aqueduct, fourth ventricle.

Congenital
1. **Aqueduct stenosis**.
2. **Colloid cyst**.

Acquired
1. **Tumours**: intraventricular and extraventricular (intra-axial and extra-axial).
2. **Haemorrhage**.
3. **Ventriculitis** (complication of meningitis or surgery; post-haemorrhagic).

Communicating

No obstruction to CSF flow but poor resorption through arachnoid granulations secondary to:

1. **Post-haemorrhagic** (esp. subarachnoid).
2. **Bacterial meningitis**.
3. **Malignant meningitis**.
4. **Increased venous pressure** (venous obstruction, vein of Galen malformation).

12.15 PNEUMOCEPHALUS

1. **Trauma**: compound fractures of vault, fractures involving paranasal sinuses or mastoid air cells.
2. **Post-operative**.
3. **Osteoma of paranasal sinus** (esp. ethmoid) may erode through sinus wall.
4. **Other sinus or skull base erosive tumours**.
5. **Empty sella**: rare complication = development of communication between sella and sphenoid sinus.

12

12.16 CT ATTENUATION OF CEREBRAL MASSES

Relative to normal brain (masses with variable appearances not included).

Hyperdense

1. **Tumour**
   (a) Meningioma (95%).
   (b) Medulloblastoma (80%).
   (c) Metastases (renal, thyroid, melanoma, mucinous adenocarcinoma).
   (d) Lymphoma (highly cellular, often deep mass, does not cavitate unless on treatment or immunocompromised).
   (e) Pituitary adenoma (25%).
   (f) Craniopharyngioma (if predominantly solid).
   (g) Ependymoma.
   (h) Choroid plexus tumour.
2. **Haematoma** (up to around 7–10 days old).
3. **Giant aneurysm**.
4. **Colloid cyst** (50%).

Isodense

1. **Tumour**
   (a) Vestibular schwannoma (95%).
   (b) Pituitary adenoma (65%).
2. **Haematoma (around 2–3 weeks old)**.
3. **Colloid cyst (50%)**.
4. **Tuberculoma**.

Hypodense

1. **Tumour**
   (a) Glioma.
   (b) Craniopharyngioma (if predominantly cystic).
   (c) Metastasis (usually).
   (d) Fat-containing tumour.
       (i) Lipoma.
       (ii) Epidermoid/dermoid.
2. **Haematoma** (over 3 weeks old).
3. **Abscess**.
4. **Cyst**.
   (a) Arachnoid.
   (b) Porencephalic.
   (c) Hydatid.

12.17 DIFFERENTIAL DIAGNOSIS OF A SOLITARY INTRACEREBRAL MASS

1. **Primary brain tumour**: high grade tumours tend to have most mass effect (tumour and surrounding oedema), heterogeneous with areas of necrosis (glioblastoma); may infiltrate and involve/cross corpus callosum; variable enhancement but *tends* to increase with increased grade.
2. **Metastasis**: appearance variable on scans depending on primary; often considerable associated oedema (vasogenic, white matter), multiple/solitary, often located grey-white junction.
3. **Arterial infarct**: developing low attenuation (CT), high T_2 signal (MR) wedge-shaped lesion with variable mass effect; various enhancement patterns if contrast given.
4. **Venous infarct**: area of low attenuation (CT), high signal (MR) not in arterial distribution, often associated mass, often haemorrhagic.
5. **Abscess**: homogeneous, thin enhancing rim, usually considerable vasogenic oedema.
6. **Acute demyelinating plaque**: may be very large with minimal clinical signs; low attenuation (CT) and high T_2 signal (MRI); variable enhancement.
7. **Haematoma**: subacute to chronic.
8. **Encephalitis**: poorly defined area of low attenuation (CT); HSV predilection for limbic system; variable enhancement.
9. **Aneurysm**: may give rise to mass effect by itself but also often associated oedema in surrounding brain; appearance varies according to whether patent or associated intramural thrombus $\pm$ calcification.

Further Reading

Omuro AM, Leite CC, Mokhtari K et al. Pitfalls in the diagnosis of brain tumours. Lancet Neurol 2006;5(11):937–48.

12

12.18 INTRACRANIAL CALCIFICATION

Normal variant

1. **Pineal**: after 10 years of age on SXR, earlier on CT.
2. **Choroid plexus**: trigones of lateral ventricles; unusual in third and fourth ventricles.
3. **Dura**: falx and tentorium.
4. **Basal ganglia**: globus pallidus; usually bilateral.
5. **Habenular commissure**: C-shaped calcification in tela choroidea of third ventricle.
6. **Dentate nuclei of cerebellum.**
7. **Parasellar ligaments.**
8. **Arachnoid granulations.**

Vascular

1. **Vertebrobasilar and carotid vessels at skull base.**
2. **AVM.**
3. **Cavernoma.**
4. **Aneurysms**: mural calcification in giant aneurysms.
5. **Chronic subdural membranes.**
6. **Old infarct or haematoma.**

Tumours

1. **Meningioma.**
2. **Oligodendroglioma** (50% calcify).
3. **Astrocytoma** (lower incidence of calcification than oligo but much more common than oligo).
4. **Low grade glioma.**
5. **Craniopharyngioma.**
6. **Metastases**: adenocarcinoma (GI and breast – especially after therapy in breast).
7. **Pineal region tumours**: teratoma and germinoma.
8. **Chordoma and chondrosarcoma.**
9. **Fatty midline tumours**: dermoid and lipoma of corpus callosum.
10. **Choroid plexus papilloma.**
11. **Dysembryoplastic neuroepithelial tumour** (DNET).
12. **Central neurocytoma.**

Infection

1. **TORCH infections.**
2. **Cysticercosis**: commonest cause of epilepsy worldwide; periventricular, cisternal and nodules at grey-white junction with nidus of calcification.
3. **TB**: basal cisterns, ventricles and parenchyma.

Neurocutaneous syndromes

1. **Sturge–Weber syndrome**: subcortical tramline calcification of pial vascular malformation with focal atrophy, ipsilateral enlargement of choroid plexus.
2. **Tuberous sclerosis**: periventricular and parenchymal.
3. **Neurofibromatosis**: choroid plexus, subependymal and basal ganglia.

12.19 BASAL GANGLIA CALCIFICATION

1. **Normal variant.**
2. **Endocrine**: hypoparathyroidism, pseudohypoparathyroidism, hypothyroidism.
3. **Metabolic**: mitochondrial disorders (Leigh's disease), Fahr's disease, Cockayne's syndrome.
4. **Toxins**: carbon monoxide, lead, post-hypoxic.
5. **Post-therapeutic**: mineralizing angiopathy following chemotherapy or radiation in basal ganglia, dentate nuclei of cerebellum and cortico-medullary junction.

12.20 MENINGEAL ENHANCEMENT ON CT AND MRI

Pachymeningeal = dural.
Leptomeningeal = pia and arachnoid.

Normal

1. **Some degree of dural enhancement** seen of falx, tentorium and cavernous sinus.
2. **Leptomeninges**: scattered smooth areas of enhancement common.
3. **Vessels**: intracranial arteries and veins; intraspinal veins.

12

Dural

1. **Infection**: skull base osteomyelitis, paranasal sinuses.
2. **Tumour**: meningioma (dural tail); metastasis (esp. breast); lymphoma.
3. **Post-operative.**
4. **Following lumbar puncture.**
5. **Intracranial hypotension**: also often subdural effusions, dural sinus engorgement and brain stem descent.
6. **Venous thrombosis.**

7. **Idiopathic pachymeningitis.**
8. **Extramedullary haematopoiesis.**
9. **Sarcoidosis.**
10. **Rheumatoid arthritis.**

Leptomeningeal

1. **Infection**: all types.
2. **Tumour**: metastases, leukaemia, lymphoma, meningeal seeding of primary brain tumours, Langerhans cell histiocytosis.
3. **Infarcts**: surface enhancement often seen.
4. **Subarachnoid haemorrhage in subacute phase.**
5. **Sarcoidosis.**
6. **Rheumatoid arthritis.**
7. **Neurocutaneous syndromes**, esp. Sturge–Weber.

12.21 ENHANCEMENT OF EPENDYMAL AND SUBARACHNOID SPACE ON CT AND MRI

Ependymal

1. **Infective ventriculitis.**
2. **Tumour**: metastases (esp. breast and lung), leukaemia, lymphoma, ependymal seeding of primary brain tumours.
3. **Post-intraventricular haemorrhage.**
4. **Sarcoidosis.**
5. **Enlarged ependymal veins**: AVM, venous angioma, venous thrombosis.
6. **Iatrogenic**: intrathecal therapy, intraventricular drainage devices.

Subarachnoid space

1. **Meningitis.**
2. **Tumour.**
3. **Post-angiogram.**

12.22 MULTIPLE RING-ENHANCING LESIONS

1. **Metastases**: solid/ring-enhancing (usually thicker irregular wall than abscess); grey-white junction; commonest primary tumours = lung, breast, kidney, colon, melanoma; multiple in 80%; commonest infratentorial mass in adults.
2. **Abscess**: usually thin, uniform wall; homogeneous centre; high signal on DWI and low signal ADC (cystic tumours in absence of haemorrhage usually low signal DWI and high signal ADC).
3. **Demyelination**: acute demyelinating plaques may enhance (breakdown of blood–brain barrier).
4. **Multifocal glioma.**
5. **Lymphoma**: solid tumour (pre-treatment) in immunocompetent patients; may be ring enhancing in immunocompromised.
6. **Infarcts**: multiple suggest emboli.
7. **Contusion/haematoma**: breakdown of blood–brain barrier can lead to peripheral enhancement.

12.23 BASAL GANGLIA: BILATERAL ABNORMALITIES

Caudate nucleus; putamen; globus pallidus; subthalamic nucleus, substantia nigra, ventral tegmentum.
Head of caudate nucleus + putamen = corpus striatum.
Putamen + globus pallidus = lentiform nucleus.

Normal

1. **Age related**: incidence of calcification of globus pallidus increases with age (high attenuation CT; increased T_1 signal MR); increased iron deposition causes reduced T_2 signal on MRI in globus pallidus and putamen.
2. **Enlarged perivascular spaces**: CSF signal on all sequences.

Vascular

1. **Lacunar (small, deep) infarcts**: well defined low attenuation lesions (CT), high T_2 signal (MR).
2. **Acute near total hypoxic insults** (esp. in perinatal period); high T_2 signal in posterior putamina, ventrolateral thalami, perirolandic white matter and cortex and hippocampal formations.
3. **Cardiac arrest, near-miss drowning and opiate overdose** can cause increased T_2 signal in globus pallidus and putamen.
4. **Deep cerebral vein thrombosis** (although thalami usually affected first/as well).

12

Neurodegenerative

1. **Parkinson's disease.**
2. **Huntington's disease** (atrophy of heads of caudate nuclei).
3. **Extrapyramidal disorders**: multisystem atrophy, progressive supranuclear palsy.

Toxins

1. **Kernicterus**: increased signal in globus pallidus on T_1 and T_2 (MRI).
2. **Hepatocellular degeneration**: high T_1 signal.
3. **Prolonged total parenteral nutrition** can lead to excess manganese deposition in basal ganglia: increased signal on T_1.
4. **Exogenous toxins**: carbon monoxide, methanol, cyanide, hydrogen sulphide.

Acquired metabolic disease

1. **Hypoglycaemia**: putamina and parieto-occipital cortex and subcortical regions.
2. **Osmotic myelinolysis.**
3. **Haemolytic-uraemic syndrome.**

Inherited metabolic disease

1. **Wilson's disease** (striatum).
2. **Kearns–Sayre disease** (globus pallidus).
3. **Mitochondrial cytopathies** (Leigh's disease): striatum and globus pallidus primarily.
4. **Leukodystrophies**: Krabbe's (thalami and periventricular white matter).
5. **Amino acid disorders**: methylmalonic aciduria (globus pallidus).
6. **Lipidoses**: Tay–Sachs disease (striatum, thalami).
7. **Neurodegeneration with brain iron accumulation** (NBIA, formerly called Hallervorden–Spatz syndrome); low signal in central globus pallidus on T_2 (MRI) with surrounding high signal: 'eye of the tiger'.

12.24 BASAL GANGLIA: BRIGHT ON T_1

Deposition of paramagnetic substances
1. **Haemorrhage.**
2. **Haemorrhagic infarction.**
3. **Wilson's disease.**
4. **Long-term parenteral nutrition** (manganese deposition).

Calcification
Usually hypo- or isointense on spin echo sequences; may be hyperintense depending on crystalline structure.

Hamartomas
1. **Neurofibromatosis type 1**: may be high signal on T_1 as well as T_2; globus pallidus, internal capsule, brainstem and cerebellum.

Indeterminate
1. **Chronic liver disease with porto-caval shunt.**

12.25 THALAMUS: BILATERAL ABNORMALITIES

Vascular
1. **Lacunar** (small, deep) infarcts.
2. **Arterial infarct** (perforating arteries from tip of basilar artery may supply both thalami).
3. **Venous ischaemic and infarction**: thrombosis of straight sinus/vein of Galen/deep cerebral veins: bilateral symmetrical low attenuation (CT) or high T_2 signal (MRI) $\pm$ haemorrhagic transformation.
4. **Profound hypoxia**, esp. perinatal.

Infection
1. **Variant CJD**: pulvinar sign.
2. **Japanese encephalitis.**

Metabolic
1. **Carbon monoxide poisoning** (basal ganglia esp. globus pallidus also involved).
2. **Wernicke's encephalopathy**: thiamine deficiency in chronic alcoholism: involvement of mesial thalamic nuclei, mamillary

12

bodies, midbrain and floor of third ventricle with increased T_2 signal.
3. **Inherited metabolic conditions**: mitochondrial cytopathies (Leigh's disease); certain leukodystrophies (Krabbe's disease).

12.26 INHERITED METABOLIC WHITE MATTER DISEASE

Low attenuation of white matter on CT; low signal T_1, high signal T_2 on MRI, FLAIR sequence increases visibility of periventricular changes. Active disease (myelin breakdown) may show contrast enhancement adjacent to normal tissue. Distribution of abnormalities may give some indication of underlying condition.

Two basic types: dysmyelination (primary abnormalities of myelin formation); demyelination (myelin loss after it has been formed).

Dysmyelination

Enzyme deficiencies in various organelles prevent normal formation of myelin or prevent its maintenance once formed, thereby increasing its fragility.

Lysosomal disorders
1. **Metachromatic leukodystrophy**: arylsulphatase-A deficiency; autosomal recessive; presentation aged 2–3 years (usually), can be later; MR: diffuse symmetrical increased white matter signal sparing subcortical U fibres; may involve cerebellum; cerebral atrophy later.
2. **Krabbe's (globoid) leukodystrophy**: galactosylceramide β-galactosidase deficiency; autosomal recessive; early presentation (within 6 months) usually; MR: symmetrical increased T_2 signal posteriorly with involvement of thalami and caudate; severe atrophy late

Peroxisomal disorders
1. **Adrenoleukodystrophy**: different phenotypes
   (a) Cerebral ALD (40%).
   (b) Adrenomyeloneuropathy (46%): progressive spastic diplegia in adults.
   (c) Primary adrenocortical deficiency without CNS involvement.

   MR: majority (80%) high signal posterior white matter, splenium and posterior body of callosum, visual and auditory pathways and corticospinal tracts. Minority (15%) anterior white matter involvement initially with genu and anterior body of splenium.

MR spectroscopy may show abnormalities (reduced NAA and increased chlorine) prior to changes on standard sequences which is important in terms of planning possible intervention = bone marrow transplantation.

2. **Zellweger's (cerebrohepatorenal) syndrome**: presents in neonatal period with extensive white matter changes and cortical dysplasia (polymicrogyria type).

Mitochondrial disorders

Respiratory chain enzyme disorders causing myopathies or multisystem disorders with encephalopathy.

1. **Leigh's disease**: usually increased T_2 signal in central grey matter (mainly corpus striatum) but white matter can be involved and any pattern of abnormality can be seen.
2. **MELAS** (mitochondrial myopathy, encephalopathy, lactic acidosis and stroke-like episodes): focal cortical and brain stem white matter changes with basal ganglia calcification; atrophy later.
3. **MERRF**: myoclonic epilepsy with ragged red fibres.
4. **Kearns–Sayre syndrome**: progressive external ophthalmoplegia and pigmentary retinal degeneration ± heart block, elevated CSF protein and cerebellar dysfunction. White matter abnormalities seen in association with cerebral and/or cerebellar atrophy and calcification in deep grey and deep white matter.

Amino organic acid abnormalities

1. **Canavan's disease**: autosomal recessive; primarily children of Ashkenazi Jewish descent; progressive increase in head size and neurological deterioration. MR: increased signal in subcortical white matter and globus pallidus; characteristic increased NAA peak on MR spectroscopy.
2. **Maple syrup urine disease.**

Others

1. **Pelizaeus–Merzbacher disease**: X-linked recessive. Lack of myelination.
2. **Alexander's disease**: microcephaly and progressive neurological deterioration; MR: increased signal in frontal white matter.

12

12.27 MULTIPLE SCLEROSIS AND ITS DIFFERENTIAL DIAGNOSIS

Commonest demyelinating condition. MR more sensitive than CT; callosal and pericallosal lesions commonest, pericallosal lesions perivenular therefore perpendicular to ventricle; other sites = optic nerves and pathway, brainstem and middle cerebellar peduncles. Grey matter and peripheral white matter lesions much less common. Acute lesions may be large, have mass effect, show target lesions and contrast enhancement. MR: high T_2 signal; old gliotic lesions may be low signal on T_1.

Normal features mimicking MS

1. **Prominent perivascular (Virchow–Robin) spaces**: peripheral spaces perpendicular to ventricles but CSF signal on all sequences; may be very large, esp. in basal ganglia.
2. **Age-related lesions**: small peripheral high T_2 signal lesions; not all due to small vessel ischaemia.

Vascular

1. **Small vessel ischaemia**: usually deep and subcortical white matter; discrete or confluent; commoner if hypertension and/or diabetes.
2. **Infarct**: solitary abnormality with little mass effect involving white matter and adjacent cortex may be difficult to distinguish from solitary plaque MS; acute infarct will have high signal on DWI and low signal ADC.

Other demyelinating conditions

1. **ADEM** (acute disseminated encephalomyelitis): monophasic autoimmune disorder, usually follows viral infection or immunization; ADEM usually fewer, larger lesions than MS and more often also affects grey matter; mass effect unusual.
2. **Central pontine (osmotic) myelinolysis**: MR low T_1, high T_2 signal in central pons with sparing of periphery, pons swollen; clinically most usually follows intravenous fluid correction of chronic hyponatraemia.
3. **Post chemo or radiotherapy.**
4. **Other toxins**: alcohol, organic solvents.

Infection

1. **Encephalitis**: viral, HIV and PML.
2. **Lyme disease**: white matter lesions resemble MS but abnormalities also in basal ganglia and brainstem.

Tumour

1. **Glioma**: large solitary MS plaque may closely mimic intrinsic tumour.
2. **Multifocal glioma.**

Further Reading

Matthews P. An update on neuroimaging of multiple sclerosis. Curr Opin Neurol 2004;17(4):453–8.

12.28 CEREBRAL ATROPHY

Generalized

1. **Normal ageing.**
2. **Cerebrovascular disease.**
3. **End-stage multiple sclerosis.**
4. **Alcohol.**
5. **Post-traumatic** (if severe and esp. if widespread DAI).
6. **Drugs.**
7. **Post-infective**: encephalitis and meningitis; HIV.
8. **Neurodegenerative.**

Focal

1. **Post ischaemia/infarction.**
2. **Post-trauma**: contusion, haematoma.
3. **Post-infective**: encephalitis and meningitis.
4. **Alzheimer's disease**: commonest dementia; hippocampal atrophy usually most severe but may be generalized.
5. **Frontotemporal dementia.**
6. **Parkinson's disease**: generalized atrophy and atrophy of substantia nigra; increased putaminal iron (reduced T_2 signal).
7. **Progressive supranuclear palsy**: atrophy of tectum, globus pallidus and frontal lobes.
8. **Pick's disease**: severe frontal and anterior temporal atrophy.
9. **Huntington's disease**: atrophy of caudate heads.
10. **Corticobasal degeneration**: atrophy of posterior parietal ± frontal lobes.

Further Reading

Whitwell JL, Jack CR Jr. Neuroimaging in dementia. Neurol Clin 2007;25(3): 843–57.
Keyserling H, Mukundan S Jr. The role of conventional MR and CT in the work up of dementia patients. Neuroimaging Clin N Am 2005;15(4):789–802.

12

12.29 DIFFUSE CEREBELLAR ATROPHY

1. **Normal ageing.**
2. **Alcohol.**
3. **Long-term anticonvulsants** (esp. phenytoin).
4. **Paraneoplastic syndromes** (lung, ovary).
5. **Post-radiotherapy.**
6. **Ataxia telangiectasia.**
7. **Neurodegenerative,** e.g. olivopontocerebellar degeneration.
8. **Hereditary spinocerebellar ataxias:** e.g. Friedrich's.
9. **Gluten sensitivity.**
10. **Idiopathic.**

12.30 INTRACRANIAL MANIFESTATIONS OF WELL-KNOWN NEUROCUTANEOUS DISORDERS

Neurofibromatosis type 1

1. **Hamartomatous lesions:** high T_2 signal in globus pallidus, visual pathway, brain stem, cerebellum.
2. **Optic pathway glioma.**
3. **Non-optic glioma:** tectum, brainstem.
4. **Plexiform neurofibroma.**
5. **Absent or dysplastic sphenoid wing, calvarial defects, dural ectasia.**
6. **Vascular abnormalities:** aneurysm, ectasia, occlusion, Moya-Moya, AV fistula.

Neurofibromatosis type 2

1. **Cranial nerve schwannomas** (bilateral acoustic schwannomas diagnostic).
2. **Multiple meningiomas.**
3. **Intrinsic tumours** (ependymomas).
4. **Non-neoplastic choroid plexus lesions.**

Tuberous sclerosis

1. **Cortical tubers.**
2. **Transmantle white matter dysplasia:** high T_2 signal on MR.
3. **Subependymal nodules** (disorganized glial cells NOT heterotopic grey).
4. **Giant cell astrocytoma:** (large glial nodules related to foramina of Munro).

Sturge–Weber syndrome

1. **Gyriform subcortical calcification.**
2. **Gyriform enhancement post-contrast** (pial angioma).
3. **Focal atrophy related to angioma.**
4. **Hyperpneumatization of frontal sinuses.**
5. **Ipsilateral enlargement of choroid plexus.**
6. **Facial angioma.**
7. **Buphthalmos, orbital angiomas.**

Von-Hippel–Lindau

1. **Haemangioblastoma:** usually cerebellar cystic tumour of variable size with avidly enhancing solid mural nodule; smaller tumours solid; may involve cord.
2. **Retinal angioma, microphthalmia** ± dystrophic calcification.

Hereditary haemorrhagic telangiectasia (Osler–Weber–Rendu)

1. **Embolic infarcts** (emboli through pulmonary AV shunts).
2. **Cerebral abscess** (septic emboli through pulmonary AV shunts).
3. **Vascular malformations:** telangiectasia, cavernomas, AVM and AVF.

12.31　CAUSES OF HIGH T_1 SIGNAL

Normal

1. **Posterior pituitary** (whole pituitary may be high signal up to 6 months of age).
2. **Moving blood** (and sometimes CSF; flow-related enhancement).
3. **Calcification** (certain crystalline forms of calcium).
4. **Fat.**
5. **Rathke's cleft cyst.**

Pathological

1. **Methaemoglobin** (haematoma, microhaemorrhage, thrombus): intracellular = low signal on T_2; extracellular = high signal on T_2.
2. **Fat:** lipomas and fatty components of dermoids.
3. **Proteinaceous fluids:** colloid cyst; craniopharyngioma.
4. **Melanin.**
5. **Heavy metals.**

12

12.32 CAUSES OF LOW T_2 SIGNAL

Normal

1. **Flowing blood.**
2. **Bone.**
3. **Calcification.**
4. **Air.**
5. **CSF flow** (esp. foramina of Munro and cerebral aqueduct).

Pathological

1. **Cerebral aneurysms**: small aneurysms show flow void, giant aneurysms may show complex flow signal $\pm$ mural thrombus.
2. **Arteriovenous malformations**: enlarged feeding vessels and draining veins.
3. **Blood**: acute: deoxyhaemoglobin and intracellular methaemoglobin; chronic: haemosiderin.

12.33 ENLARGED PITUITARY FOSSA

Normal range = height: 6.5–11mm; length: 9–16mm; width 9–19mm.

1. **Apparent**
   (a) Double floor (normal variant or intrasellar tumour).
   (b) Elevation/erosion of clinoid processes.
   (c) Loss of lamina dura.
2. **Real**
   (a) Intra/parasellar mass.
   (b) Raised intracranial pressure.
   (c) Empty sella.
   (d) Nelson's syndrome (post-adrenalectomy for Cushing's syndrome).

12.34 J-SHAPED SELLA

Flattened tuberculum sellae with a prominent sulcus chiasmaticus.

1. **Normal variant.**
2. **Optic chiasm glioma** (if chiasmatic sulcus very depressed [W or omega shaped sella], glioma may be bilateral).
3. **Neurofibromatosis.**
4. **Achondroplasia.**
5. **Mucopolysaccharidoses.**
6. **Chronic hydrocephalus** (enlarged anterior aspect of third ventricle).

12.35 INTRASELLAR MASS

Neoplastic

1. **Pituitary microadenoma**: (<10mm); enhance more slowly than normal pituitary therefore low signal on enhanced studies (will show enhancement if imaged late); often different signal to normal gland on unenhanced scans; distort outline of gland.
2. **Pituitary macroadenoma**: >10mm; solid/cystic enhancing mass; MR most sensitive for diagnosis and demonstration of tumour spread: suprasellar (chiasm), parasellar (cavernous sinus; significant if >50% of carotid encased), retroclival.
3. **Meningioma**: usually extend into sella; origin in sella very rare.
4. **Craniopharyngioma**.
5. **Chordoma/chondrosarcoma**: clival tumours.
6. **Pituitary metastasis**: rare.

Non-neoplastic

1. **Pituitary** (pars intermedia) cyst: similar to microadenoma but may be lower T_1, higher T_2 signal.
2. **Pituitary hyperplasia**: peripubertal, pregnancy.
3. **Internal carotid aneurysm** (medially placed flow void).
4. **Ectatic carotid**.
5. **Rathke's cleft cyst**: may be intrasellar, suprasellar or involve both compartments.
6. **Lymphocytic hypophysitis**: lymphocytic infiltration of anterior pituitary, infundibulum and floor of hypothalamus; typically during pregnancy and peripartum period but also occurs in males; enhances post-contrast with hypothalamic tail.
7. **Langerhans cell histiocytosis**: typically enlarged enhancing infundibulum.
8. **Pituitary abscess**: rare.

12

12.36 INFUNDIBULAR MASS

Neoplastic

1. **Germinoma**: involvement of infundibulum, anterior recesses of third ventricle and hypothalamic region; homogeneous avidly enhancing mass; check for pineal region involvement; transependymal spread common.
2. **Lymphoma.**
3. **Leukaemia.**
4. **Glioma.**
5. **Metastasis.**

Non-neoplastic

1. **Sarcoidosis**: involvement of optic pathways, floor of third ventricle and infundibulum very suggestive of sarcoidosis.
2. **Lymphocytic hypophysitis.**
3. **Langerhans cell histiocytosis.**

12.37 SUPRASELLAR MASS

Neoplastic

1. **Extension of pituitary macroadenoma.**
2. **Meningioma**: arising in and extending from anterior cranial fossa, sphenoid wing or diaphragma sella: homogeneous mass with uniform enhancement (unless cystic); pituitary should be visible as separate structure.
3. **Craniopharyngioma**: sellar/suprasellar/both; solid/cystic.
4. **Chiasmatic glioma.**
5. **Infundibular mass.**
6. **Hypothalamic hamartoma**: uniform mass in patients with precocious puberty or gelastic seizures.

Non-neoplastic

1. **Ectatic or aneurysmal carotid artery.**
2. **Arachnoid cyst.**
3. **Epidermoid cyst**: non-enhancing lobulated mass; signal usually higher than that of CSF on T_1, FLAIR and DWI.
4. **Dermoid**: midline mass with fat and calcification; rupture gives rise to disseminated small areas of high T_1 signal in subarachnoid space.
5. **Rathke's cleft cyst.**
6. **Lymphocytic hypophysitis.**
7. **Langerhans cell histiocytosis.**
8. **Sarcoidosis.**

12.38 CAVERNOUS SINUS/PARASELLAR MASS

Neoplastic

1. **Trigeminal schwannoma**: if large may involve cerebello-pontine angle, Meckel's cave, cavernous sinus and pterygo-maxillary fissure; extension through foramen ovale if present helps differentiate between schwannoma and meningioma.
2. **Meningioma.**
3. **Pituitary adenoma.**
4. **Metastasis.**
5. **Lymphoma.**
6. **Direct extension of skull base or nasopharyngeal tumour.**

Non-neoplastic

1. **Ectatic or aneurysmal carotid artery.**
2. Cavernous sinus thrombosis: sinus expanded, abnormal signal; usually secondary to perifacial/orbital sepsis.
3. **Carotico-cavernous fistula**: direct (via internal carotid artery) or indirect (via dura) causes enlargement of sinus and draining veins (esp. superior ophthalmic vein) leading to ophthalmoplegia, proptosis and chemosis. Drainage routes other than orbit may predominate (therefore normal orbit does not exclude CC fistula).
4. **Invasive sinusitis**: Aspergillus in immunocompromised patients.
5. **Dermoid/epidermoid.**
6. **Lymphocytic hypophysitis.**
7. **Sarcoidosis.**
8. **Tolosa–Hunt syndrome**: painful ophthalmoplegia caused by non-specific granulomatous infiltration of cavernous sinus and superior orbital fissure; usually steroid responsive.

12

12.39 PINEAL REGION MASS

Pineal gland

1. **Simple pineal cyst**: <1cm, often slightly higher signal than CSF; no enhancement; common incidental finding of no significance if no mass effect or symptoms.
2. **Germinoma**: commonest pineal germ cell tumour; M:F = 10:1; check infundibulum/suprasellar region for synchronous tumour (10%); CT: hyperdense, calcification; MR: image whole neuraxis for spread; serum markers often positive (α-fetoprotein); tend to occur first two decades.
3. **Teratoma**: second commonest pineal germ cell tumour: heterogeneous mass (fat, calcification, cystic change); spectrum of malignant potential.
4. **Parenchymal pineal tumours**:
    (a) Pineocytoma: commoner in older adults; slow growing.
    (b) Pineoblastoma: usually larger heterogenous mass; local spread and CNS dissemination more likely.

Posterior brainstem

1. **Tectal glioma**: commonest; other causes rare.
2. **Infarct**.
3. **Cavernoma**.
4. **Metastasis**.
5. **Demyelination**.
6. **Post-traumatic contusion**.

Posterior third ventricle

1. **Glioma**.
2. **Metastasis**.
3. **Choroid plexus tumour**.

Perimesencephalic cistern

1. **Arachnoid cyst**.
2. **Dermoid**.
3. **Lipoma**.
4. **Meningioma**.
5. **Metastasis**.
6. **AV malformation** (inc. vein of Galen).
7. **Posterior cerebral artery aneurysm**.

12.40 INTRAVENTRICULAR MASS IN ADULTS

Lateral ventricles

1. **Glioblastoma.**
2. **Oligodendroglioma.**
3. **Central neurocytoma**: low grade, usually applied to septum pellucidum.
4. **Lymphoma.**
5. **Metastasis.**
6. **Subependymoma**: benign, usually attached to septum pellucidum.
7. **Meningioma.**
8. **Choroid plexus tumour/cyst.**
9. **AV malformation.**
10. **Subependymal heterotopia.**

Foramen of Munro

1. **Colloid cyst.**
2. **Giant cell astrocytoma.**

Third ventricle

1. **Craniopharyngioma.**
2. **Germinoma.**
3. **Metastasis.**
4. **Subependymoma.**
5. **Sarcoidosis.**

Fourth ventricle

1. **Metastasis.**
2. **Subependymoma.**
3. **Haemangioblastoma.**
4. **Choroid plexus tumour.**
5. **Inflammatory cyst** (e.g. cysticercosis).

12

12.41 CEREBELLO-PONTINE ANGLE MASS

1. **Vestibular schwannoma** (acoustic neuroma) commonest (90%); intracanalicular component often expands porus acousticus of internal auditory meatus but may be all extracanalicular; may cause distortion of brainstem (middle cerebellar peduncle) and obstructive hydrocephalus (but hydrocephalus may be present in absence of obstruction).
2. **Meningioma** (9%): broad base against petrous bone, may extend into but usually do not expand porus.
3. **Epidermoid** (1%): low attenuation (CT); lobulated mass (MRI) of similar signal to CSF on most sequences but increased signal on FLAIR and DWI. Growing epidermoids insinuate themselves around surroundings vessels and nerves.
   Rest all very rare:
4. **Trigeminal schwannoma.**
5. **Aneurysms** (vertebrobasilar system).
6. **Metastases.**
7. **Skull base tumours:** glomus, cholesterol granulomas, metastases.
8. **Skull base infection.**

12.42 INTERNAL AUDITORY CANAL ABNORMALITY

Neoplastic

1. Vestibular schwannoma.
2. Meningioma.
3. Facial nerve schwannoma.
4. Metastasis.
5. Haemangioma.
6. Lipoma.

Non-neoplastic

1. **Bell's palsy:** may see enhancement of facial nerve on MRI.
2. **Post-operative:** dural following acoustic surgery.
3. **Sarcoidosis.**
4. **Langerhans cell histiocytosis.**

12.43 MIDDLE EAR MASS

Inflammatory

1. **Acquired cholesteatoma**: expanding mass of epithelial debris in epitympanum of middle ear cavity; erodes and invades surrounding bone leading to:
   (a) Cerebral abscess/meningitis by erosion of tegmen.
   (b) Conductive deafness by erosion of ossicles.
   (c) Facial palsy.
   (d) Vertigo and deafness by labyrinthine erosion and endolymph leak.
2. **Acute otitis media** – may result in mastoiditis.
3. **Malignant otitis externa**: acute osteomyelitis of temporal bone in elderly, diabetics, immunocompromised: local bone erosion and extensive soft tissue swelling.
4. **Cholesterol granuloma**: non-specific chronic inflammation of middle ear and mastoid; high signal T_1 and T_2.
5. **Serous otitis media**: sterile fluid in middle ear cavity.
6. **Middle ear effusion**: secondary to blockage of Eustachian tube, e.g. nasopharyngeal carcinoma.
7. **Tympanosclerosis**: deposits of fibrotic/calcified tissue in middle ear, epitympanum, tympanic membrane; areas of high density on high resolution CT.

Neoplastic

1. **Glomus tympanicum**: CT/MR shows soft tissue mass on cochlear promontory; may be quite small as present early with pulsatile tinnitus.
2. **Glomus jugulare**: glomus tumour extending from jugular foramen.
3. **Facial nerve schwannoma**.
4. **Temporal bone mass**.

Vascular

1. **Aberrant internal carotid artery**.
2. **High riding (dehiscent) jugular bulb**.

12

12.44 TEMPORAL BONE MASS

Neoplastic

1. **Glomus tumour**: jugulare and tympanicum.
2. **Meningioma**.
3. **Metastasis**: breast, lung, renal, prostate.
4. **Myeloma**.
5. **Lymphoma**: but more commonly involves orbits or paranasal sinuses.
6. **Nasopharyngeal carcinoma**: direct extension.
7. **Rhabdomyosarcoma**: commonest soft tissue sarcoma in children; usually involves orbit, paranasal sinuses and pharynx.
8. **Carcinoma of the parotid**: direct extension into floor of external auditory meatus/mastoid; infiltration along facial nerve.
9. **Chordoma/chondrosarcoma**.
10. **Carcinoma of the external auditory canal**.

Non-neoplastic

1. **Cholesteatoma**.
2. **Cholesterol granuloma**.
3. **Apical petrositis**.
4. **Aneurysm of petrous carotid**.
5. **Langerhans cell histiocytosis**.

12.45 TEMPORAL BONE SCLEROSIS

1. **Otosclerosis**: condition characterized by periods of demineralization followed by sclerotic repair; ill defined bone resorption around oval window or cochlea (lucent halo around cochlea) followed by irregular bone deposition; both processes may be simultaneous rather than sequential.
2. **Paget's disease**: initial changes at petrous apex with demineralization and irregular bone deposition leading to hypertrophied, irregularly mineralized bone; can involve otic capsule, labyrinth and internal auditory canal.
3. **Fibrous dysplasia**: thickening of outer table of squamous temporal bone with obliteration of mastoid air cells.
4. **Osteopetrosis**: homogeneous sclerotic temporal bone with obliteration of air cells; progressive narrowing of internal auditory meatus can cause facial palsy.
5. **Meningioma**.

12.46 PULSATILE TINNITUS

Anatomical

1. **Large/dehiscent jugular bulb**: normal flow may be perceived especially if thin plate of bone normally between wall of jugular vein and middle ear absent; may also give rise to protrusion of jugular bulb into middle ear (not to be mistaken for glomus).
2. **Aberrant carotid artery**: inferior compartment of middle ear filled by carotid running posterior and lateral to its normal course.
3. **Persistent stapedial artery**: failure of regression of embryonic stapedial artery runs through lumen of stapes.

Vascular

1. **Dural AV fistula**: common presentation of fistula in transverse or sigmoid sinus.
2. **Petrous carotid artery aneurysm**.
3. **Venous sinus thrombosis**: incomplete thrombosis of lateral sinus may lead to turbulent flow.
4. **Arterial stenosis**.

Neoplastic

1. **Glomus tumour**.

12.47 JUGULAR FORAMEN MASS

Neoplastic

1. **Glomus jugulare**: erosion/lysis and expansion of jugular foramen and surrounding structures; intratumoral vessels seen as flow voids on T_2 MRI (pepper pot appearance); arterial blush on angiography with AV shunting.
2. **Schwannoma**: foramen enlarged but no erosion or lysis; well defined, lobulated tumour which enhances post-contrast.
3. **Direct invasion from local tumour**.
4. **Metastasis**.
5. **Meningioma**.
6. **Chondrosarcoma**.
7. **Langerhans cell histiocytosis**.
8. **Lymphoma**.

Non-neoplastic

1. **Enlarged jugular bulb**.
2. **Venous thrombosis**.
3. **Skull base osteomyelitis**.

12

12.48 FORAMEN MAGNUM MASS

Intramedullary

1. **Intrinsic cord/brainstem tumour.**
2. **Hydromyelia** (syrinx).
3. **Demyelination.**

Intradural, extramedullary

1. **Chiari malformation**: descent of cerebellar tonsils and distortion of brainstem.
2. **Meningioma.**
3. **Schwannoma.**
4. **Aneurysm.**

Extradural

1. **Inflammatory arthropathies**: rheumatoid with soft tissue pannus eroding odontoid peg.
2. **Skull base tumour.**
3. **Skull base osteomyelitis.**

12.49 DIFFUSE SKULL BASE ABNORMALITY

Neoplastic

1. **Metastases**: commonest = breast, bronchus, prostate; four common clinical syndromes:
   - **(a)** Orbital: pain, diplopia, proptosis, external ophthalmoplegia.
   - **(b)** Parasellar: headache, ocular paresis, facial numbness (maxillary and mandibular divisions of fifth cranial nerve).
   - **(c)** Jugular foramen: hoarseness and dysphagia.
   - **(d)** Occipital condyle: stiffness and pain in neck worse on flexion.
2. **Myeloma.**
3. **Nasopharyngeal carcinoma.**
4. **Lymphoma.**
5. **Meningioma.**
6. **Rhabdomyosarcoma.**

Non-neoplastic

1. **Fibrous dysplasia.**
2. **Paget's disease.**
3. **Osteomyelitis.**
4. **Langerhans cell histiocytosis.**
5. **Renal osteodystrophy.**
6. **Haemoglobinopathy**: e.g. sickle cell disease.

12.50 SKULL VAULT LUCENCY WITHOUT SCLEROTIC EDGE

Normal

1. **Parietal foramina**: usually bilateral and symmetrical anterior to lambdoid suture.
2. **Venous lakes and vascular channels** (emissary veins may have sclerotic margin).
3. **Pacchionian granulations.**
4. **Normal ageing calvarium.**
5. **Prominent normal markings.**
6. **Anterior and posterior fontanelle.**

Neoplastic (adults)

1. **Myeloma**: multiple lytic lesions (pepper pot skull); can involve mandible (where metastases very rare).
2. **Metastases**: commonest breast, lung, renal, leukaemia, prostate.
3. **Sarcoma secondary to Paget's.**

Neoplastic (children)

1. **Metastases**: neuroblastoma, leukaemia.
2. **Langerhans cell histiocytosis** (acute phase).
3. **Hand–Schuller–Christian disease**: multiple lucencies covering large area.

Traumatic

1. **Leptomeningeal cyst**: skull fracture with trapped meninges; CSF pulsation causes progressive widening and scalloping (growing fracture).
2. **Burr hole.**

Metabolic

1. **Hyperparathyroidism**: solitary brown tumour or multiple lucencies (pepper pot skull).
2. **Osteoporosis.**

Infective

1. **Acute pyogenic**: complication of sinusitis, mastoiditis, penetrating head trauma, post-surgical.
2. **TB.**
3. **Hydatid.**
4. **Syphilis**: moth-eaten appearance.

12

Vascular

1. **Haemangioma**: sunburst pattern of radiating spicules.
2. **Sinus pericranii**: abnormally large communication between intracranial and extracranial venous circulations; congenital, traumatic or spontaneous; presents as:
   (a) Numerous small localized defects.
   (b) Discrete area of bone loss.
   (c) Complete absence of bone.

Others

1. **Osteoporosis circumscripta**: lytic phase of Paget's disease; usually inferior frontal and occipital bones; rarer at vertex; can cross sutures.
2. **Neurofibroma.**
3. **Intradiploic arachnoid cyst.**

12.51 SKULL VAULT LUCENCY WITH SCLEROTIC EDGE

Developmental

1. **Epidermoid.**
2. **Encephalocoele/meningocoele**: overlying soft tissue mass.

Neoplastic

1. **Langerhans cell histiocytosis**: healing phase.
2. **Treated lytic metastasis.**

Infective

1. **Chronic osteomyelitis.**
2. **Frontal sinus mucocoele.**

Other

1. **Fibrous dysplasia.**

12.52 GENERALIZED INCREASE IN DENSITY OF SKULL VAULT

1. **Paget's disease**: multiple islands of dense bone, loss of differentiation of inner and outer tables, thickening of skull vault; basilar invagination can occur.
2. **Sclerotic metastases**: breast (post-treatment), prostate.
3. **Fibrous dysplasia**: younger age group than Paget's.
4. **Myelofibrosis.**
5. **Renal osteodystrophy**: osteosclerosis in 25%; looks similar to Paget's.
6. **Acromegaly**: enlarged frontal sinuses, prognathism, enlarged sella, thickened skull vault.
7. **Chronic haemolytic anaemias.**
8. **Sclerosing bone dysplasia**
   (a) Osteopetrosis.
   (b) Pyknodysostosis: especially skull base, multiple Wormian bones, wide sutures.
   (c) Pyle's disease.
9. **Prolonged phenytoin treatment.**
10. **Fluorosis.**

12.53 LOCALIZED INCREASE IN DENSITY OF SKULL VAULT

Within bone

1. **Tumour**
   (a) Sclerotic metastasis: prostate, breast, neuroblastoma.
   (b) Osteoma.
   (c) Treated lytic metastasis.
   (d) Treated brown tumour of hyperparathyroidism.
2. **Paget's disease.**
3. **Fibrous dysplasia.**
4. **Depressed fracture.**
5. **Hyperostosis frontalis interna.**

Adjacent to bone

1. **Meningioma.**
2. **Calcified cephalhaematoma.**
3. **Calcified epidermoid cyst.**

Artefact

1. **Hairbraids.**

12

12.54 THICKENED SKULL

Generalized

1. Normal variant.
2. Prolonged phenytoin treatment.
3. Microcephaly.
4. Shunted hydrocephalus.
5. Acromegaly.
6. Extramedullary haemopoiesis.

Focal

1. Normal variant.
2. Paget's disease.
3. Hyperostosis frontalis interna.
4. Fibrous dysplasia.
5. Meningioma.
6. Osteoma.
7. Sclerotic metastasis: prostate.

12.55 THIN SKULL

Generalized

1. Hyperparathyroidism.
2. Hypophosphatasia.
3. Osteogenesis imperfecta.
4. Rickets.
5. Chronically raised intracranial pressure.
6. Lacunar skull: bone dysplasia of membranous skull; indentations or pits in frontal and parietal regions that may be full thickness; defects separated by thin rims of bone; usually disappear by 6 months; not associated with raised intracranial pressure.

Focal

1. Normal variants.
2. Osteporosis circumscripta.
3. Large intracranial cyst: arachnoid, porencephalic.
4. Slow growing cortical tumour: DNET, ganglioglioma.

12.56 BASILAR INVAGINATION

Upward extension of cervical spine into foramen magnum leading to brainstem compression. McGregor's line lies between posterior tip of hard palate and base of occiput; odontoid tip should lie less than 5mm above line.

1. **Primary developmental/segmentation anomaly:** Klippel–Feil.
2. **Rickets/osteomalacia.**
3. **Paget's disease.**
4. **Fibrous dysplasia.**
5. **Osteogenesis imperfecta.**

12.57 PLATYBASIA

Angulation between anterior cranial fossa floor and clivus = basal angle. This angle less than 140° in platybasia. May coexist with basilar invagination.

1. **Rickets/osteomalacia.**
2. **Paget's disease.**
3. **Fibrous dysplasia.**
4. **Osteogenesis imperfecta.**
5. **Hyperparathyroidism.**

12

12.58 'HAIR-ON-END' SKULL VAULT

Haemolytic anaemias

1. **Sickle cell anaemia**: initially in frontal region but can involve whole skull where diploic space present (marrow cavity) i.e. above level of internal occipital protruberance.
2. **Thalassaemia**: marrow hyperplasia more marked in this than other anaemias.
3. **Hereditary spherocytosis and elliptocytosis.**
4. **Pyruvate kinase deficiency.**
5. **Glucose-6-phosphate dehydrogenase deficiency.**

Neoplastic

1. **Haemangioma.**
2. **Meningioma.**
3. **Metastases.**

Other

1. **Cyanotic heart disease**: erythroid hyperplasia.
2. **Severe childhood iron deficiency anaemia.**

Recommended reading
Osborn A (ed). Diagnostic imaging: brain. Amirsys, Salt Lake City, 2004.

Gynaecology and obstetrics

Colin Davies

GYNAECOLOGICAL IMAGING

13.1 VAGINA

Imaging mainly of use in congenital abnormalities (ultrasound and MRI) and for staging of carcinoma (MRI), although limited data on accuracy.

Ultrasound detectable lesions

1. Haematocolpos.
2. Gartner duct cysts.
3. Urethral diverticulae.

13.2 MRI FINDINGS IN VULVAL CARCINOMA

1. Occurs in elderly women, mainly 6th/7th decade.
2. Diagnosed clinically and confirmed on biopsy.
3. Staging according to FIGO classification.
4. Useful to assess depth of invasion, particularly into adjacent organs.
5. Tumour best seen on T_2 weighted scans and is of intermediate signal.
6. Early and en plaque disease may be difficult to recognize on MR.

13.3 UTERINE CERVIX

1. Not normally primarily imaged by ultrasound.
2. Best assessed clinically and staged by MRI.
3. FIGO staging used for clinical and radiological assessment.
4. Combined assessment influences prognosis and treatment decisions.
5. MRI imaging – T_2 scans axial to cervix, T_2 scans true coronal, T_2 sagittal to cervix and uterus.
6. MRI features – Stage IA tumour may not be visible. Tumour normally hypointense compared to endometrium and hyperintense compared to myometrium and cervical stroma.

13.4 UTERINE MYOMETRIUM

Clinical and imaging features of benign disease

1. **Leiomyomata**
    (a) Very common, usually benign, smooth muscle tumour.
    (b) >20% of women over 35. More common in Afro-Caribbean women.
    (c) Often asymptomatic and incidental finding on ultrasound.
    (d) Present with menstrual disturbance, pelvic mass, pelvic heaviness, increased frequency, infertility, recurrent abortion.
    (e) May be single or multiple, large or small.
    (f) Defined by size and position – submucosal, myometrial or subserosal.
    (g) May be extra-uterine e.g. broad ligament fibroid.
    (h) Usually well defined heterogeneous but mainly hypoechoic pattern on US.
    (i) Variable pattern seen in cystic degeneration.
    (j) Check for involvement of adjacent structures e.g. endometrium, ureters.
    (k) MRI used for assessment pre-embolisation and for follow-up.
    (l) MRI also used for problem solving with indeterminate masses.
    (m) Well defined, isointense to myometrium on T_1 scans.
    (n) Hypointense on T_2 weighted scans.
    (o) Become more heterogeneous on T_2 as degeneration occurs.
    (p) Haemorrhagic degeneration (red degeneration) shows high signal areas on T_1 imaging.
2. **Adenomyosis.**
    (a) Defined as endometrial stroma and glands within myometrium.
    (b) May be focal (adenomyoma) or diffuse.
    (c) Presents later in menstrual life with pain, dyspareunia and dysfunctional bleeding.

(d) May be difficult to diagnose but can be effectively managed with a progesterone impregnated intra-uterine system.

(e) Ultrasound shows increased focal reflectivity in the myometrium with asymmetric thickening of the myometrium. May show a focal adenomyoma.

(f) MR imaging is highly accurate, sensitive and specific.

(g) T_2 weighted scans show punctuate foci of high signal within the myometrium.

(h) Associated feature but less specific is thickening of the junctional zone >12mm.

3. **Congenital uterine anomalies.**

   (a) May be identified on ultrasound.

   (b) 3D ultrasound has increasing importance as experience develops with this technique.

   (c) Best imaged on MRI with three-plane T_2 scans. A T_2 scan, coronal to plane of uterus, is useful to evaluate uterine/ endometrial abnormalities.

Clinical and imaging features of malignant disease

1. **Leiomyosarcoma**

   (a) Thought to arise from pre-existing fibroid, usually but not exclusively postmenopausal.

   (b) Lacks any specific features on US or MRI and it is impossible to accurately differentiate on imaging between benign fibroid and sarcoma.

   (c) Large tumour size, ill-defined margins and rapid increase in size are all worrying features.

2. **Uterine metastases**

   (a) Usually direct invasion from contiguous tumour.

   (b) Usually other features of metastatic malignant disease.

13

13.5 UTERINE ENDOMETRIUM

Clinical and imaging features of benign disease

1. Normal endometrium varies across the menstrual cycle with most prominent thickening in the secretory phase.
2. Postmenopausal endometrium should be thin (<5mm) and homogenous.
3. Endometrial hyperplasia can occur pre- and postmenopausally due to prolonged oestrogen exposure.
4. Endometrial polyps may be difficult to differentiate from endometrial thickening. Accuracy improved by performing sonohysterography. Power Doppler evaluation may demonstrate a stalk with a large entering vessel.
5. Endometrial thickening may be due to multiple processes:
   (a) Early pregnancy.
   (b) Ectopic pregnancy.
   (c) Retained products of conception.
   (d) Anovulatory cycles.
   (e) Tamoxifen therapy.
   (f) Hormone replacement therapy (HRT).
6. Sometimes difficult to differentiate between an endometrial polyp and a submucosal fibroid. MR useful as polyps show significant and persistent increased signal.

Clinical and imaging features of malignant disease

1. Commonest presentation is postmenopausal vaginal bleeding.
2. Endometrial carcinoma is the commonest gynaecological carcinoma.
3. Risk factors are:
   (a) HRT therapy.
   (b) Tamoxifen therapy.
   (c) Age.
   (d) FH of endometrial/colorectal carcinoma.
   (e) Past history of unopposed oestrogen exposure.
   (f) Hypertension.
   (g) Obesity in diabetes.
4. Ultrasound useful for identifying endometrial thickening in symptomatic women but not good at staging.
5. MR imaging is the modality of choice to stage endometrial carcinoma diagnosed on sampling/hysteroscopy.
6. Staging performed according to the FIGO (International Federation of Obstetrics and Gynaecology) definition.
7. High resolution scanning required using T_2 sequences in the axial, sagittal and coronal planes with a specific sequence axial to the plane of the uterus to assess the endometrium/myometrial junctional zone.

8. The depth of the myometrial invasion is critical to staging and subsequent surgical management.
9. Post-gadolinium T_1 weighted scans are sometimes useful to define the depth of myometrial invasion.
10. Staging more problematic in the presence of fibroids or adenomyosis.
11. Tumour appears slightly hypointense compared to endometrium but hyperintense compared to myometrium.
12. Lymph node status is critical to management.

13.6 OVARY

Clinical and imaging features of benign ovarian disease

1. Ultrasound is very sensitive at diagnosing ovarian lesions but is less specific at differentiating pathology.
2. Functional ovarian cysts are extremely common. Cysts less than 3cm are considered normal follicular cysts.
3. Most cysts are relatively asymptomatic until they become space occupying although torsion, haemorrhage and rupture may be very painful.
4. Haemorrhage into a cyst alters the appearance and makes it very difficult to exclude a more sinister lesion.
5. Simple cystic lesions in the pelvis:
    (a) Follicular cyst.
    (b) Cystadenoma.
    (c) Theca lutein cyst (hydatidiform mole etc).
    (d) Para-ovarian cyst.
    (e) Corpus luteal cyst (may be slightly echogenic due to blood).
    (f) Dermoid cysts may rarely be purely cystic.
    (g) Other cystic lesions e.g. lymphocoele, bladder diverticulum, urinoma, loculated fluid.
6. Polycystic ovaries. Not necessarily related to polycystic ovary syndrome. Consensus is that the ultrasound diagnosis of a polycystic ovary depends on an overall increase in size of the ovary to 10cc or greater and/or 12 or more subcapsular follicles measuring 2–9mm in diameter.
7. Ovarian remnant syndrome. Post bilateral oophorectomy a pelvic cyst may be due to a small amount of residual functioning ovarian tissue.
8. Endometriosis is not easily diagnosed in Stage 1 or 2 disease but larger endometriomas are well recognized on ultrasound. They present as well defined, diffusely hypoechoic cysts with 'low level' echoes throughout. They may contain fluid/fluid levels due to blood of different ages being present.

13

9. Complex lesions:
   (a) Haemorrhagic cyst.
   (b) Torted cyst.
   (c) Mucinous cystadenomas.
   (d) Dermoid cyst.
10. Solid benign lesions:
    (a) Fibroid – pedunculated or broad ligament.
    (b) Brenner's tumour.
    (c) Gonadal stromal tumours e.g. thecoma, fibroma.
11. Ultrasound is primary imaging tool with MRI reserved for differentiating the indeterminate mass lesion. Additional fat suppression sequences are useful for evaluating the size and extent of dermoid tumours.

Clinical and imaging features of malignant ovarian disease

1. Ovarian cancer is second most common gynaecological malignancy but with highest mortality rate due to late presentation at an advanced stage.
2. Presents in middle and old age with a pre-clinical stage of two years on average.
3. Risk factors include:
   (a) Family history.
   (b) Early menarche.
   (c) Low parity.
   (d) Late menopause.
4. No single screening programme has yet been defined although postmenopausal serum testing with CA125 and annual ultrasound screening of ovarian size and morphology are being promoted.
5. Ultrasound is currently imaging modality of choice although problems with indeterminate lesions (up to 20%) limit its effectiveness in early carcinoma.
6. Significant ultrasound features of malignancy are:
   (a) Presence of solid nodules.
   (b) Increased Doppler flow.
   (c) Presence of ascites.
   (d) Presence of thickened irregular septae.
7. Tumours of borderline malignancy are diagnosed in up to 15% of oophorectomy cases as they lack any specific features to confirm benign or malignant disease.
8. Ovarian malignancies include:
   (a) Serous cystadenocarcinoma.
   (b) Mucinous cystadenocarcinoma.
   (c) Clear cell carcinoma.

(d) Endometrioid tumours.

(e) Dysgerminoma (LDH elevated in 90%).

(f) Lymphoma.

(g) Ovarian metastases (Krukenberg tumours) usually of GIT origin (50%).

9. Yolk sac tumour is an aggressive tumour of adolescence with a good prognosis with modern treatment regimes. Associated with elevated alpha fetoprotein and used to monitor treatment.

10. CT is currently the staging investigation of choice principally to assess extent of intraperitoneal spread of disease.

11. Post contrast MRI useful to differentiate benign from malignant lesions.

13.7 ADNEXA

Clinical and imaging features

Commonest adnexal problems relate principally to the fallopian tube and infection (see 13.17 for ectopic gestation). These are best imaged with ultrasound although MRI is useful for problem solving in difficult cases.

1. Ultrasound appearance may be completely normal in acute PID.

2. Vague adnexal mass and free fluid is consistent with acute PID but the clinical and biochemical features are important discriminators.

3. Doppler is useful in the acute phase to confirm increased vascularity.

4. In the acute phase of PID there may be additional features of endometritis with fluid and even air within the endometrial cavity.

5. Chronic changes of tubal dilatation are well seen on US. This can be confirmed by MRI, hystersalpingography or laparoscopy.

6. MRI is useful to differentiate a dilated tube from a complex ovarian cyst.

OBSTETRIC IMAGING

Obstetric scanning is no longer part of the radiological core curriculum and should therefore only be practised by those individuals with a specific interest and qualification e.g. RCR/RCOG Diploma. Nonetheless knowledge of current obstetric practice is appropriate as much of routine obstetric scanning still takes place in radiology departments by experienced radiographer sonographers. Also, early pregnancy problems are an important part of the emergency gynaecological workload in all units.

13

13.8 NORMAL PREGNANCY

1st trimester imaging

Every pregnant woman should be offered an early scan to confirm viability, site of pregnancy, gestational age and number (NICE).

Ultrasound assessment of gestational age is recommended as being more accurate than LMP. This allows better management of post term pregnancies, 2nd trimester serum screening programmes and serial growth measurements where fetal growth restriction is present/suspected.

Ultrasound should not be used to routinely diagnose pregnancy.

Where 1st trimester combined Down's screening is offered then the scan should ideally be performed between 9w 0d and 13w 6d to facilitate the detection and measurement of nuchal translucency (NT).

When scanning is performed between 11 and 14 weeks there is an increased rate of detection of fetal abnormalities e.g. neural tube defects, renal, cardiac and limb abnormalities. This however is not the current rationale for 1st trimester screening.

Where a multiple pregnancy is present the chorionicity is best determined on this early scan by assessment of the intersac chorion. This assessment is less accurate in later gestation. See diagram.

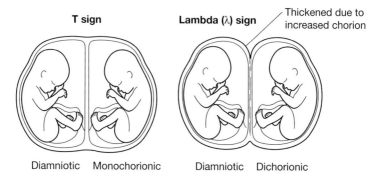

T sign

Diamniotic   Monochorionic

Lambda (λ) sign

Thickened due to increased chorion

Diamniotic   Dichorionic

2nd trimester imaging

A fetal anomaly scan should be offered to all pregnant women between 18w 0d and 20w 6d (NICE).

1. Fetal biometry assessed by measurement of head circumference (HC), biparietal diameter (BPD) and femur length (FL). Other measurements can be made as required, e.g. cerebellar diameter, humeral length etc. The recommended principal measurements are

the head circumference and femur length (BMUS). Standardized national charts are also recommended (BMUS).

2. Fetal anatomical checklist recommended along with potential abnormalities (RCOG and NSC).

3. Placental site assessed. Where placenta *crosses* the internal os a repeat scan is advised at 36 weeks gestation to assess status prior to decision making about mode of delivery (NICE).

13.9 ABNORMAL PREGNANCY

1st trimester loss

Very common problem. It is estimated that as many as 15–20% of conceptions will end in early pregnancy failure. Many of these patients are now assessed in dedicated 'early pregnancy loss' units but they will still make up a significant percentage of ultrasound departmental workload.

Features of early pregnancy failure

1. **Gestational sac:**
   (a) Deformity of sac.
   (b) Mean sac diameter >18mm without a yolk sac.
   (c) Mean sac diameter >20mm without a fetal pole.
   (d) Abnormally low position of sac.

2. **Fetal pole:**
   (a) CRL of >6mm without detectable cardiac activity.

All of these features are seen better and earlier on transvaginal scanning.

13

13.10 FETAL GROWTH RESTRICTION

≤ 5th centile for growth parameters.

Risk factors

1. **Idiopathic.**
2. **Maternal:**
   (a) Hypertension (essential or of pregnancy).
   (b) Renal disease.
   (c) Cardiac disease.
   (d) Diabetes.
   (e) Collagen vascular disease (SLE).
   (f) Cigarette/alcohol abuse.
   (g) Drug abuse.
   (h) Infection.
3. **Multiple gestation.**
4. **Placental causes.**

Assessment

1. **Fundus symphysis height measurement** (by palpation).
2. **Ultrasound measurement of:**
   (a) Head circumference (HC).
   (b) Abdominal circumference (AC).
   (c) Femur length (FL).
   (d) Amniotic fluid volume (usually decreased).
   (e) Umbilical artery Doppler (increasing vascular resistance).
   (f) Fetal vascular Doppler (middle cerebral artery, ductus venosus).

13.11 FETAL HYDROPS

Many causes. Defined as fluid in the subcutaneous tissues and one other potential space, e.g. pleural cavity, peritoneal cavity.

1. **Immune hydrops**:
   (a) Rhesus incompatibility.
   (b) Other blood group incompatibility.
2. **Non-immune hydrops**:
   (a) Cardiovascular disease.
   (b) Pulmonary.
   (c) Chromosomal.
   (d) Syndromic.
   (e) Haematological.
   (f) Infections.
   (g) Neoplasia.
   (h) Genitourinary.
   (i) Hepatic.
   (j) GI tract.
   (k) Metabolic.
   (l) Musculoskeletal.
   (m) Multiple pregnancies.

13.12 MULTIPLE PREGNANCY

1. Chorionicity best assessed on early pregnancy scan (see above).
2. Importance of careful assessment and management of twins is emphasized by the increased fetal loss of twins generally and monochorionic twins in particular. IU loss is 7× greater in twins than in singleton pregnancies and is highest in monochorionic, monoamniotic pregnancy.
3. Monochorionic twins have an increased rate of fetal anomalies, increased shared vascular connections leading to twin–twin transfusion and acardiac twinning, increased cord entanglement and increased complications in the event of the death of one of the twins.
4. Major issues with Down's screening in multiple pregnancy as serum screening is not effective. Nuchal translucency assessment is likely to be the way forward although multiple issues arise when interventional assessment is required both for diagnostic and therapeutic purposes, e.g. amniocentesis and subsequent fetocide.

13

13.13 PLACENTA

Ultrasound appearance of placenta varies throughout pregnancy:

Gestational age (weeks)	Sonographic appearance
8	Focal isoechoic thickening of gestational sac wall
12	Placenta is clearly visible; increasing echogenicity
16	Placenta and fetus similar in size
20+	Placenta usually 2–3cm thick; >5cm considered abnormal
29	Placental calcification becomes visible
33	50% of normal placentas now show foci of calcification

13.14 ABNORMALITIES OF THE PLACENTA

Placenta praevia

Defined as a portion of the placenta covering the internal os.

Ultrasound diagnosis of placenta praevia at 18–20 week scan is far greater than incidence at term due to differential growth of uterus and in particular the lower segment (20% cf 0.5%). 'Low lying placenta' and 'touching the os' are terms no longer advised on the 18–20 week scan. Placenta must cross the internal os to initiate a follow-up scan (NICE).

Other placental abnormalities

1. **Placental abruption** – premature separation of a normal sited placenta. Associated with maternal hypertension, vascular disease, smoking, drug abuse, trauma and presence of fibroids.
2. **Placental lakes** – normal variant.
3. **Succenturiate lobe** – accessory lobe attached to main placental vessels.
4. **Placenta accreta/increta/percreta** – varying degrees of direct placental invasion of the myometrium by chorionic villi. Frequency increased in placenta praevia and increases further in the presence of previous caesarean section. Repeated caesarean section significantly increases the risk further.
5. Chorioangioma of placenta – benign tumour of placenta. May be associated with pregnancy complications if greater than 5cm or diffuse in nature. Vascular shunting in large tumours may cause hydrops, restricted fetal growth, etc.

13.15 GESTATIONAL TROPHOBLASTIC DISEASE

Neoplastic disease arising from trophoblastic tissue. Spectrum of presentation from benign hydatidiform mole to malignant choriocarcinoma. The trophoblastic tissue shows an abnormal chromosomal karyotype.

Hydatidiform mole (classic mole/molar pregnancy)

1. Diagnosed during early pregnancy with US features of a large echogenic vesicular mass filling the uterus.
2. Associated with hyper-emesis, early pre-eclampsia, and vaginal loss of cystic material.
3. In early pregnancy, appearance may be confused with hydropic degeneration of the placenta in a failed pregnancy for other reasons. Differential diagnosis also includes retained products.
4. Mole usually associated with abnormally raised hCG levels and may have abnormal ovarian stimulation with large theca lutein ovarian cysts (30–50%).
5. May rarely have a normal fetus with a coexistent molar pregnancy. This is due to molar degeneration of a dizygotic twin.

Incomplete mole (partial mole)

1. Coexistent abnormal fetus with a mole.
2. Fetal IUGR present and usually abnormal fetal karyotype.
3. Ultrasound appearance as for a classic mole with a vesicular mass associated with abnormal fetal parts.

Invasive mole

1. Locally invasive molar tissue.
2. Molar tissue demonstrated to invade myometrium on ultrasound.
3. Often a previous history of molar pregnancy (up to 75%).

Choriocarcinoma

1. Most malignant form.
2. Half are associated with previous molar pregnancy.
3. Also associated with spontaneous abortion (25%), normal pregnancy (22%) and ectopic pregnancy (3%).
4. Present with persistently elevated hCG after successful or failed pregnancy.
5. Uterine mass as with molar pregnancy but likelihood of myometrial invasion and distant metastases to liver, lung, brain, bone and GIT.

13

13.16 EARLY PREGNANCY BLEEDING

Causes and features

All ultrasound appearances are seen earlier and more clearly on transvaginal (TV) rather than transabdominal (TA) scanning. Presumed early pregnancy failures should be offered a second scan after minimum of 7 days to confirm the diagnosis (RCR/RCOG).

1. **Implantation bleed.**
    (a) Normally no ultrasound features. Usually settle spontaneously.
2. **Pregnancy failure** – threatened/missed/incomplete abortion.
    (a) Viable fetus identified in up to 50%. Remainder have a variable size fetal pole but with no fetal heart activity or movement. An irregular sac is often present.
    (b) Fetal pole >6mm in length with no fetal heart pulsation.
3. **Pregnancy failure** – anembryonic gestation ('blighted ovum').
    (a) Large empty sac with no fetal pole (sac diameter >30mm) or yolk sac (sac diameter >20mm). Failed development of the fertilized ovum is usually due to a chromosomal abnormality.
4. **Ectopic gestation.**
    (a) See next section.

13.17 ECTOPIC GESTATION

Over last decade the incidence of ectopic gestation has remained static at 11.0 per 1000 pregnancies in the UK.

Risk factors

1. **Previous ectopic pregnancy.**
2. **IUCD in situ.**
3. **Previous tubal surgery.**
4. **Previous known or unknown PID** (particularly Chlamydia).
5. **IVF.**

Clinical features

The classic presentation of pain, vaginal bleeding and pelvic mass is neither common nor specific and not all women have missed a period. Ultrasound (preferably TV) and serum hCG are therefore vital to the early diagnosis of this condition.

Ultrasound findings

1. No evidence of an intrauterine pregnancy (but beware early gestation).
2. Endometrial thickening – pseudogestational sac.
3. Fluid in pelvis (often slightly echogenic as usually blood).
4. Adnexal mass – often complex.
5. Live fetus/fetal cardiac activity outside uterus occurs in about 10%.
6. No ultrasound abnormality does not exclude ectopic gestation.
7. Live intra-uterine gestation normally excludes the diagnosis of ectopic pregnancy but beware the coincidental ectopic twin gestation (approx 1:30,000 in unstimulated population).
8. Empty uterus with hCG >1800 iu/l is highly suggestive of ectopic.

Further Reading

Adusimilli HK, Caoili EM, Weadcock WJ et al. MRI of sonographically indeterminate adnexal masses. Am J Roentgenol 2006;187:732–40.

Bates J. Practical gynaecological ultrasound. Cambridge University Press, Cambridge, 2006.

Bisset RAL, Khan AN, Thomas NB. Differential diagnosis in obstetric & gynaecological ultrasound. WB Saunders, Philadelphia, 2002.

Brown MA. MR Imaging of the female pelvis. Magnetic resonance imaging clinics of North America. Elsevier Saunders, New York, 2006.

Callen PW. Ultrasonography in obstetrics and gynaecology. WB Saunders, Philadelphia, 2000.

National Collaborating Centre for Women's and Children Health. Antenatal care: routine care for the healthy pregnant woman. Commissioned by the National Institute for Clinical Excellence. NCCWCH, London, 2003.

Sohaib SA, Mills TD, Webb JAW et al. The role of magnetic resonance imaging and ultrasound in patients with adnexal masses. Clin Radiol 2005;60:340–8.

Standing Joint Committee on Obstetric Ultrasound of the Royal College of Radiologists/Royal College of Obstetricians & Gynaecologists, Guidance on ultrasound procedures in early pregnancy. RCR/RCOG, London, 1995.

Twining P, McHugo J, Pilling D. Textbook of fetal abnormality. Churchill Livingstone, Edinburgh, 2006.

13

Paediatrics

Paul Humphries and Alistair Calder

14.1 RETARDED SKELETAL MATURATION

Chronic ill health

1. **Congenital heart disease** – particularly cyanotic.
2. **Renal failure**.
3. **Inflammatory bowel disease**.
4. **Malnutrition**.
5. **Rickets***.
6. **Maternal deprivation**.
7. **Any other chronic illness**.

Endocrine disorders

1. **Hypothyroidism*** – with granular, fragmented epiphyses. This causes severe retardation (five or more standard deviations below the mean).
2. **Steroid therapy and Cushing's disease** – see Cushing's syndrome*.
3. **Hypogonadism** – including older patients with Turner's syndrome.
4. **Hypopituitarism** – panhypopituitarism, growth hormone deficiency and Laron dwarfism.

Chromosome disorders

1. **Trisomy 21**.
2. **Most other chromosome disorders** – severely depressed in trisomy 18.

Other congenital disorders

1. **Most bone dysplasias**.
2. **Most malformation syndromes**.

Further Reading

Poznanski AK. The hand in radiologic diagnosis, Ch 3. WB Saunders, Philadelphia, 1984, p67–96.

14.2 GENERALIZED ACCELERATED SKELETAL MATURATION

Endocrine disorders

1. Idiopathic sexual precocity.
2. Intracranial masses in the region of the hypothalamus (hamartoma, astrocytoma and optic chiasm glioma), hydrocephalus and encephalitis.
3. Adrenal and gonadal tumours.
4. Hyperthyroidism.

Congenital disorders

1. **McCune–Albright syndrome** – polyostotic fibrous dysplasia with precocious puberty.
2. **Cerebral gigantism (Soto's syndrome).**
3. **Lipodystrophy.**
4. **Pseudohypoparathyroidism.**
5. **Acrodysostosis.**
6. **Weaver (Weaver–Smith) syndrome.**
7. **Marshall (Marshall–Smith) syndrome.**

Others

1. Large or obese children.

Further Reading
Fahmy JL, Kaminsky CK, Kaufman F et al. The radiological approach to precocious puberty. Br J Radiol 2000;73(869):560–7.
Poznanski AK. The hand in radiologic diagnosis, Ch 3. WB Saunders, Philadelphia, 1984, p67–96.
Rieth KG, Comite F, Dwyer AJ et al. CT of cerebral abnormalities in precocious puberty. Am J Roentgenol 1987;148:1231–8.

14

14.3 PREMATURE CLOSURE OF A GROWTH PLATE

1. **Local hyperaemia** – juvenile idiopathic arthritides, infection, haemophilia or arteriovenous malformation.
2. **Trauma.**
3. **Vascular occlusion** – infarcts and sickle-cell anaemia.
4. **Radiotherapy.**
5. **Thermal injury** – burns, frostbite.
6. **Multiple exostoses and enchondromatosis (Ollier's disease).**
7. **Hypervitaminosis A** – now more usually via vitamin A analogue treatment for dermatological conditions rather than dietary overdosage.

Further Reading
Piddo C, Reed MH, Black GB. Premature epiphyseal fusion and degenerative arthritis in chronic recurrent multifocal osteomyelitis. Skeletal Radiol 2000;29(2):94–6.

Rothenberg AB, Bedon WE, Woodard JC et al. Hypervitaminosis A-induced premature closure of epiphyses (physeal obliteration) in humans and calves (hyena disease): a historical review of the human and veterinary literature. Ped Rad 2007;37(12):1264–67.

14.4 ASYMMETRICAL MATURATION

1. **Normal children** – minor differences only.

Hemihypertrophy or localized gigantism

1. **Vascular anomalies**
   (a) Haemangioma and AVM.
   (b) Klippel–Trenaunay–Weber syndrome – hypertrophy of the skeleton and soft tissues of one limb or one side of the body in association with an angiomatous malformation.
   (c) Maffucci's syndrome – enchondromas + haemangiomas.
2. **Chronic hyperaemia** – e.g. chronic arthritides (juvenile chronic arthritis or haemophilia).
3. **Hemihypertrophy** – M>F; R>L. May be a presenting feature of Beckwith–Wiedemann syndrome (hemihypertrophy, macroglossia, hypoglycaemia and umbilical hernia). Increased incidence of Wilms' tumour.
4. **Neurofibromatosis** – type 1*.
5. **Macrodystrophia lipomatosa.**

6. **Russell–Silver dwarfism** – evident from birth. Triangular face with down-turned corners of the mouth, frontal bossing, asymmetrical growth and skeletal maturation.
7. **Proteus syndrome** – hamartomatous disorder with multiple and varied manifestations including vascular and lymphatic malformations, macrocephaly and cranial hyperostoses.
8. **WAGR syndrome** – Wilms tumour, Aniridia, Genitourinary abnormalities and mental Retardation.

Hemiatrophy or localized atrophy
1. **Paralysis** – with osteopenia and overtubulation of long bones.
2. **Radiation treatment in childhood.**

14.5 SHORT LIMB SKELETAL DYSPLASIAS

Rhizomelic (proximal limb shortening)
1. **Hypochondroplasia** – resembles a mild form of achondroplasia.
2. **Achondroplasia*.**
3. **Chondrodysplasia punctata** – see 14.17.
4. **Pseudoachondroplasia** – see 14.6.

Mesomelic (middle segment limb shortening)
1. **Dyschondrosteosis (Leri–Weil disease)** – limb shortening with a Madelung deformity.
2. **Mesomelic dysplasia**
   (a) Type Langer.
   (b) Type Reinhardt–Pfeiffer.

Acromesomelic (middle and distal segment limb shortening)
1. **Chondroectodermal dysplasia (Ellis–van Creveld syndrome)** – similar to asphyxiating thoracic dysplasia but: (a) hexadactyly is a constant finding, (b) there is severe hypoplasia of the fingers and nails, (c) congenital heart disease is common and (d) hypoplastic lateral tibial plateau is characteristic in childhood.
2. **Acromesomelic dysplasia.**

14

3. **Mesomelic dysplasia**
   (a) Type Nievergelt.
   (b) Type Robinow.
   (c) Type Werner.

Acromelic (distal segment shortening)

1. **Asphyxiating thoracic dysplasia (Jeune's syndrome)** – narrow thorax with short ribs leading to respiratory distress. Spur-like projections of the acetabular roof. Premature ossification of the femoral capital epiphyses. Occasional postaxial hexadactyly. Cone-shaped epiphyses in childhood.
2. **Peripheral dysostosis.**

14.6 SHORT SPINE SKELETAL DYSPLASIAS

1. **Pseudoachondroplasia** – short limb and short spine dwarfism, marked joint laxity, platyspondyly with exaggerated grooves for the ring apophyses, C1/2 dislocation.
2. **Spondyloepiphyseal dysplasia** – ovoid or 'pear-shaped' vertebral bodies in infancy → severe platyspondyly in later life; normal metaphyses; retarded development of the symphysis pubis and femoral heads; coxa vara, which may be severe; ± odontoid hypoplasia and C1/2 instability.
3. **Spondylometaphyseal dysplasias**
   (a) Type Kozlowski.
   (b) Other types.
4. **Diastrophic dwarfism** – progressive kyphoscoliosis, hitch-hiker thumb, delta-shaped epiphyses, interpedicular narrowing of the lumbar spine.
5. **Metatropic dwarfism** – short-limbed dwarfism in infancy → short spine dwarfism in later childhood, severe progressive scoliosis, dumbbell-shaped long bones, hypoplastic odontoid.
6. **Kniest syndrome** – dumbbell-shaped long bones, irregular epiphyses, kyphoscoliosis, platyspondyly, interpedicular narrowing of the lumbar spine, limited and painful joint movements.

14.7 LETHAL NEONATAL DYSPLASIA

1. **Osteogenesis imperfecta*** – usually type II.
2. **Thanatophoric dwarfism** – small thorax, severe platyspondyly with 'H'-shaped or 'inverted U'-shaped vertebral bodies, 'telephone handle'-shaped long bones ± 'clover-leaf' skull deformity.
3. **Chondrodysplasia punctata** – rhizomelic form. See 14.17.
4. **Asphyxiating thoracic dysplasia (Jeune's syndrome)** – see 14.5.
5. **Campomelic dwarfism** – bowed long bones.
6. **Achondrogenesis** – types I and II.
7. **Short rib syndromes ± polydactyly**
   (a) Type I (Saldino–Noonan).
   (b) Type II (Majewski).
   (c) Type III (lethal thoracic dysplasia).
8. **Homozygous achondroplasia*.**
9. **Hypophosphatasia*** – lethal type.

14.8 DUMBBELL-SHAPED LONG BONES

Short narrow diaphyses with marked metaphyseal widening.

1. **Metatropic dwarfism** – see 14.6.
2. **Pseudoachondroplasia** – see 14.6.
3. **Kniest syndrome** – see 14.6.
4. **Diastrophic dwarfism** – see 14.6.
5. **Osteogenesis imperfecta (type III)*.**
6. **Chondroectodermal dysplasia (Ellis–van Creveld syndrome)** – see 14.5.

14.9 CONDITIONS EXHIBITING DYSOSTOSIS MULTIPLEX

Dysostosis multiplex is a constellation of radiological signs which are exhibited, in total or in part, by a number of conditions caused by defects of complex carbohydrate metabolism. These signs include: (a) abnormal bone texture, (b) widening of diaphyses, (c) tilting of distal radius and ulna towards each other, (d) pointing of the proximal ends of the metacarpals, (e) large skull vault with calvarial thickening, (f) anterior beak of upper lumbar vertebrae, and (g) 'J-shaped' sella.

14

Mucopolysaccharidoses

Type	Eponym	Inheritance	Onset	Osseous and visceral abnormalities	Neurological features
IH	Hurler*	AR	By 1–2 years	Marked. Severe dwarfism. Skeletal abnormalities ++. Corneal clouding	Severe
IS	Scheie	AR	Childhood	Carpal tunnel syndrome	Mild
II	Hunter	XR	2–4 years	Marked. Severe dwarfism. Dysostosis multiplex similar to Hurler but less severe. No corneal clouding	Mild to moderate
III	Sanfilippo	AR	Childhood	Mild	Severe
IV	Morquio*	AR	1–3 years	Severe skeletal abnormalities	Absent (but may be neurological complications of spinal abnormalities)
VI	Maroteaux–Lamy	AR	Childhood	Severe dwarfism and skeletal abnormalities	Absent (except as a complication of meningeal involvement)
VII	Sly	AR		Mild to severe	Absent to severe

Mucolipidoses
1. MLS I (neuraminidase deficiency).
2. MLS II (I-cell disease).
3. MLS III (pseudopolydystrophy of Maroteaux).

Oligosaccharidoses
1. Fucosidosis I.
2. Fucosidosis II.
3. GM1 gangliosidosis.
4. Mannosidosis.
5. Aspartylglucosaminuria.

14.10 GENERALIZED INCREASED BONE DENSITY

NB Infants in the first few months of life can exhibit 'physiological' bone sclerosis which regresses spontaneously.

Dysplasias

1. **Osteopetrosis*.**
2. **Pyknodysostosis** – short stature, hypoplastic lateral ends of clavicles, hypoplastic terminal phalanges, bulging cranium and delayed closure of the anterior fontanelle. AR.
3. **The craniotubular dysplasias** – abnormal skeletal modelling ± increased bone density.
   (a) Metaphyseal dysplasia (Pyle).
   (b) Craniometaphyseal dysplasia.
   (c) Craniodiaphyseal dysplasia.
   (d) Frontometaphyseal dysplasia.
   (e) Osteodysplasty (Melnick–Needles).
4. **The craniotubular hyperostoses** – overgrowth of bone with alteration of contours and increased bone density.
   (a) Endosteal hyperostosis, Van Buchem type.
   (b) Endosteal hyperostosis, Worth type.
   (c) Sclerosteosis.
   (d) Diaphyseal dysplasia (Camurati–Engelmann).

Metabolic

1. **Renal osteodystrophy*** – rickets + osteosclerosis.

Poisoning

1. **Lead** – dense metaphyseal bands. Cortex and flat bones may also be slightly dense. Modelling deformities later, e.g. flask-shaped femora.
2. **Fluorosis** – more common in adults. Usually asymptomatic but may present in children with crippling stiffness and pain. Thickened cortex at the expense of the medulla. Periosteal reaction. Ossification of ligaments, tendons and interosseous membranes.
3. **Hypervitaminosis D** – slightly increased density of skull and vertebrae early, followed later by osteoporosis. Soft-tissue calcification. Dense metaphyseal bands and widened zone of provisional calcification.

14

4. **Chronic hypervitaminosis A** – not before 1 year of age. Failure to thrive, hepatosplenomegaly, jaundice, alopecia and haemoptysis. Cortical thickening of long and tubular bones, especially in the feet. Subperiosteal new bone. Normal epiphyses and reduced metaphyseal density. The mandible is not affected (cf. Caffey's disease).

Idiopathic

1. **Caffey's disease (infantile cortical hyperostosis)** – see 14.13.
2. **Idiopathic hypercalcaemia of infancy** – probably a manifestation of hypervitaminosis D. Elfin facies, failure to thrive and mental retardation. Generalized increased density or transverse dense metaphyseal bands. Increased density of the skull base.

Further Reading

Beighton P, Cremin BJ. Sclerosing bone dysplasias. Springer-Verlag, Berlin, 1980.

Herman TE, McAlister WH. Inherited diseases in bone density in children. Radiol Clin North Am 1991;29(1):149–64.

Vanhoenacker FM, De Beuckeleer LH, Van Hul W et al. Sclerosing bone dysplasias: genetic and radioclinical features. Eur Radiol 2000;10:1423–33.

14.11 PAEDIATRIC TUMOURS THAT METASTASIZE TO BONE

1. **Neuroblastoma.**
2. **Leukaemia** – although not truly metastases.
3. **Lymphoma*.**
4. **Clear cell sarcoma (Wilms' variant).**
5. **Rhabdomyosarcoma.**
6. **Retinoblastoma.**
7. **Ewing's sarcoma** – lung metastases much more common.
8. **Osteosarcoma*** – lung metastases much more common.

Further Reading

Parker BR. Leukaemia and lymphoma in childhood. Radiol Clin North Am 1997;35(6):1495–516.

14.12 'MOTH-EATEN BONE' IN A CHILD

See Figure 1.18

Neoplastic

1. **Neuroblastoma metastases*.**
2. **Leukaemia** – consider when there is diffuse involvement of an entire bone or a neighbouring bone with low signal on T_1W and high signal on T_2W and short tau inversion recovery (STIR) MRI.
3. **Long-bone sarcomas**
   (a) Primitive neuroectodermal tumour (PNET)/Ewing's sarcoma*.
   (b) Lymphoma of bone.
   (c) Osteosarcoma*.
4. **Langerhans cell histiocytosis*.**

Infective

1. **Acute osteomyelitis.**

Further Reading
Sammak B, Abd El Bagi M, Al Shahed M et al. Osteomyelitis: a review of currently used imaging techniques. Eur Radiol 1999;9:894–900.

14.13 PERIOSTEAL REACTIONS – BILATERALLY SYMMETRICAL IN CHILDREN

1. **Normal infants** – diaphyseal, not extending to the growth plate, bilaterally symmetrical and a single lamina. Very unusual beyond 4 months of age.
2. **Juvenile idiopathic arthritis*** – in approximately 25% of cases. Most common in the periarticular regions of the phalanges, metacarpals and metatarsals. When it extends into the diaphysis it will eventually result in enlarged, rectangular tubular bones.
3. **Acute leukaemia** – associated with prominent metaphyseal bone resorption ± a dense zone of provisional calcification. Osteopenia. Periosteal reaction is due to cortical involvement by tumour cells. Metastatic neuroblastoma can look identical.
4. **Rickets*** – the presence of uncalcified subperiosteal osteoid mimics a periosteal reaction because the periosteum and ossified cortex are separated.
5. **Caffey's disease** – first evident before 5 months of age. Mandible, clavicles and ribs show cortical hyperostosis and a diffuse periosteal reaction. The scapulae and tubular bones are less often affected and tend to be involved asymmetrically.

14

6. **Scurvy*** – subperiosteal haemorrhage is most frequent in the femur, tibia and humerus. Periosteal reaction is particularly evident during the healing phase. Age 6 months or older.
7. **Prostaglandin E1 therapy** – in infants with ductus-dependent congenital heart disease. Severity is related to duration of therapy. Other features include fever, flushing, diarrhoea, skin oedema, pseudowidening of cranial sutures and bone-in-bone appearance.
8. **Congenital syphilis** – an exuberant periosteal reaction can be due to infiltration by syphilitic granulation tissue or the healing (with callus formation) of osteochondritis. The former is essentially diaphyseal and the latter around the metaphyseal/epiphyseal junction.

Further Reading

Matzinger MA, Briggs VA, Dunlap HJ et al. Plain film and CT observations in prostaglandin-induced bone changes. Pediatr Radiol 1992;22: 264–6.
Shopfner CE. Periosteal bone growth in normal infants. Am J Roentgenol 1966;97:154–63.
Swischuk LE, John SD. Differential diagnosis in pediatric radiology, 2nd edn. Williams and Wilkins, Baltimore, 1995, p318–26.

14.14 SYNDROMES AND BONE DYSPLASIAS WITH MULTIPLE FRACTURES AS A FEATURE

With reduced bone density

1. Osteogenesis imperfecta*.
2. Achondrogenesis.
3. Hypophosphatasia.
4. Mucolipidosis II (I-cell disease).
5. Cushing's syndrome.

With normal bone density

1. Cleidocranial dysplasia.
2. Fibrous dysplasia.

With increased bone density

1. Osteopetrosis*.
2. Pyknodysostosis – see 14.10.

14.15 PSEUDARTHROSIS IN A CHILD

1. **Non-union of a fracture** – including pathological fracture.
2. **Congenital** – in the middle to lower third of the tibia ± fibula. 50% present in the first year. Later there may be cupping of the proximal bone end and pointing of the distal bone end.
3. **Neurofibromatosis*.**
4. **Osteogenesis imperfecta*.**
5. **Cleidocranial dysplasia*** – congenitally in the femur.
6. **Fibrous dysplasia*.**

Further Reading
Boyd HB, Sage FP. Congenital pseudarthrosis of the tibia. J Bone Joint Surg 1958;40A:1245–70.

14.16 'BONE WITHIN A BONE' APPEARANCE

1. **Normal neonate** – especially in the spine.
2. **Growth arrest/recovery lines.**
3. **Bisphosphonate therapy.**
4. **Sickle-cell anaemia*.**
5. **Osteopetrosis*.**
6. **Acromegaly*.**
7. **Gaucher's disease.**
8. **Heavy metal poisoning.**
9. **Prostaglandin E1 therapy** – see 14.13.

Further Reading
Brill PW, Baker DH, Ewing ML. Bone within bone in the neonatal spine. Radiology 1973;108:363–6.
Frager DH, Subbarao K. The 'bone within a bone'. J Am Med Assoc 1983;249:77–9.
Matzinger MA, Briggs VA, Dunlap HJ et al. Plain film and CT observations in prostaglandin-induced bone changes. Pediatr. Radiol 1992;22:264–6.
O'Brien JP. The manifestations of arrested bone growth: the appearance of a vertebra within a vertebra. J Bone Joint Surg 1969;51A:1376–8.

14

14.17 IRREGULAR OR STIPPLED EPIPHYSES

1. **Normal** – particularly in the distal femur.
2. **Avascular necrosis** (q.v.) – single, e.g. Perthes' disease (although 10% are bilateral), or multiple, e.g. sickle-cell anaemia.
3. **Congenital hypothyroidism*** – not present at birth. Delayed appearance and growth of ossification centres. Appearance varies from slightly granular to fragmentation. The femoral capital epiphysis may be divided into inner and outer halves.
4. **Morquio's syndrome*** – irregular ossification of the femoral capital epiphyses results in flattening.
5. **Multiple epiphyseal dysplasia** – onset 5–14 years. May be familial. Delayed appearance and growth of epiphyses but the time of fusion is normal. ± Metaphyseal irregularity. Carpal and tarsal bones, hips, knees and ankles are most commonly affected. Tibio-talar slant. Short, stubby digits and metacarpals. Spine usually, but not always, normal. Early and severe osteoarthritis.
6. **Meyer dysplasia** – an epiphyseal dysplasia resembling MED but confined to the femoral heads.
7. **Chondrodysplasia punctata** – autosomal dominant and (rarer) autosomal recessive types are recognized.
   (a) **Autosomal dominant type (Conradi–Hünerman)** – in the newborn stippling is evident in the long bone epiphyses, spine and larynx. ± Malsegmentation of vertebral bodies. Stippling disappears by 2 years of age. Asymmetrical shortening of limbs. Usually survive to adulthood.
   (b) **Autosomal recessive (severe rhizomelic) type** – marked symmetrical rhizomelia with humeri more severely affected than femora. Spinal stippling is mild. Stillborn or perinatal death.
8. **Trisomy 18 and 21**.
9. **Prenatal infections**.
10. **Warfarin embryopathy** – stippling of uncalcified epiphyses, particularly of the axial skeleton, proximal femora and calcanei. Disappears after first year.
11. **Zellweger syndrome (cerebrohepatorenal syndrome)**.
12. **Fetal alcohol syndrome** – mostly calcaneum and lower extremities.

14.18 SOLITARY RADIOLUCENT METAPHYSEAL BAND

Apart from point 3, this is a non-specific sign which represents a period of poor endochondral bone formation.

1. **Normal neonate.**
2. **Any severe illness.**
3. **Metaphyseal fracture** – especially in non-accidental injury*. Depending on the radiographic projection there may be the additional appearance of a 'corner' or 'bucket-handle' fracture.
4. **Healing rickets.**
5. **Leukaemia, lymphoma* or metastatic neuroblastoma.**
6. **Congenital infections.**
7. **Intrauterine perforation.**
8. **Scurvy*.**

Further Reading

Kleinman PK, Marks SC, Blackbourne B. The metaphyseal lesion in abused infants: a radiologic-histopathologic study. Am J Roentgenol 1986;146:895–905.
Wolfson JJ, Engel RR. Anticipating meconium peritonitis from metaphyseal bands. Radiology 1969;92:1055–60.

14.19 ALTERNATING RADIOLUCENT AND DENSE METAPHYSEAL BANDS

1. **Growth arrest** (Harris or Park's lines).
2. **Bisphosphanate therapy**
3. **Rickets*** – especially those types that require prolonged treatment such as vitamin D-dependent rickets.
4. **Osteopetrosis*.**
5. **Chemotherapy.**
6. **Chronic anaemias** – sickle-cell and thalassaemia.
7. **Treated leukaemia.**

Further Reading

Harris HA. Lines of arrested growth in the long bones in childhood. Correlation of histological and radiographic appearances in clinical and experimental conditions. Br J Radiol 1931;4:561–622.
Follis RH, Park EA. Some observations on bone growth, with particular respect to zones and transverse lines of increased density in the metaphysis. Am J Roentgenol 1952;68:709–24.
Roebuck DJ. Skeletal complications in pediatric oncology patients. Radiographics 1999;19:873–85.
Grissom LE, Harcke HT. Radiographic features of bisphosphonate therapy in pediatric patients. Pediatr Radiol; 2003;33:226–9.

14

14.20 SOLITARY DENSE METAPHYSEAL BAND

1. **Normal infants.**
2. **Lead poisoning** – dense line in the proximal fibula is said to differentiate from normal. Other poisons include bismuth, arsenic, phosphorus, mercury fluoride and radium.
3. **Radiation.**
4. **Congenital hypothyroidism*.**
5. **Osteopetrosis*.**
6. **Hypervitaminosis D.**

Further Reading
Mitchell MJ, Logan PM. Radiation induced changes in bone. Radiographics 1998;18:1125–36.
Raber SA. The dense metaphyseal band sign. Radiology 1999;211:773–4.

14.21 DENSE VERTICAL METAPHYSEAL LINES

1. **Congenital rubella** – celery stalk appearance. Less commonly in congenital CMV.
2. **Osteopathia striata** – $\pm$ exostoses.
3. **Hypophosphatasia*.**
4. **Localized metaphyseal injury.**

14.22 FRAYING OF METAPHYSES

1. **Rickets*.**
2. **Hypophosphatasia*.**
3. **Chronic stress** (in the wrists of young gymnasts) – with wide, irregular, asymmetrical widening of the distal radial growth plate and metaphyseal sclerosis.
4. **Copper deficiency.**

Further Reading
Carter SR, Aldridge MJ, Fitzgerald R et al. Stress changes of the wrist in adolescent gymnasts. Br J Radiol 1988;61:109–12.
Grünebaum M, Horodniceanu C, Steinherz R. The radiographic manifestations of bone changes in copper deficiency. Paed Radiol 1980;9:101–4.

14.23   CUPPING OF METAPHYSES

Often associated with fraying.

1. **Normal** – especially of the distal ulna and proximal fibula of young children. No fraying.
2. **Rickets*** – with widening of the growth plate and fraying.
3. **Trauma** – to the growth plate and/or metaphysis. Asymmetrical and localized changes.
4. **Bone dysplasias** – a sign in a large number, e.g. achondroplasia*, pseudoachondroplasia, metatropic dwarfism, diastrophic dwarfism, the metaphyseal chondrodysplasias and hypophosphatasia*.
5. **Scurvy*** – usually after fracture.

14.24   ERLENMEYER FLASK DEFORMITY

An Erlenmeyer flask is a wide-necked glass container used in chemical laboratories and named after the German chemist Richard August Carl Emil Erlenmeyer (1825–1907). The shape of the flask is also used to describe the distal expansion of the long bones, particularly the femora, that is observed in a number of the sclerosing skeletal dysplasias and in other afflictions of bone.

Dysplasias

1. **Pyle's disease** (metaphyseal dysplasia).
2. **Craniometaphyseal dysplasia.**
3. **Osteodysplasty (Melnick–Needles syndrome).**
4. **Osteopetrosis.***

Haematological

1. **Thalassaemia.**

Depositional disorders

1. **Gaucher's disease.**
2. **Niemann–Pick Disease.**

Poisoning

1. **Lead poisoning** – thick transverse dense metaphyseal bands are the classic manifestation of chronic infantile and juvenile lead poisoning. Additionally there may be flask-shaped femora which may persist for years before resolving.

14

Further Reading

Beighton P, Cremin BJ. Sclerosing bone dysplasias. Springer-Verlag, Berlin, 1980.

Goldblatt J, Sacks S, Beighton P. Orthopaedic aspects of Gaucher disease. Clin Orthop Rel Res 1978;137:208–14.

Myer HS, Cremin BJ, Beighton P et al. Chronic Gaucher's disease: radiological findings in 17 South African cases. Br J Radiol 1975;48:465–9.

Pease CN, Newton GG. Metaphyseal dysplasia due to lead poisoning in children. Radiology 1962;79:233.

14.25 FOCAL RIB LESION (SOLITARY OR MULTIPLE) IN A CHILD

Neoplastic

Secondary more common than primary. Primary malignant more common than benign.

1. **Metastases**
   (a) Neuroblastoma.
2. **Primary malignant**
   (a) peripheral PNET including Ewing's sarcoma* and Askin tumour.
3. **Benign**
   (a) Osteochondroma*.
   (b) Enchondroma*.
   (c) Langerhans cell histiocytosis*.

Non-neoplastic

1. **Healed rib fracture**.
2. **Fibrous dysplasia**.
3. **Osteomyelitis** – bacterial, tuberculous or fungal.

Further Reading

Guttentag AR, Salwen JK. Keep your eyes on the ribs: the spectrum of normal variants and diseases that involve the ribs. Radiographics 1999;19: 1125–42.

Omell GH, Anderson LS, Bramson RT. Chest wall tumours. Radiol Clin North Am 1973;11:197–214.

14.26   WIDENING OF THE SYMPHYSIS PUBIS

>10mm in the newborn.
>9mm at age 3 years.
>8mm at 7 years and over.

Acquired

1. **Trauma.**
2. **Infection** – low-grade osteomyelitis shows similar radiological features to osteitis pubis.

Congenital

With normal ossification

1. **Exstrophy of the bladder.**
2. **Cloacal exstrophy.**
3. **Epispadias** – the degree of widening correlates well with the severity of the epispadias.
4. **Hypospadias.**
5. **Imperforate anus with rectovaginal fistula.**
6. **Urethral duplication.**
7. **Prune belly syndrome.**
8. **Sjögren–Larsson syndrome.**
9. **Goltz syndrome.**

Poorly ossified cartilage

1. **Achondrogenesis.**
2. **Campomelic dysplasia.**
3. **Chondrodysplasia punctata (Conradi–Hünermann syndrome).**
4. **Chromosome 4p– syndrome (Wolf's syndrome).**
5. **Chromosome 9(p+) trisomy syndrome.**
6. **Cleidocranial dysplasia*.**
7. **Hypochondrogenesis.**
8. **Hypophosphatasia.**
9. **Hypothyroidism*.**
10. **Larsen syndrome.**
11. **Pyknodysostosis.**
12. **Spondyloepimetaphyseal dysplasia.**
13. **Spondyloepiphyseal dysplasia congenita.**

14

Further Reading

Cortina H, Vallcanera A, Andres V et al. The non-ossified pubis. Pediatr Radiol 1979;8:87–92.

Muecke EC, Currarino G. Congenital widening of the symphysis pubis. Associated clinical disorders and roentgen anatomy of affected bony pelves. Am J Roentgenol 1968;103:179–85.

Patel K, Chapman S. Normal symphysis pubis width in children. Clin Radiol 1993;47:56–7.

Taybi H, Lachman RS. Radiology of syndromes, metabolic disorders, and skeletal dysplasias, 4th edn. Mosby, St Louis, 1996, p1045.

14.27 'SHEETS' OF CALCIFICATION IN A CHILD

1. **Congenital myositis ossificans progressiva** – manifest in childhood. Initially neck and trunk muscles involved. Short first metacarpal and metatarsal.
2. **Juvenile dermatomyositis**.

14.28 ABNORMAL THUMBS – CONGENITAL

Broad

1. **Acrocephalopolysyndactyly (Carpenter type)** – two ossification centres for the proximal phalanx in childhood → duplication in adulthood.
2. **Acrocephalosyndactyly (Apert type)** – partial or complete duplication of the proximal phalanx. Complete syndactyly of digits II–V – 'mitten hand' and 'sock foot'.
3. **Diastrophic dysplasia** – short, ovoid thumb metacarpal with proximally located thumb.
4. **Rubinstein–Taybi syndrome** – terminal phalanx + 'hitch-hiker thumb'.
5. **Oto-palato-digital syndrome** – large cone epiphysis of the distal phalanx.

Large

1. **Klippel–Trenaunay–Weber syndrome**.
2. **Macrodystrophia lipomatosa**.
3. **Maffucci's syndrome**.
4. **Neurofibromatosis***.

Short or small

1. **Fanconi's anaemia** – ± other radial ray abnormalities. Onset of pancytopaenia at 5–10 years of age.
2. **Holt–Oram syndrome** – finger-like, absent, hypoplastic or triphalangeal thumb + congenital heart disease (ASD, VSD).
3. **Brachydactyly C or D.**
4. **Cornelia de Lange syndrome** – hypoplastic metacarpal.
5. **Fetal hydantoin** – finger-like thumb with hypoplasia of all the distal phalanges.
6. **Fibrodysplasia ossificans progressiva.**

Absent

1. **Fanconi's anaemia.**
2. **Poland syndrome** – partial or complete absence of pectoralis muscles + abnormalities of the ipsilateral upper limb.
3. **Thalidomide.**
4. **Trisomy chromosome 18.**

Triphalangeal

1. **Fanconi's anaemia.**
2. **Holt–Oram syndrome.**
3. **Blackfan–Diamond syndrome** – pure red cell aplasia. Musculoskeletal abnormalities in 30%.
4. **Poland syndrome.**
5. **Trisomy chromosome 13 and 21.**
6. **Thalidomide.**

Abnormally positioned

1. **Cornelia de Lange syndrome** – proximally placed.
2. **Diastrophic dysplasia** – 'hitch-hiker thumb'.
3. **Rubinstein–Taybi syndrome** – 'hitch-hiker thumb' + broad terminal phalanx.

Further Reading
De Kerviler E, Guermazi A, Zagdanski A-M et al. The clinical and radiological features of Fanconi's anaemia. Clin Radiol 2000;55:340–5.
Taybi H, Lachman RS. Radiology of syndromes, metabolic disorders, and skeletal dysplasias, 4th edn. Mosby, St Louis, 1996, p1042–3.

14

14.29 DIFFERENTIAL DIAGNOSIS OF SKELETAL LESIONS IN NON-ACCIDENTAL INJURY*

Disease	Shaft fractures	Abnormal metaphysis	Osteopenia	Periosteal reaction	Comments
Non-accidental injury*	+	+	–	+	
Accidental trauma	+	–	–	Callus	
Birth trauma	+	±	–	±	Clavicle, humerus and femur are most frequent fractures
Osteogenesis imperfecta*	+	±	+	–	Highly unlikely in the absence of osteopenia, wormian bones dentinogenesis imperfecta and a relevant family history
Osteomyelitis	–	+	Localized	+	May be multifocal
Rickets*	+	+	+	+	↑ Alkaline phosphatase
Scurvy*	–	+	+	+	Not before 6 months age
Congenital syphilis	–	+	–	+	
Congenital insensitivity to pain	+	+	–	+	
Paraplegia	+	+	+	With fractures	Lower limb changes only
Prostaglandin E₁ therapy	–	–	–	+	
Menke's syndrome	–	+	+	+	Males only. Abnormal hair. Retardation. Wormian bones
Copper deficiency	+	+	+	±	See note 1

¹Copper deficiency. Rare. Unlikely in the absence of at least one risk factor — prematurity, total parenteral nutrition, malabsorption or a low copper diet. Unlikely in full-term infants less than 6 months age. Microcytic, hypochromic anaemia. Leukopenia. Normal serum copper and caeruloplasmin does not exclude the diagnosis. Skull fracture never recorded in copper deficiency. Rib fractures only recorded in

Further Reading
Carty H, Pierce A. Non-accidental injury: a retrospective analysis of a large cohort. Eur Radiol 2002;12(12):2919–25.
Chapman S, Hall CM. Non-accidental injury or brittle bones. Pediatr Radiol 1997;27:106–10.
Kleinman P. Diagnostic imaging of child abuse, 2nd edn. Mosby, St Louis, 1998.
Shaw JCL. Copper deficiency and non-accidental injury. Arch Dis Childhood 1988;63:448–55.

14.30 PLATYSPONDYLY IN CHILDHOOD

This sign describes a uniform decrease in the distance between the upper and lower vertebral end-plates and should be differentiated from wedge-shaped vertebrae. Platyspondyly may be generalized, affecting all the vertebral bodies, multiple, affecting some of the vertebral bodies, or localized, involving one vertebral body (also termed vertebra plana).

Congenital platyspondyly

1. **Thanatophoric dwarfism** – inverted 'U'- or 'H'-shaped vertebrae with a markedly increased disc space: body height ratio. Telephone handle-shaped long bones.
2. **Metatropic dwarfism.**
3. **Osteogenesis imperfecta*** – type IIA.
4. **Homozygous achondroplasia.**

Platyspondyly in later childhood

1. **Morquio's disease*.**
2. **Spondyloepiphyseal dysplasia congenita.**
3. **Spondyloepiphyseal dysplasia tarda.**
4. **Kniest syndrome.**

Acquired platyspondyly

1. **Scheuermann's disease** – irregular end-plates and Schmorl's nodes in the thoracic spine of children and young adults. Disc-space narrowing. May progress to a severe kyphosis.
2. **Langerhans cell histiocytosis*** – the spine is more frequently involved in eosinophilic granuloma and Hand–Schüller–Christian disease than in Letterer–Siwe disease. Most common in young people. The thoracic and lumbosacral spine are the usual sites of disease. Disc spaces are preserved.
3. **Sickle-cell anaemia*** – characteristic step-like depression in the central part of the end-plate.

14

Further Reading
Kozlowski K. Platyspondyly in childhood. Pediatr Radiol 1974;2(2):81–7.

14.31 ANTERIOR VERTEBRAL BODY BEAKS

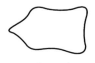

Central

Lower third

Involves 1–3 vertebral bodies at the thoracolumbar junction and usually associated with a kyphosis. Hypotonia is probably the common denominator which leads to an exaggerated thoracolumbar kyphosis, anterior herniation of the nucleus pulposus and subsequently an anterior vertebral body defect.

1. **Mucopolysaccharidoses** (with platyspondyly in Morquio's: this is probably a more useful distinguishing characteristic than the position of the beak, inferior or middle, which is variable)*.
2. **Achondroplasia***.
3. **Mucolipidoses**
4. **Pseudoachondroplasia.**
5. **Congenital hypothyroidism/cretinism***.
6. **Down's syndrome***.
7. **Neuromuscular diseases.**

Further Reading
Levin TL, Berdon WE, Lachman RS et al. Lumbar gibbus in storage diseases and bone dysplasias. Pediatr Radiol 1997;27(4):289–94.
Swischuk LE. The beaked, notched or hooked vertebra. Its significance in infants and young children. Radiology 1970;95:661–4.

14.32 ACUTE UPPER AIRWAY OBSTRUCTION IN A CHILD

Most commonly in infants, because of the small calibre of the airways. Small or normal volume lungs with distension of the upper airway proximal to the obstruction during inspiration.

1. **Laryngo-tracheobronchitis** – narrowing of the glottic and subglottic regions. Indistinct tracheal margin because of oedema.
2. **Acute epiglottitis** – the epiglottis is swollen and may be shortened. Other components of the supraglottic region – aryepiglottic folds, arytenoids, uvula and prevertebral soft tissues – are also swollen. The hypopharynx and pyriform sinuses are distended with air.
3. **Retropharyngeal abscess** – enlargement of the prevertebral soft tissues which may contain gas or an air fluid level.
4. **Oedema** – caused by angio-oedema (allergic, anaphylactic or hereditary), inhalation of noxious gases or trauma. Predominantly laryngeal oedema.
5. **Foreign body** – more commonly produces a major bronchial occlusion rather than upper airway obstruction.
6. **Choanal atresia** – bilateral (33%) or unilateral, bony (90%) or membranous, complete or incomplete. When bilateral and complete, presentation is with severe respiratory distress at birth. Incomplete obstruction is associated with respiratory difficulty during feeding. Diagnosis is by failure to pass a catheter through the nose, and nasopharyngography or CT.
7. **Retropharyngeal haemorrhage** – due to trauma, neck surgery, direct carotid arteriography and bleeding disorders. Widening of the retropharyngeal soft-tissue space.

Further Reading
Cohen LF. Stridor and upper airway obstruction in children. Pediatr Rev 2000;21(1):4–5.
John SD, Swischuk LE. Stridor and upper airway obstruction in infants and children. Radiographics 1992;12(4):625–43.

14

14.33 CHRONIC UPPER AIRWAY OBSTRUCTION IN A CHILD

May be associated with overinflation of the lungs.

Nasal

1. **Choanal atresia** – See 14.32.
2. **Nasal angiofibroma** – adolescent males. Symptoms of nasal obstruction and/or epistaxis. Plain films may show:
   (a) anterior bowing of the posterior wall of the maxillary antrum.
   (b) deviation of the nasal septum.
   (c) a nasopharyngeal soft-tissue mass with erosion of contiguous bony structures. CT/MRI to assess full extent. Originates in sphenoid sinus, maxillary antrum or at inferior turbinate.
3. **Antrochoanal polyp**.

Supraglottic

1. **Grossly enlarged tonsils and adenoids**.
2. **Laryngomalacia** – presents at or shortly after birth, persists for several months and usually resolves by 2 years. Diagnosis is confirmed by direct laryngoscopy, but fluoroscopy reveals anterior motion of the aryepiglottic folds and distension of the hypopharynx.
3. **Micrognathia** – in the Pierre Robin syndrome.
4. **Cysts** – of the epiglottis or aryepiglottic folds. The degree of obstruction depends on the size and location.

Glottic

1. **Laryngeal polyp, papilloma or cyst**.

Subglottic and tracheal

1. **Tracheomalacia** – weakness of tracheal wall which may be primary or secondary:
   (a) Primary
      (i) Premature infants. Also in cartilage disorders e.g. polychondritis, chondromalacia and mucopolysaccharidoses.
   (b) Secondary
      (i) following prolonged intubation.
      (ii) with tracheo-oesophageal fistula/oesophageal atresia.
      (iii) with vascular ring or other extrinsic vascular compression.
      (iv) with long standing external compression by tumour, etc.

2. **Vascular ring**
   (a) Double arch.
   (b) Right arch with left sided duct/ductal ligament.
   (c) Pulmonary artery sling (frequently co-existent intrinsic narrowing).
   (d) Innominate artery compression.
3. **Subglottic haemangioma** – the most common subglottic soft-tissue mass in infancy. Occurs before 6 months. 50% have associated cutaneous haemangiomas. Characteristically it produces an asymmetrical narrowing of the subglottic airway.
4. **Following prolonged tracheal intubation** – may be fixed stenosis or malacia.
5. **External compression from other mediastinal structures** – e.g. lymphadenopathy.
6. **Congenital tracheal stenosis** – usually due to presence of complete cartilaginous rings. Associated with pulmonary artery sling.
7. **Respiratory papillomatosis** – occurs anywhere from the nose to the lungs. Irregular soft-tissue masses which may cavitate around the glottis or in the trachea mostly.

Further Reading

Cohen LF. Stridor and upper airway obstruction in children. Pediatr Rev 2000;21(1):4–5.
John SD, Swischuk LE. Stridor and upper airway obstruction in infants and children. Radiographics 1992;12(4):625–43.

14.34 NEONATAL RESPIRATORY DISTRESS

Pulmonary causes

A. With no mediastinal shift

1. **Hyaline membrane disease (surfactant deficiency disease)** – in premature infants. Infants are symptomatic soon after birth but maximum radiographic findings develop at 12–14 hours. Fine granular pattern throughout both lungs, air bronchograms and, later, obscured heart and diaphragmatic outlines. Small lung volume due to diffuse micro-atelectasis. Often cardiomegaly. May progress to a complete 'white-out'. Interstitial emphysema, pneumomediastinum and pneumothorax are frequent complications of ventilator therapy. Patchy clearing of infiltrate occurs following surfactant therapy. As oxygenation improves, bidirectional or left-to-right shunting through the ductus arteriosus may lead to pulmonary oedema, cardiomegaly and occasionally pulmonary haemorrhage.

14

2. **Transient tachypnoea of the newborn** – prominent interstitial markings and vessels, thickened septa, small effusions and occasionally mild cardiomegaly. May resemble hyaline membrane disease, meconium aspiration or neonatal pneumonia. Resolves within 2–3 days.

3. **Meconium aspiration syndrome** – predominantly postmature infants. Coarse linear and irregular opacities of uneven size, generalized hyperinflation and focal areas of collapse and emphysema. Spontaneous pneumothorax and effusions in 20%. Pleural effusion in up to two-thirds; never in hyaline membrane disease. No air bronchograms.

4. **Pneumonia** – in <1% of newborns. Risk factor – prolonged rupture of membranes. Most commonly Group B Streptococcus. Segmental or lobal consolidation. Pleural effusions may be large and suggest diagnosis. May resemble hyaline membrane disease or meconium aspiration syndrome, but should be suspected if unevenly distributed.

5. **Pulmonary haemorrhage** – 75% are less than 2.5 kg. Onset at birth or delayed several days. May occur following surfactant therapy probably due to left to right shunting. Resembles meconium aspiration syndrome or hyaline membrane disease.

6. **Upper airway obstruction** – e.g. choanal atresia and micrognathia.

7. **Abnormal thoracic cage**
   (a) Neuromuscular abnormalities – often with thin ribs and clavicles.
   (b) Skeletal dysplasias – e.g. Jeune's asphyxiating thoracic dysplasia, thanatophoric dwarfism, osteogenesis imperfecta and metatropic dwarfism.
   (c) Pulmonary hypoplasia: e.g. due to fetal renal failure (Potter sequence) or primary (rare).
   (d) Major abdominal wall defects (exomphalos/gastroschisis). Short down-sloping ribs with 'long' chest.

8. **Alveolar capillary dysplasia** – often normal radiographic appearances despite severe respiratory distress. Microscopic misalignment of capillaries pulmonary veins. Universally poor prognosis.

B. With mediastinal shift away from the abnormal side

1. **Diaphragmatic hernia** – six times more common on the left side. Multiple lucencies due to gas containing bowel in the chest. Herniated bowel may appear solid if x-rayed too early but there will still be a paucity of gas in the abdomen.

2. **Congenital lobar overinflation** – involves the left upper, right upper and right middle lobes (in decreasing order of frequency) with compression of the lung base (cf. pneumothorax which produces symmetrical lung compression). CT is useful, particularly to exclude external compression of a bronchus by an aberrant vessel.

3. **Congenital pulmonary airway malformation** (previously termed congenital cystic adenomatoid malformation) – translucencies of various shapes and sizes scattered throughout an area of opaque lung with well-defined margins.
4. **Pneumothorax** – may complicate resuscitation or positive pressure ventilation, or may be spontaneous. Spontaneous pneumothorax is associated with pulmonary hypoplasia e.g. in Potter sequence. In the supine neonate, pleural air collects anteriorly and may not collapse the lung medially. In the absence of a lung edge, other signs which suggest the presence of a pneumothorax are:
   (a) Sharp ipsilateral heart border.
   (b) Depression or inversion of the ipsilateral hemidiaphragm.
   (c) Sharp ipsilateral parietal pleura in the upper medial part of the hemithorax. If there is tension this may herniate across the superior mediastinum.
   (d) Medial deviation of the ipsilateral compressed thymic lobe.
   (e) Mediastinal shift to the contralateral side.
5. **Pleural effusion** (empyema, chylothorax) – rare.

C. With mediastinal shift towards the abnormal side
1. **Atelectasis** – most commonly due to incorrect placement of an endotracheal tube down a major bronchus. Much less commonly, primary atelectasis may occur without any other abnormality.
2. **Agenesis/aplasia** – rare. May be difficult to differentiate from collapse but other congenital defects, especially hemivertebrae, are commonly associated. Agenesis = no bronchus, aplasia = rudimentary bronchus present
3. **Unilateral pulmonary hypoplasia**. Most commonly due to compression e.g. by diaphragmatic hernia. May also be associated with vascular anomalies, e.g. absent pulmonary artery, anomalous venous drainage (=scimitar syndrome).

Cardiac causes (q.v.)
Cerebral causes
Haemorrhage, oedema and drugs. After cardiopulmonary causes these account for 50% of the remainder.

Metabolic causes
Metabolic acidosis, hypoglycaemia and hypothermia.

14

Abdominal causes

Massive organomegaly, e.g. polycystic kidneys, elevating the diaphragms.

Further Reading

Agrons GA, Courtney SE, Stocker JT et al. From the archives of the AFIP: Lung disease in premature neonates: radiologic-pathologic correlation. Radiographics 2005;25(4):1047–73.

Cleveland RH. A radiologic update on medical diseases of the newborn chest. Pediatr Radiol 1995;25:631–7.

Donoghue VP (ed). Radiological imaging of the neonatal chest. Springer-Verlag, Berlin, 2007.

Markowitz RI, Fellows KE. The effects of congenital heart disease on the lungs. Semin Roentgenol 1998;33(2):126–35.

Newman B. Imaging of medical disease of the newborn lung. Radiol Clin North Am 1999;37(6):1049–65.

Schwartz DS, Reyes-Mugica M, Keller MS. Imaging of surgical diseases of the newborn chest. Radiol Clin North Am 1999;37(6):1067–78.

14.35 RING SHADOWS IN A CHILD

Neonate

1. **Diaphragmatic hernia** – unilateral.
2. **Interstitial emphysema** – secondary to ventilator therapy. May be unilateral or bilateral. Usually transient, but may persist.
3. **Congenital pulmonary airway malformation** (previously termed congenital cystic adenomatoid malformation) – unilateral.
4. **Bronchopulmonary dysplasia** – 'bubbly lung' appearances with air-trapping.

Older child

1. **Cystic bronchiectasis** (q.v.).
2. **Cystic fibrosis***.
3. **Pneumatocoeles** (q.v.).
4. **Langerhans cell histiocytosis***.
5. **Respiratory papillomatosis**.
6. **Neurofibromatosis***

14.36 INTERSTITIAL LUNG DISEASE UNIQUE TO CHILDHOOD

1. **Persistent tachypnoea of the newborn** – ground glass opacities and air-trapping. Disorder of pulmonary neuroendocrine cells.
2. **Bronchopulmonary dysplasia** – patchy atelectasis and air-trapping, interstitial opacities with triangular subpleural opacities.
3. **Cellular interstitial pneumonitis of infancy**. Interstitial infiltrates. Relatively good prognosis.
4. **Infantile pulmonary haemosiderosis**. Recurrent pulmonary haemorrhage leading to fibrotic changes.
5. **Chronic pneumonitis of infancy** (CPI). Interstitial changes. High mortality.
6. **Surfactant protein B deficiency** – AR. Similar appearance to hyaline membrane disease but in a full-term newborn infant. May account for some cases of CPI and alveolar proteinosis.
7. **Familial desquamative interstitial pneumonitis** – worse prognosis than typical desquamative interstitial pneumonitis.

Further Reading

Copley SJ, Padley SP. High-resolution CT of paediatric lung disease. Eur Radiol 2001;11:2564–75.

Koh DM, Hansell DM. Computed tomography of diffuse interstitial lung disease in children. Clin Radiol 2000;55:659–67.

Lynch DA, Hay T, Newell JD et al. Pediatric diffuse lung disease: diagnosis and classification using high-resolution CT. Am J Roentgenol 1999;173: 713–8.

Owens C.M. Radiology of diffuse interstitial pulmonary disease in children. Eur Radiol 2004;14(Suppl 4):L2–12.

Schaefer-Prokop C, Prokop M, Fleischmann D et al. High-resolution CT of diffuse interstitial lung disease: key findings in common disorders. Eur Radiol 2001;11:373–92.

14.37 THE NORMAL THYMUS

The normal thymus is a bilobed anterosuperior mediastinal structure. It is only visible on plain films of infants and young children, and is inconstantly visible after 2–3 years of age. On plain films three radiological signs aid diagnosis – the 'sail' sign (a triangular projection to one (usually right) or both sides of the mediastinum), the 'wave' sign (a rippled thymic contour due to indentations by the anterior rib ends) or the 'notch' sign (an indentation at the junction of thymus with heart). A large normal thymus may be seen in:

(a) Well nourished children.
(b) Following recovery from illness (rebound overgrowth in 25% following previous involution).
(c) Hyperthyroidism and euthyroid children following treatment for hypothyroidism.

It has the following CT characteristics:

1. **Incidence** – identifiable in 100% <30 years of age, decreasing to 17% >49 years. However, <10 years of age the distinction from great vessels is very difficult without the use of contrast enhancement.
2. **Shape** – quadrilateral shape in childhood with, usually, convex, undulating margins. After puberty two separate lobes (ovoid, elliptical, triangular or semilunar) or an arrowhead (triangle). The normal thymus is never multilobular.
3. **Size** – progressive enlargement during childhood. Maximum absolute size is in the 12–19-year age group but relative to body size it is largest in infancy. Left lobe nearly always larger than right lobe. Becomes narrower with increasing age. Maximum thickness (the perpendicular to the long axis) of one lobe in those >20 years is 1.3cm. In those >40 years there may be linear or oval soft-tissue densities but they are never >7mm in size and never alter the lateral contour of the mediastinal fat.
4. **Density** – homogeneous, isodense or hyperdense when related to chest wall musculature in childhood. After puberty becoming inhomogeneous and progressively lower in attenuation due to fatty infiltration. In those >40 years the majority will have total fatty involution.

On MRI the normal thymus is:

1. Larger than is seen by CT (probably because the study is undertaken during quiet respiration rather than with suspended full inspiration).
2. Homogeneous in childhood (T_1W slightly greater than muscle, T_2W similar to fat).
3. Heterogeneous in adults (T_1W and T_2W similar to fat).

14.38 ANTERIOR MEDIASTINAL MASSES IN CHILDHOOD

The anterior mediastinum is bounded by the clavicles (superiorly), the diaphragm (inferiorly), the sternum (anteriorly) and the anterior surfaces of the heart and great vessels (posteriorly). 45% of paediatric mediastinal masses occur at this site.

Congenital

1. **Normal thymus** – see 14.37.
2. **Lymphatic malformation** (previously termed cystic hygroma) – 5% of anterior mediastinal masses but the majority are extensions from the neck with only 1% being purely mediastinal.
3. **Morgagni hernia**.

Neoplastic

1. **Hodgkin lymphoma (HL), non-Hodgkin lymphoma (NHL) and leukaemia** – the majority of neoplastic anterior mediastinal masses are due to Hodgkin's disease. At presentation, mediastinal lymph nodes are seen in 23% of HD, 14% of NHL and 5–10% of leukaemics. Comparing mediastinal involvement in HD with NHL:

Hodgkin lymphoma	Non-Hodgkin lymphoma
Usually >10 years old	Any age in children
Mostly localized. Mediastinal lymphadenopathy (LN) in 85% of those with cervical LN	Disseminated disease in >75% at presentation
Histology usually nodular sclerosing	Histology usually lymphoblastic
Displacement of other mediastinal structures rather than compression	Tracheal compression is more likely
Paratracheal > hilar > subcarinal LN. Hilar LN without mediastinal LN is rare	
Lung involvement in 10% at diagnosis – direct spread from LNs	Pulmonary involvement is higher
	Pleural effusion is more common but may be 2° to ascites or lymphatic obstruction

14

After treatment for lymphoma a residual anterior mediastinal mass may present a diagnostic difficulty. If CT shows this to be homogeneous and there is no other lymphadenopathy then tumour is unlikely to be present. PET scanning has evolving role in this scenario.

2. **Germ cell tumours** – 5–10% of germ cell tumours arise in the mediastinum. Two age peaks: at 2 years and during adolescence. Majority (80%) are teratomas and benign. Endodermal sinus (yolk sac) tumours are more aggressive. Seminomas rare. Tumours may contain calcification (including teeth), fat and cystic/necrotic areas. Radiological appearance does not accurately correlate with histology but large size, marked mass effect and local infiltration suggest an aggressive lesion.

3. **Thymoma** – 5–8% of mediastinal tumours in childhood. Most occur after 10 years of age. 50% discovered incidentally. Calcification in 10% – linear. Only rarely associated with myasthenia gravis.

Inflammatory

1. **Lymphadenopathy** – inflammatory lymph node masses are less common than neoplasia. Most frequent causes are tuberculosis and histoplasmosis.

Further Reading

Crisci KL, Greenberg SB, Wolfson BJ. Cardiopulmonary and thoracic tumours of childhood. Radiol Clin North Am 1997;35(6):1341–66.

Franco A, Mody NS, Meza MP. Imaging evaluation of pediatric mediastinal masses. Radiol Clin North Am 2005;43(2):325–53.

14.39 MIDDLE MEDIASTINAL MASSES IN CHILDHOOD

The middle mediastinum is bordered by the anterior and posterior mediastinum. 20% of paediatric mediastinal masses occur at this site.

Neoplastic

1. Most middle mediastinal tumours are extensions of those which arise primarily in the anterior mediastinum (see 14.38).

Inflammatory

1. **Lymphadenopathy** – tuberculosis, histoplasmosis and sarcoidosis.

Congenital

1. **Foregut duplication cysts** – account for 10–20% of paediatric mediastinal masses. The spectrum of abnormalities includes bronchogenic cysts, oesophageal duplication cysts and neurenteric cysts.
   (a) *Bronchogenic cyst* – round or oval, unilocular, homogeneous, water-density mass (usually 0–20 HU, but up to 100 HU due to mucus or milk of calcium contents) with well-defined borders. There may be airway obstruction and secondary infection, both within the cyst and in the surrounding lung. Communication with the tracheobronchial tree, resulting in a cavity, is rare, and may indicate infection. Four groups may be defined according to location:
      (i) Paratracheal cysts are attached to the tracheal wall above the carina.
      (ii) Carinal cysts are the most common and are attached to the carina ± anterior oesophageal wall.
      (iii) Hilar cysts are attached to a lobar bronchus and appear to be intrapulmonary.
      (iv) Para-oesophageal cysts may be attached or communicate with the oesophagus but have no communication with the bronchial tree.
   (b) *Oesophageal duplication cyst* – 10-15% of intestinal duplications. Less common than bronchogenic cysts, usually larger and usually situated to the right of the midline extending into the posterior mediastinum. May be an incidental finding or produce symptoms related to oesophageal or tracheobronchial tree compression. May contain ectopic gastric mucosa (positive ^{99m}Tc-pertechnetate scan) which causes ulceration, haemorrhage or perforation. Communication with the oesophageal lumen is rare.

14

    (c) *Neurenteric cyst* – located in the middle or posterior mediastinum, contains neural tissue and maintains a connection with the spinal canal. More commonly right-sided. Vertebral body anomalies (hemivertebra, butterfly vertebra and scoliosis) are usually superior to the cyst.

2. **Lymphatic malformation** (previously termed cystic hygroma) – 5% of cystic hygromas extend into the mediastinum from the neck. Most present at birth. Cystic with some solid components on all imaging modalities.

3. **Hiatus hernia.**

4. **Achalasia.**

5. **Cardiomegaly or vena caval enlargement** – see Chapter 5.

Further Reading

Berrocal T, Torres I, Gutierrez J et al. Congenital anomalies of the upper gastrointestinal tract. Radiographics 1999;19:855–72.

Franco A, Mody NS, Meza MP. Imaging evaluation of pediatric mediastinal masses. Radiol Clin North Am 2005;43(2):325–53.

Jaggers J, Balsara K. Mediastinal masses in children. Semin Thorac Cardiovasc Surg 2004;16(3):201–8.

Merten DF. Diagnostic imaging of mediastinal masses in children. Am J Roentgenol 1992;158:825–32.

14.40 POSTERIOR MEDIASTINAL MASSES IN CHILDHOOD

The posterior mediastinum is bounded by the thoracic inlet (superiorly), the diaphragm (inferiorly), the bodies of the thoracic vertebrae and paravertebral gutters (posteriorly), and the pericardium (anteriorly). In children, 30–40% of mediastinal masses lie in the posterior mediastinum and 95% of these are of neurogenic origin.

Left-sided paravertebral soft tissues greater than the width of the adjacent pedicle (particularly on radiographs taken in the upright position) and any right-sided paravertebral soft-tissue shadows are abnormal.

Neoplastic

1. **Ganglion cell tumours** – neuroblastoma (most malignant, usually <5 years), ganglioneuroblastoma (age 5–10 years) and ganglioneuroma (benign, usually >10 years). Imaging features of all three types are similar but metastases do not occur with ganglioneuroma. Plain films show a paravertebral soft-tissue mass with calcification in 30%. Thinning of posterior ribs, separation of ribs and enlargement of intervertebral foramina. CT shows calcification in 90%. Both CT and MRI may show extradural extension.

Congenital

1. **Bochdalek hernia** – most present at, or shortly after, birth with respiratory distress, but 5% present after the neonatal period. Rarely it may complicate Group B streptococcal infection. Bochdalek hernias include:
   - **(a)** Persistence of the pleuroperitoneal canal with a posterior lip of diaphragm.
   - **(b)** Larger defects with no diaphragm.
   - **(c)** Herniation through the costolumbar triangles.

The appearance of herniated liver may provoke thoracentesis and herniated bowel may mimic pneumothorax, pneumatocoeles or cystic adenomatoid malformation.

Further Reading

Berman L, Stringer DA, Ein S et al. Childhood diaphragmatic hernias presenting after the neonatal period. Clin Radiol 1988;39:237–44.
Donnelly LF, Frush DP, Zheng J-Y et al. Differentiating normal from abnormal inferior thoracic paravertebral soft tissues on chest radiography in children. Am J Roentgenol 2000;175:477–83.

14

14.41 SOLITARY PULMONARY MASS IN CHILDHOOD

Unlike in adults, solitary pulmonary mass lesions in children are rarely malignant.

Pseudo-mass lesions

1. **Round pneumonia** – may contain air-bronchograms. Rare over age 8.
2. **Encysted pleural effusion** – usually elliptiform mass in right mid zone. Lateral film confirms.
3. **Mucus plug in cystic fibrosis** – can be large. CT confirms location.

Non-neoplastic lesions

1. **Pulmonary sequestration** – most commonly in medial basal segment of right lower lobe.
2. **Intrapulmonary bronchogenic cyst** – well defined rounded lesion that may contain air-fluid level, particularly if previous infection.
3. **Granuloma** – most commonly following TB.
4. **Inflammatory pseudotumour** – synonyms include plasma cell granuloma and inflammatory myofibroblastic tumour. Variable size and may be large. Usually peripheral. Calcified in 25%.
5. **Pulmonary AVM** – may visualise draining vessel.
6. **Ectopic kidney** – well defined cranial aspect.

Neoplastic lesions

1. **Solitary metastasis** – most commonly Wilms tumour and sarcomas.
2. **Bronchial adenoma/carcinoid** – usually malignant, despite name. Frequently endobronchial causing lobar collapse or overinflation.
3. **Pleuropulmonary blastoma** – embryonal tumour. May be solid, cystic or mixed. May be very large peripheral and locally invasive mass.
4. **Bronchogenic carcinoma** – very rare in childhood. Most commonly bronchoalveolar cell carcinoma.
5. **Hamartoma** – occasionally calcified. Slow growing, well defined mass.

Further Reading
McCahon E. Lung tumours in children. Paediatr Respir Rev 2006;7(3):191–6.

14.42 MULTIPLE PULMONARY NODULES IN A CHILD

1. **Miliary TB/other granulomatous infection** – miliary pattern of haematogenous spread should be distinguished from 'tree-in-bud' pattern of endobronchially disseminated TB
2. **Septic emboli** – frequently cavitary.
3. **Langerhans cell histiocytosis** – initial nodular pattern 1–10mm, developing cavitation or cysts.
4. **Multiple pulmonary metastases** – Wilms and sarcomas most common primary sites.
5. **Wegener's granulomatosis** – may cavitate.
6. **Respiratory papillomatosis** – represents pulmonary seeding of laryngeal papillomata, occurring in 1% of cases. Nodular and cystic lesions present. Poor prognosis. Risk of malignant transformation.
7. **Multiple arteriovenous malformations** – 2/3 associated with hereditary haemorrhagic telangiectasia. Multiple in most cases. Usually lower lobes

14.43 SITUS AND CARDIAC MALPOSITIONS

Assess the positions of the cardiac apex, aortic arch, left and right main bronchi, stomach bubble, liver and spleen.

1. **Situs solitus** – normal. All structures are concordant.
2. **Situs inversus** – cardiac apex, aortic arch and stomach are on the right; visceral organs are on the opposite side to normal. Slight increase in the incidence of congenital heart disease. Patients have sinusitis and bronchiectasis (Kartagener's syndrome).
3. **Situs solitus with dextrocardia** – cardiac apex on right with stomach bubble on left. Caused by failure of rotation of the embryonic cardiac loop and > 90% of cases are associated with congenital heart disease, usually cyanotic (corrected TGA, VSD and pulmonary stenosis). Scimitar syndrome is dextrocardia, hypoplastic right lung and partial anomalous pulmonary venous drainage into the inferior cava.
4. **Levoversion with abdominal situs inversus** – incidence of congenital heart disease 100%.
5. **Situs ambiguous with bilateral 'right-sidedness': asplenia syndrome** – absent spleen, bilateral trilobed lungs, right and left lobes of liver are similar size. Cardiac apex left, right or midline. Complex cardiac anomalies ± small bowel malrotation.

14

6. **Situs ambiguous with bilateral 'left-sidedness':**
   polysplenia syndrome – bilateral bilobed lungs, absent hepatic
   segment of IVC and enlarged azygos and hemiazygos veins.
   Intracardiac anomalies, but less complex than in bilateral
   'right-sidedness'.

Further Reading
Applegate KE. Situs revisited: imaging of the heterotaxy syndrome.
   Radiographics 1999;19:837–52.

14.44 NEONATAL PULMONARY VENOUS CONGESTION

1. **Prominent interstitial markings.**
2. **Indistinct vessels.**
3. **Perihilar haze.**
4. **Pleural effusions.**
5. **Cardiomegaly** – in all except the infradiaphragmatic type of TAPVD.

1st week

1. **Overhydration** – delayed clamping of the cord and twin–twin
   transfusion.
2. **Asphyxia** – the most common cause of cardiomegaly on the first day.
3. **Hypoplastic left heart** – heart size normal to mild cardiomegaly.
   Pulmonary vasculature normal or mild oedema. Often a marked
   discrepancy between the 'near normality' of the CXR and severity of
   clinical symptoms.
4. **Critical aortic stenosis.**
5. **TAPVD (obstructed).**

2nd–3rd weeks

1. **Coarctation of the aorta.**
2. **Interrupted aortic arch.**
3. **Critical aortic stenosis.**

4th–6th weeks

1. **Coarctation.**
2. **Critical aortic stenosis.**
3. **Endocardial fibroelastosis.**
4. **Anomalous left coronary artery.**

NB. Left-to-right shunts are usually asymptomatic during the
neonatal period because of the high pulmonary vascular resistance.
However, pulmonary vascular resistance in premature infants is

lower, so shunts may present earlier in this particular group. PDA is the commonest shunt to cause heart failure in premature infants.

Further Reading
Strife JL, Sze RW. Radiographic evaluation of the neonate with congenital heart disease. Radiol Clin North Am 1999;37(6):1093–107.

14.45 NEONATAL CYANOSIS

With increased pulmonary vascularity

Cyanosis and congestive cardiac failure – either may predominate.

1. **Transposition of the great arteries** – CXR may be normal and classic findings seen in only 50%:
   (a) Narrow mediastinum because of the abnormal relationship of the great vessels and a small thymus.
   (b) Poor visualization of the aorta and main pulmonary artery.
   (c) Asymmetrical pulmonary flow, R > L. The lungs show only mild pleonaemia or may be normal.
2. **Truncus arteriosus.**
3. **TAPVD.**
4. **Single ventricle.**
5. **Hypoplastic left ventricle** } predominantly congestive cardiac
6. **Interrupted aortic arch** } failure, but may be cyanosed.

With oligaemia and cardiomegaly

1. **Pulmonary stenosis.**
2. **Ebstein's anomaly.**
3. **Pulmonary atresia with an intact ventricular septum.**
4. **Tricuspid atresia.**

With oligaemia but no cardiomegaly

Signs appear towards the end of the first week due to closure of the ductus arteriosus.

1. **Fallot's tetralogy** – small PA segment; large aorta; right-sided aortic arch in 25%.
2. **Pulmonary atresia with a VSD.**
3. **Tricuspid atresia.**

See also 'Neonatal respiratory distress' (14.34).

14

Further Reading
Ferguson EC, Krishnamurthy R, Oldham SA. Classic imaging signs of congenital cardiovascular abnormalities. Radiographics 2007;27(5):1323–34.

14.46 CARDIOVASCULAR INVOLVEMENT IN SYNDROMES

Syndrome	Involvement
Cri-du-chat	Variable
Down's*	AV canal, VSD, PDA, ASD, and aberrant right subclavian artery
Ehlers–Danlos	Mitral valve prolapse, aortic root dilatation, dissecting aortic aneurysm and intracranial aneurysm
Ellis–Van Creveld	ASD and common atrium
Friedreich's ataxia	Hypertrophic cardiomyopathy
Holt–Oram	ASD and VSD
Homocystinuria*	Medial degeneration of the aorta and pulmonary artery causing dilatation. Arterial and venous thromboses
Hurler's/Hunter's*	Intimal thickening of coronary arteries and valves
Kartagener's	Situs inversus ± septal defects
Marfan's	Cystic medial necrosis of the wall of the aorta, and less commonly the pulmonary artery, leading to dilatation and predisposing to dissection. Aortic and mitral regurgitation.
Morquio's*	Late onset of aortic regurgitation
Noonan's	Pulmonary valve stenosis, and branch stenosis of pulmonary arteries, septal defects
Osteogenesis imperfecta*	Aortic and mitral regurgitation. Ruptured chordae.
Rubella	Septal defects, PDA, pulmonary artery branch stenoses and myocardial disease
Trisomy 13	VSD, ASD, PDA and dextroposition
Trisomy 18	VSD, ASD and PDA
Tuberous sclerosis*	Cardiomyopathy and rhabdomyoma of the heart
Turner's	Coarctation, aortic and bicuspid aortic valve stenosis

14.47 ABDOMINAL MASS IN A CHILD

(After Kirks et al 1981)

Renal (55%)

1. **Renal tumour** – see 14.52.
2. **Hydronephrosis** (20%) – see 14.53.
3. **Cysts** – see 8.20.

Non-renal retroperitoneal (23%)

1. **Neuroblastoma** (21%).
   - (a) *Age*: 75% <5 years; 15–30% <1 year. Accounts for 50% of all neonatal tumours.
   - (b) *Site*: adrenal (40%), abdominal sympathetic chain (25%), posterior mediastinal sympathetic chain (15%), neck (5%), pelvis (5%), unknown (10%).
   - (c) *Staging*: In addition to staging along conventional lines, stage IVS (or 4S) is defined as localized primary tumour not crossing the midline and with remote disease confined to liver, subcutaneous tissues and bone marrow but without evidence of cortical bone involvement. This group invariably presents in the first year of life and has an excellent prognosis.
   - (d) *Clinical presentation*: 70% have metastases at presentation and a similar percentage has systemic symptoms. There may be local effects: pain, mass, spinal cord compression, dyspnoea or dysphagia, the effects of metastases (scalp masses, pain, weight loss, anaemia, fatigue etc.), or other effects due to hormone secretion (opsomyoclonus [cerebellar ataxia and jerky eye movements]; 50% have neuroblastoma), hypertension, diarrhoea (due to vasoactive intestinal peptide, VIP), flushing and sweating).
   - (e) *Plain films*: calcification in two-thirds, loss of psoas outline, bony metastases, enlargement of intervertebral foramina and, in the chest, abnormal posterior ends of ribs.
   - (f) *Ultrasound*: heterogeneous, echogenic mass.
   - (g) *CT*: soft-tissue mass with calcification in nearly all. Encasement rather than displacement of major vessels.
   - (h) *MRI*: Prolonged T_1 and T_2 relaxation times. Calcification is not as readily recognized as on CT but MRI is superior for lymph node metastases, liver metastases and extradural spread of tumour.
   - (i) *Radionuclide scanning*: bone scanning (for cortical disease) and meta-iodo-benzyl-guanidine (MIBG) scanning (for medullary disease) are complementary techniques for the demonstration of skeletal metastases. MIBG is superior for follow-up of disease.

14

Gastrointestinal (18%)

1. **Appendix abscess** (10%) – particularly spreads to pouch anterior to rectum.
2. **Hepatoblastoma** – more commonly in right lobe, but 40% in both lobes. 40% calcify. See 14.58.
3. **Haemangioma** – commonly multiple, involving entire liver. Rarely calcify. ± Associated with congestive heart failure and cutaneous haemangiomas.
4. **Choledochal cyst** – the classic triad of mass, pain and jaundice is only present in 10%. Dynamic radionuclide scintigraphy with ^{99}Tc-TBIDA is diagnostic. See 14.60.
5. **Enteric duplication cyst.**
6. **Mesenteric cyst.**

Genital (4%)

1. **Ovarian cysts or teratoma.**

Further Reading

Abramson SJ. Adrenal neoplasms in children. Radiol Clin North Am 1997;35 (6):1415–53.

Cohen MD. Imaging of children with cancer, Ch. 6. Mosby, St Louis, 1992, p134–76.

Haddad MC, Birjawa GA, Hemadeh MS et al. The gamut of abdominal and pelvic cystic masses in children. Eur Radiol 2001;11:148–66.

Hiorns MP, Owens CM. Radiology of neuroblastoma in children. Eur Radiol 2001;11:2071–81.

Hoffer FA. Magnetic resonance imaging of abdominal masses in the pediatric patient. Semin Ultrasound CT MR 2005;26(4):212–23.

Kirks DR, Merten DF, Grossman H et al. Diagnostic imaging of paediatric abdominal masses: an overview. Radiol Clin North Am 1981;19:527–45.

14.48 INTESTINAL OBSTRUCTION IN A NEONATE

1. It is usually impossible to differentiate small from large bowel.
2. Not all gaseously distended bowel is obstructed. Resuscitation and infants on positive pressure ventilation may lead to significant abdominal distension. A rule of thumb is that bowel that is wider than the width of a lumbar vertebral body is dilated.
3. Ileus is characterized by uniform dilatation of bowel. It is found in sepsis, NEC and electrolyte imbalance. Infants with sepsis and NEC are sick; those with uncomplicated bowel obstruction are usually otherwise well.
4. Bowel obstruction should be considered as 'high' (as far as the jejunum) or 'low' (for more distal obstructions). The former present with vomiting and are investigated by upper GI contrast study while the lower present with delayed passage of meconium and may require a contrast enema.

High intestinal obstruction

1. **Pyloric atresia** – rare.
2. **Pyloric or prepyloric membrane/antral web** – gastric outlet obstruction in the presence of a normal pylorus and the appearance of two duodenal caps. The web may be identified by US.
3. **Duodenal atresia/stenosis/web** – marked dilatation of the proximal duodenum with the 'double bubble' sign, which may also be seen by ultrasound of the fetus (50% have a history of polyhydramnios). No gas distally when there is atresia, but a variable amount of gas in the distal bowel when there is stenosis. Duodenal web may produce 'windsock' appearance as web balloons into distal duodenum. Bile-stained vomiting in the majority. Associated with annular pancreas (20%), Down's syndrome (30%), cardiac abnormalities (25%), oesophageal atresia (10%) and other abnormalities of gastrointestinal tract (60%).
4. **Preduodenal portal vein** – identified on US, CT or MRI. Associated with an intrinsic duodenal obstruction; the vein is not the direct cause of the obstruction.
5. **Malrotation and volvulus** – sudden onset of bile-stained vomiting. Few radiological signs if the obstruction is recent, intermittent or incomplete. Because of the acute nature of the condition, the duodenum is not dilated. If not recognized, obstruction progresses to bowel ischaemia, infarction and death. A contrast study should demonstrate the normal C-shaped duodenal loop which terminates to the left of the left-sided pedicle at the same level as the duodenal cap. In malrotation without volvulus the duodenojejunal flexure is to the right of and below its normal position. Volvulus with incomplete obstruction

14

is identified by a corkscrew pattern of the jejunum. When there is complete obstruction the distal duodenum terminates as a beak.

6. **Congenital fibrous band (of Ladd)** – connects caecum to posterolateral abdominal wall and commonly crosses the duodenum. Associated with malrotation and midgut volvulus.

7. **Jejunal atresia** – 50% of small bowel atresias and 50% are associated with other atretic sites distally (ileum > colon). AXR demonstrates three ('triple bubble') or more dilated, air-filled loops. Colon usually normal in calibre.

Low intestinal obstruction

1. **Meconium ileus** – mottled lucencies ('soap bubble' appearance) due to gas trapped in meconium but only few fluid levels (since it is very viscous). Bowel loops of variable calibre. Rapid appearance of fluid levels suggests volvulus. Peritoneal calcification due to perforation occurring in utero is seen in 30%. Secondary microcolon on contrast enema which also shows meconium pellets in the distal ileum. Cystic fibrosis in the majority.

2. **Ileal atresia** – 50% of small bowel atresia, may be multiple and may coexist with jejunal atresia. Multiple dilated loops with fluid levels. Secondary microcolon.

3. **Incarcerated inguinal hernia**.

4. **Small left colon syndrome** – 50% associated with maternal diabetes. Small colon on enema up to level of splenic flexure, sometimes with meconium plugging. Infants should be followed up to exclude Hirschsprung's disease.

5. **Hirschsprung's disease** – multiple dilated loops of bowel. Diagnosis is made by contrast enema which demonstrates normal size, aganglionic distal bowel with a transition zone at the junction with proximal dilated ganglionic bowel.

6. **Meconium plug syndrome** – plugged meconium present in distal colon. May be a feature of Hirschsprung's, small left colon syndrome and a presenting feature of cystic fibrosis (but NB this is not the same as meconium ileus).

7. **Inspissated milk** – presents from 3 days to 6 weeks of age. Dense, amorphous intraluminal masses frequently surrounded by a rim of air, ± mottled lucencies within them. Usually resolves spontaneously.

8. **Colonic atresia** – 5–15% of intestinal atresias. AXR may be similar to other distal bowel obstructions but some infants show a huge, disproportionately dilated loop (between the atretic segment and a competent ileocaecal valve).

9. **Anorectal malformation/imperforate anus**
   (a) High – ± sacral agenesis/hypoplasia and gas in the bladder (due to a rectovesical or recto-urethral fistula).
   (b) Low – ± perineal or urethral fistula.

Further Reading

Applegate KE, Anderson JM, Klatte EC. Intestinal malrotation in children: a problem-solving approach to the upper gastrointestinal series. Radiographics 2006;(5):1485–500.

Berrocal T, Torres I, Gutierrez J et al. Congenital anomalies of the upper gastrointestinal tract. Radiographics 1999;19:855–72.

Berrocal T, Lamas M, Gutierrez J et al. Congenital anomalies of the small intestine, colon, and rectum. Radiographics 1999;19:1219–36.

Carty H, Brereton RJ. The distended neonate. Clin Radiol 1983;34:367–80.

Hernanz-Schulman M. Imaging of neonatal gastrointestinal obstruction. Radiol Clin North Am 1999;37(6):1163–86.

14.49 INTRA-ABDOMINAL CALCIFICATIONS IN THE NEWBORN

1. **Meconium peritonitis** – antenatal bowel perforation results in aseptic peritonitis which rapidly calcifies. Calcification occurs in the peritoneum itself most commonly, but also in the bowel wall and in the scrotum. Commonest causes are meconium ileus and ileal atresia, but any cause of bowel obstruction may be associated.
2. **Meconium pseudocyst** – cyst-like mass with peripheral calcification resulting from walling off of extruded meconium following perforation.
3. **Intraluminal meconium calcification** – may occur in association with distal obstruction, particularly meconium ileus and anorectal malformations.
4. **Hepatic calcification** – neonatal liver calcification occasionally occurs with congenital infections.
5. **Adrenal calcification**.

Further Reading

Beasley SW, de Campo M. Intraluminal calcification in the newborn: diagnostic and surgical implications. Pediatr Surg 1986;1:249.

Berdon WE, Baker DH, Wigger HJ et al. Calcified intraluminal meconium in newborn males with imperforate anus. Am J Roentgenol 1975;125:449–55.

Lang I, Daneman A, Cutz E et al. Abdominal calcification in cystic fibrosis with meconium ileus: radiologic-pathologic correlation. Pediatr Radiol 1997;27:523–7.

Miller JP, Smith SD, Sukarochana K. Neonatal abdominal calcification: is it always meconium peritonitis? J Pediatr Surg 1988;23:555.

Yousefzadeh DK, Jackson JH Jr, Smith WL et al. Intraluminal meconium calcification without distal obstruction. Pediatr Radiol 1984;14:23–27.

14

14.50 ABNORMALITIES OF BOWEL ROTATION

1. **Exomphalos** – total failure of the bowel to return to the abdomen from the umbilical cord. Bowel is contained within a sac. To be differentiated from gastroschisis, in which bowel protrudes through a defect in the abdominal wall.
2. **Non-rotation** – usually an asymptomatic condition with the small bowel on the right side of the abdomen and the colon on the left side. Small and large bowel lie on either side of the superior mesenteric artery (SMA) with a common mesentery. CT or transverse US scans show the superior mesenteric vein (SMV) lying to the left of the SMA, cf. the normal arrangement in which the SMV lies to the right of the SMA.
3. **Malrotation** – the duodenojejunal flexure lies to the right and caudad to its usual position which is to the left of the left-sided pedicle on a true AP projection and approximately in the same axial plane as the first part of the duodenum. The caecum is usually more cephalad than normal but is normally sited in 5%. Malrotation is a frequent feature of diaphragmatic hernia and abdominal wall defects. Also associated with visceral heterotaxy. US or CT shows the SMV to the left of the SMA. A normal US does not however exclude malrotation (3% false negative rate): upper GI contrast examination remains the gold standard. At risk of volvulus, which is life-threatening.
4. **Reverse rotation** – rare. Colon lies dorsal to the SMA with jejunum and duodenum anterior to it.
5. **Paraduodenal hernia** – rare.
6. **Cloacal extrophy** – rare. No rotation of the bowel, and the ileum and colon open separately onto the extroverted area in the midline below the umbilical cord.

Further Reading

Applegate KE, Anderson JM, Klatte EC. Intestinal malrotation in children: a problem-solving approach to the upper gastrointestinal series. Radiographics 1992;26(5):1485–500.

Dufour D, Delaet MH, Dassonville M et al. Midgut malrotation, the reliability of sonographic diagnosis. Pediatr Radiol 1992;22:21–3.

Gaines PA, Saunders AJ, Drake D. Midgut malrotation diagnosed by ultrasound. Clin Radiol 1987;38:51–3.

Strouse PJ. Disorders of intestinal rotation and fixation ('malrotation'). Pediatr Radiol 2004;34:837–51.

14.51　ADRENAL MASS IN CHILDHOOD

1. **Cystic disease** – usually the result of haemorrhage which may be secondary to birth trauma, infection, haemorrhagic disorders or arterial or venous thromboses. Partial or complete ring-like calcification is observed initially but this later becomes compact as the cyst collapses. Frequently asymptomatic.
2. **Neuroblastoma** – in 50% of cases on plain films; 90% calcified on CT. Ill-defined, stippled and non-homogeneous. Lymph node and liver metastases can also calcify.
3. **Ganglioneuroma** – similar appearance to neuroblastoma, but only 20% are within the adrenal.
4. **Wolman's disease** – a rare AR lipoidosis. Hepatomegaly, splenomegaly and adrenomegaly with punctate cortical adrenal calcification is pathognomonic.

14.52　PRIMARY RENAL NEOPLASMS IN CHILDHOOD

1. **Wilms' tumour** – $8/10^6$ children. 80% present in the first 3 years. Bilateral in 5%. Associated abnormalities: cryptorchidism (3%), hypospadias (2%), hemihypertrophy (2%), sporadic aniridia (1%) (30% of those with aniridia and 10% of those with Beckwith–Wiedemann syndrome [macroglossia, organomegaly, exomphalos $\pm$ hemihypertrophy] develop Wilms' tumour). 90% have favourable histology. $2° \rightarrow$ lungs and liver. 5% have tumour thrombus in the IVC or right atrium. Hypertension in 25%.
   - (a) *Plain film:* bulging flank (75%), loss of renal outline (66%), enlargement of renal outline (33%), displacement of bowel gas (50%), loss of psoas outline (33%), calcification (10%).
   - (b) *Ultrasound:* large well-defined mass, greater echogenicity than liver. Solid with haemorrhage/necrosis. Lack of IVC narrowing on inspiration suggests occlusion.
   - (c) *CT:* large, well-defined, low attenuation, heterogeneous with foci of even lower attenuation due to necrosis. Minimal enhancement compared with the residual rind of functioning renal tissue.
   - (d) *MRI:* inhomogeneous, low signal (T_1W), high signal (T_2W). Inhomogeneous enhancement compared with residual renal tissue.

14

2. **Nephroblastomatosis** – nephrogenic rests which maintain the potential for malignant induction to Wilms' tumour. Nephrogenic rests in 40% of unilateral and 99% of bilateral Wilms' tumours. May be: *perilobar*: most common, at the lobar surface; *intralobar*: anywhere in the cortex or medulla, or combined.
   (a) *Ultrasound:* hypoechoic.
   (b) *CT:* low attenuation and non-enhancing (therefore best shown on contrast-enhanced images).
   (c) *MRI:* similar signal to renal cortex. Non-enhancing (therefore best shown on contrast-enhanced images).

3. **Congenital mesoblastic nephroma** – most common solid renal tumour in the newborn. Mean age at diagnosis is 3.5 months. No recurrence when diagnosed in first 3 months. Indistinguishable from Wilms' tumour but some demonstrate function.

4. **Clear cell sarcoma** – 4–6% of childhood renal tumours. Presentation at 3–5 years. Poor prognosis with early 2° (to bone; usually lytic but may be sclerotic). Never bilateral. No specific imaging features of the primary tumour.

5. **Rhabdoid tumour of kidney** – 2% of childhood renal tumours. Presentation at 3 months to 4.5 years (50% in first year). Most malignant renal tumour with extrarenal extension or haematogenous 2° (to brain or bone) often present at diagnosis. Association with midline posterior fossa tumours. Hypercalcaemia sometimes present. Imaging of the primary tumour is similar to Wilms' tumour.

6. **Multilocular cystic nephroma** – presents 3 months to 4 years. Multiple cysts of varying size. Thin septae. Thick septae, nodules or a large solid component suggest Wilms' tumour with cystic degeneration. Resection is curative and local recurrence is rare. Differential diagnosis is a multicystic dysplastic kidney but this affects the entire kidney.
   (a) *Ultrasound and CT:* cystic with thin septae.
   (b) *MRI:* round collections of variable signal intensity suggesting haemorrhage or proteinaceous material.

7. **Renal cell carcinoma** – rare. Differentiating features from Wilms' tumour are: older age at presentation (mean 11–12 years), calcification is more common (25%) and more homogeneous, smaller at the time of diagnosis and haematuria is more common. Poorer prognosis compared with Wilms' tumour. Similar imaging findings. Association with von Hippel–Lindau disease and tuberous sclerosis*.

8. **Angiomyolipoma** – in 50–80% of patients with tuberous sclerosis*. 50% of patients with angiomyolipomas have tuberous sclerosis. Multiple bilateral tumours, which are usually small.
   (a) *Ultrasound, CT and MRI:* fat densities within the tumours. NB Fat may occasionally be identified within Wilms' tumour.

Further Reading

Geller E, Smergel EM, Lowry PA. Renal neoplasms of childhood. Radiol Clin North Am 1997;34(6):1081–100.

Lowe LH, Isuani BH, Heller RM et al. Pediatric renal masses: Wilms tumor and beyond. Radiographics 2000;20:1585–603.

McHugh K. Renal and adrenal tumours in children. Cancer Imaging 2007;7:41–51.

Riccabona M. Imaging of renal tumours in infancy and childhood. Eur Radiol 2003;13(Suppl 4):L116–29.

Scott DJ, Wallace WH, Hendry GM. With advances in medical imaging can the radiologist reliably diagnose Wilms' tumours? Clin Radiol 1999;54: 321–7.

14.53 HYDRONEPHROSIS IN A CHILD

1. **Pelviureteric junction obstruction** – more common on the left side. 20% bilateral. Due to stricture, neuromuscular inco-ordination or aberrant vessels. Contralateral kidney is dysplastic in 25% of cases and absent in 12%.
2. **Bladder outflow obstruction** (q.v.) – bilateral upper tract dilatation.
3. **Ureterovesical obstruction** – more common in males and more common on the left side. May be bilateral.
4. **Reflux without obstruction.**
5. **Associated with urinary tract infection** – but no obstruction or reflux? Represents atony.
6. **Neurogenic.**

Further Reading

Riccabona M. Assessment and management of newborn hydronephrosis. World J Urol 2004;22(2):73–8.

14

14.54 RENAL MASS IN THE NEWBORN AND YOUNG INFANT

1. **Hydronephrosis** (q.v.) – unilateral or bilateral. The most common cause of an abdominal mass in the first 6 months of life.
2. **Multicystic kidney** – unilateral, but 30% have an abnormal contralateral kidney (mostly pelviureteric junction obstruction). Non-functioning, multilobulated kidney. Rarely, nephrographic crescents and late pooling of contrast medium in cysts is observed. Curvilinear calcification is characteristic but only seen occasionally. US reveals multiple cysts of unequal size. The commonest renal mass in the first year of life.
3. **Polycystic kidneys** (see Polycystic disease*) – bilateral. Poor renal excretion. Striated nephrogram with no visualization of calyces. Highly echogenic on US.
4. **Renal vein thrombosis** (q.v.) – unilateral or bilateral.
5. **Congenital mesoblastic nephroma** – see 14.52.
6. **Nephroblastomatosis or mesoblastic nephroma.**
7. **Renal ectopia.**

Further Reading
Merten DF, Kirks DR. Diagnostic imaging of paediatric abdominal masses. Pediatr Clin North Am 1985;32:1397–425.

14.55 BLADDER OUTFLOW OBSTRUCTION IN A CHILD

1. Distended bladder with incomplete emptying or reduced bladder volume with trabeculation if long-standing obstruction.
2. ± Bilateral upper tract dilatation.
3. ± Upper tract cystic disease.

Causes (from proximal to distal)

1. **Vesical diverticulum** – posteriorly behind the bladder base. It fills during micturition and compresses the bladder neck and proximal urethra. More common in males.
2. **Bladder neck obstruction** – probably not a distinct entity and only occurs as part of other problems such as ectopic ureterocoele and rhabdomyosarcoma.

3. **Ectopic ureterocoele** – 80% are associated with the upper moiety of a duplex kidney. 15% are bilateral. More common in females. Opens into the urethra, bladder neck or vestibule. May be largely outside the bladder and the bladder base may be elevated. 'Drooping lily' appearance of lower moiety. May prolapse into the urethra.

4. **Posterior urethral valves** – posterior urethra is dilated and the distal urethra is small. Almost exclusively males.

5. **Urethral stricture** – post-traumatic strictures are most commonly at the penoscrotal junction and follow previous instrumentation or catheterization.

6. **Cowper's syringocoele** – a dilatation of Cowper's gland ducts. Filling of Cowper's ducts may be a normal finding. When dilated, occasionally presents with haematuria, infection or urethral obstruction.

7. **Anterior urethral diverticulum** – a saccular wide-necked, ventral expansion of the anterior urethra, usually at the penoscrotal junction. The proximal lip of the diverticulum may show as an arcuate filling defect and during micturition the diverticulum expands with urine and obstructs the urethra.

8. **Prune-belly syndrome**.

9. **Calculus or foreign body**.

10. **Meatal stenosis** – usually a clinical diagnosis, but may be detected on MCUG: voiding images should include the meatus.

11. **Phimosis**.

NB The commonest cause in males is posterior urethral valves and in females is ectopic ureterocoele.

14

14.56 VESICOURETERIC REFLUX

CONGENITAL = Primary reflux

Renal scarring with UTI in 50%.

1. **Simple congenital reflux** – due to incompetence of vesicoureteric junction secondary to abnormal tunnelling of distal ureter through bladder. 10% of normal Caucasian babies and 30% of children with a first episode of ITI. Renal scars in up to 50%. Usually disappears in 80% but can cause end-stage renal disease in 10% adults.
2. **Reflux associated with duplex kidneys** – usually occurs into lower moiety ureter, which has a normal position but abnormal tunnelling. Reflux may also occur into a ureterocoele if this everts during filling or voiding.

ACQUIRED = Secondary reflux

1. **Hutch diverticulum.**
2. **Cystitis** – in 50%.
3. **Neurogenic bladder.**
4. **Urethral obstruction** – most commonly posterior urethral valves: see 14.55. More commonly on L side.
5. **Prune-Belly syndrome** – almost exclusively males. High mortality. Bilateral hydronephrosis and hydroureters with a distended bladder are associated with undescended testes, hypoplasia of the anterior abdominal wall and urethral obstruction.

Further Reading

Buckley O, Geoghegan T, O'Brien J, Torreggiani WC. Vesicoureteric reflux in the adult. Br J Radiol 2007;80:392–400.

Fernbach SK, Feinstein KA, Schmidt MB. Pediatric voiding cystourethrography: a pictorial guide. Radiographics 2000;20(1):155–71.

14.57 GAS IN THE PORTAL VEINS

See Figure 7.4

1. **Necrotizing enterocolitis** – 10% develop gas in the portal vein. Necrotic bowel wall allows gas or gas-forming organisms into the portal circulation.
2. **Umbilical vein catheterization** – with the inadvertent injection of air.
3. **Erythroblastosis fetalis.**

14.58 HEPATIC TUMOURS IN CHILDREN

Feature	Hepatoblastoma	Hepatocellular carcinoma
Age	Usually < 5 years old	Usually > 5 years old
Sex	M >> F	M > F
Associated conditions	Beckwith–Wiedemann syndrome, hemihypertrophy	
Associated liver disease	No	↑ incidence (cirrhosis, glycogen storage disease 1, tyrosinaemia, biliary atresia and chronic hepatitis)
Presentation	Mass ± pain. Hormone production may lead to male sexual precocity, polycythaemia, hypoglycaemia, hyperlipidaemia or hypercalcaemia. ± Signs of chronic liver disease	
↑ Serum alpha-fetoprotein	Almost all	Most
Multifocal	Less likely	More likely
Location	Right lobe >> left lobe	Right lobe > left lobe, but in most both lobes are involved
Resectability at diagnosis	More likely	Less likely
Relative prognosis	Better	Worse
Ultrasound	Very variable; usually non-homogeneous increased echoes	
CT	Non-homogeneous low attenuation with some enhancement	
MRI	↓ Signal on T_1W and ↑ signal on T_2W. Tumour invasion of vessels is seen best by this modality	
Metastases	Lungs (in 10% at diagnosis), abdominal lymph nodes and skeleton	

Modified from Cohen (1992).

1. **Hepatoblastoma**.
2. **Hepatocellular** carcinoma.
3. **Haemangioendothelioma** – often present in the newborn period with hepatomegaly and congestive cardiac failure. ± Skin haemangiomas (50%) ± consumptive coagulopathy (thrombocytopenia). Unifocal or multifocal, well-defined or diffuse.

14

Typical pattern of enhancement on CT with early rim enhancement and variable delayed 'filling-in' of the centre of the tumour over next 30 minutes. On MRI the lesions have a non-specific hypointense T_1W and hyperintense T_2W appearance with variable areas of T_1W hypointensity corresponding to fibrosis and haemosiderin deposition. 99mTc-labelled red cells will accumulate in this tumour. In the neonate, this and cavernous haemangioma may be considered together.

4. **Stage IV-S/M-S neuroblastoma** – diffuse and infiltrating. Lesions in bone and bone marrow, ↑ urinary VMAs and positive MIBG scan.

5. **Adenoma** – solitary or multiple, occurring spontaneously or complicating glycogen storage disease, Fanconi's anaemia treated with anabolic steroids, and teenagers on the oral contraceptive pill. Hypodense on CT. Variable appearance on MRI.

Differential diagnosis

1. **Focal nodular hyperplasia** – a wide spectrum of appearances.
2. **Simple cyst.**
3. **Choledochal cyst.**
4. **Abscess.**

Further Reading

Burrows PE, Dubois J, Kassarjian A. Pediatric hepatic vascular anomalies. Pediatr Radiol 2001;3:533–45.

Cheon J-E, Kim WS, Kim I-O et al. Radiological features of focal nodular hyperplasia of the liver in children. Pediatr Radiol 1998;28:878–83.

Cohen MD. Imaging of children with cancer, Ch. 3. Mosby, St Louis, 1992, p20–42.

Donnelly LF, Bissett GS III. Pediatric hepatic imaging. Radiol Clin North Am 1998;36(2):413–27.

Helmberger TK, Ros PR, Mergo PJ et al. Pediatric liver neoplasms: a radiologic-pathologic correlation. Eur Radiol 1999;9:1339–47.

Pobiel RS, Bisset GS III. Pictorial essay: imaging of liver tumours in the infant and child. Pediatr Radiol 1995;25:495–506.

14.59 FETAL OR NEONATAL LIVER CALCIFICATION

Peritoneal

1. **Meconium peritonitis** – the commonest cause of neonatal abdominal calcification. US reveals intra-abdominal solid or cystic masses with calcified walls.
2. **Plastic peritonitis due to ruptured hydrometrocolpos** – similar appearance to meconium peritonitis but US may demonstrate a dilated, fluid-filled uterus and vagina.

Parenchymal

1. **Congenital infections** – TORCH complex (toxoplasmosis, rubella, cytomegalovirus, herpes simplex) and varicella. Randomly scattered nodular calcification. Often calcification elsewhere and other congenital abnormalities.
2. **Tumours** – haemangioma, hamartoma, hepatoblastoma, teratoma and metastatic neuroblastoma. Complex mass on US.

Vascular

1. **Portal vein thromboemboli** – subcapsular branching calcification.
2. **Ischaemic infarcts** – branching calcifications but distributed throughout the liver.

Further Reading

Brugman SM, Bjelland JJ, Thomason JE et al. Sonographic findings with radiologic correlation in meconium peritonitis. J Clin Ultrasound 1979;7:305–6.

Friedman AP, Haller JO, Boyer B et al. Calcified portal vein thromboemboli in infants: radiography and ultrasonography. Radiology 1981;140:381–2.

Nguyen DL, Leonard JC. Ischaemic hepatic necrosis: a cause of fetal liver calcification. Am J Roentgenol 1986;147:596–7.

Schackelford GD, Kirks DR. Neonatal hepatic calcification secondary to transplacental infection. Radiology 1977;122:753–7.

14

14.60 JAUNDICE IN INFANCY

Anatomical abnormalities

1. **Biliary atresia** – 1 in 15000 live births. Three types: I (fCBD atresia), extremely rare; II (intrahepatic), uncommon; III (extrahepatic), which is subdivided into subtype 1 (66%) with a bile duct remnant at the porta hepatis and subtype 2 (34%) with no bile duct. Subtype 2 is associated with multiple congenital abnormalities (polysplenia, intestinal malrotation, azygos continuation of the IVC, situs inversus and preduodenal portal vein).

   US:
   (a) A normal-sized gallbladder that contracts following a fatty meal excludes the diagnosis.
   (b) Absence of, or a small or irregular gallbladder or thin walled gallbladder (gallbladder 'ghost' triad), favours the diagnosis but a normal gallbladder may be seen in 10% of cases.
   (c) Liver echogenicity is normal or heterogeneously increased.
   (d) A triangular or tubular echogenic structure (due to fibrous tissue) at the porta hepatis is highly specific for extrahepatic biliary atresia (triangular cord sign).
   (e) A prominent hepatic artery may also support the diagnosis, but cannot be used in isolation to make the diagnosis.

   TBIDA scan:
   (a) Normal uptake by hepatocytes but no excretion into the bowel suggests the diagnosis but is not diagnostic since alpha-1-antitrypsin may show similar appearances. Operative cholangiography is indicated.

2. **Choledochal cyst** – may present in the neonatal period or at a later age. Classification is:

   I   (80–90%) Fusiform or focal dilatation of the common bile duct ± common hepatic duct.
   II (2%) Diverticulum of the common bile duct.
   III (2–5%) Outpouching of the common bile duct in the wall of the second part of the duodenum – a choledochocoele.
   IVa Dilatation of the common bile duct and focal dilatations of the intrahepatic ducts.
   IVb Focal dilatations of the common bile duct.
   V   Focal dilatations of the intrahepatic bile ducts (Caroli's disease).

   US:
   (a) Anechoic structure which communicates with the biliary tree and is separate from the gallbladder.

   TBIDA scan:
   (a) Photopenic area which accumulates tracer on delayed images.

   Complications:
   (a) Calculi.
   (b) Pancreatitis.

(c) Intrahepatic abscesses.
(d) Biliary cirrhosis.
(e) Portal hypertension.
(f) Malignancy – 4–28%; in the cyst in 3%.
3. **Alagille syndrome** – AD with variable expressivity. Dysmorphic facies, eye abnormalities, cardiovascular abnormalities, especially peripheral pulmonary stenosis or hypoplasia, hypoplasia of intrahepatic bile ducts, butterfly vertebrae, radioulnar synostosis.

Metabolic defects

e.g. Alpha-1-antitrypsin deficiency, galactosaemia, tyrosinaemia.

Infections

1. **Neonatal hepatitis** – possibly secondary to reovirus.
   US:
   (a) Liver echogenicity and size normal or increased.
   (b) Normal bile ducts and gallbladder, although gallbladder may be small when hepatocellular function is poor and bile flow is reduced.
   TBIDA scan:
   (a) May have delayed uptake by hepatocytes.
   (b) Normal excretion into bowel but may be little, if any, if hepatocyte function is severely impaired.

Further Reading

Humphrey TM, Stringer MD. Biliary atresia: US diagnosis. Radiology 2007;244:845–51.
Gubernick JA, Rosenburg HK, Ilaslan H et al. US approach to jaundice in infants and children. Radiographics 2000;20:173–95.
Kim OH, Chung HJ, Choi BG. Imaging of the choledochal cyst. Radiographics 1995;15:69–88.

14

14.61 DIFFERENTIAL DIAGNOSIS OF RETINOBLASTOMA

	Clinical features	Age	Radiology
Persistent hyperplastic primary vitreous	Unilateral leukokoria	At or soon after birth	Microphthalmia. Small irregular lens; shallow anterior chamber. No calcification. Increased attenuation of the vitreous. Enhancement of abnormal intravitreal tissue. Triangular retrolental density with its apex on the posterior lens and base on the posterior globe. Fluid level on decubitus scanning
Coat's disease	A vascular anomaly of telangiectatic vessels which leak proteinaceous material into the subretinal space. Usually boys; unilateral. Present at birth but usually asymptomatic until the retina detaches and vision deteriorates	4–8 years	Appearances of retinal detachment. Indistinguishable from non-calcified retinoblastoma on CT. High signal subretinal effusion on T_1W and T_2W MRI
Retinopathy of prematurity	Uni- or bilateral leukokoria. Appropriate previous medical history of oxygen therapy and prematurity	7–10 weeks	No calcification (but may calcify in the older child). Microphthalmia
Toxocariasis	Close contact with dogs. No systemic symptoms. Positive ELISA test	Mean 6 years	Opaque vitreous or a localized, irregular retinal mass. No contrast enhancement
Chronic retinal detachment	Rare. Presentation late. More common in developmentally abnormal eyes and dysmorphic syndromes		No enhancement or calcification
Retinal astrocytoma (astrocytic hamartoma)	In 40% of patients with tuberous sclerosis or, less commonly, neurofibromatosis, retinitis pigmentosa or as an isolated abnormality		May be bilateral. Multiple, small retinal masses. May calcify in the older child
Retinal dysplasia	Bilateral leukokoria	At or soon after birth	Bilateral retrolental masses. No calcification

More than 50% of children presenting with a clinical diagnosis of retinoblastoma may have another diagnosis. Ocular toxocariasis, persistent hyperplastic primary vitreous (PHPV) and Coat's disease are the three commonest conditions confused with retinoblastoma. Under the age of 3 years, which is when retinoblastoma usually presents, none of the conditions shown in the table show calcification, but above that age some, e.g. retinal astrocytoma, retrolental fibroplasia and toxocariasis, may do so.

Further Reading

Chung EM, Specht CS, Schroeder JW. From the archives of the AFIP: pediatric orbit tumors and tumorlike lesions: neuroepithelial lesions of the ocular globe and optic nerve. Radiographics 2007;27(4):1159–86.

Edward DP, Mafee MF, Garcia-Valenzuela E et al. Coat's disease and persistent hyperplastic primary vitreous. Radiol Clin North Am 1998;36(6):1119–31.

Kaufman LM, Mafee MF, Song CD. Retinoblastoma and simulating lesions. Role of CT, MR imaging and use of Gd-DTPA contrast enhancement. Radiol Clin North Am 1998;36:1101–17.

14.62 PREVERTEBRAL SOFT-TISSUE MASS ON THE LATERAL CERVICAL X-RAY

NB Anterior bucking of the trachea with an increase in the thickness of the retropharyngeal tissues may occur as a normal phenomenon in expiration during the first 2 years of life and is due to laxity of the retropharyngeal tissues. These soft tissues may contain a small collection of air, trapped in the inferior recess of the laryngeal pharynx above the contracted upper oesophageal sphincter. An ear lobe may also mimic a prevertebral mass.

1. **Trauma/haematoma** – ± an associated fracture.
2. **Abscess** – ± gas lucencies within it. Unlike the normal variant described above these lucencies are constant and persist during deep inspiration.
3. **Neoplasms**
   (a) Lymphatic malformation.
   (b) Lymphoma*.
   (c) Nasopharyngeal rhabdomyosarcoma.
   (d) Neuroblastoma.

Further Reading

Brenner GH. Variations in the depth of the cervical prevertebral tissues in normal infants studied by cine fluorography. Am J Roentgenol 1964;91:573–7.

Currarino G, Williams B. Air collection in the retropharyngeal soft tissues observed in lateral expiratory films of the neck in 9 infants. Pediatr Radiol 1993;23:186–8.

14

14.63 NECK MASSES IN INFANTS AND CHILDREN

Ultrasound is a valuable first imaging modality. MRI is generally preferred to CT.

Soft

1. Lipoma.
2. Vascular malformation.
3. Lymphatic malformation.

Firm

1. Cyst
   (a) Thyroglossal – midline position.
   (b) Branchial cleft – lateral position.
   (c) Lingual.
   (d) Thymic.
2. Abscess.
3. Haematoma.
4. Lymphadenopathy.
5. Fibromatosis coli.
6. Rhabdomyosarcoma.
7. Thyroid
   (a) Diffuse enlargement – Graves' disease, multinodular goitre, thyroiditis.
   (b) Focal mass – cyst, benign adenoma. Malignancy is rare.

Further Reading

Swischuk LE, John SD. Neck masses in infants and children. Radiol Clin North Am 1997;35(6):1329–40.

14.64 CAUSES OF STROKE IN CHILDREN AND YOUNG ADULTS

1. **Emboli** – cyanotic heart disease (secondary to right-to-left intracardiac shunt), cardiomyopathies, mitral valve prolapse, Osler–Weber–Rendu (secondary to pulmonary arteriovenous malformations).
2. **Arterial dissection** – trauma, spontaneous, fibromuscular dysplasia (also vessel stenoses and saccular dilatations, intracranial aneurysms), Marfan's syndrome, Ehlers–Danlos syndrome and homocystinuria (see 12.4).
3. **Venous thrombosis** – pregnancy, postpartum, oral contraceptive pill, skull base/intracranial sepsis, inflammatory bowel disease, systemic lupus erythematosus*, Behçet's disease and malignancy (see 12.3).
4. **Infection** – purulent meningitis may cause arterial and venous strokes. Viral infection is a well-recognized cause of arterial stroke due to a 'vasculitis' that usually involves the proximal MCA (infarction of basal ganglia with sparing of the cortical territories).
5. **Trauma** – arterial dissection and hypoxia.
6. **Drugs** – cocaine, amphetamines.
7. **Blood disorders** – sickle-cell anaemia*, polycythaemia, protein C and S deficiency.
8. **Migraine** – usually posterior circulation.
9. **Vasculopathy, vasculitis** – neurofibromatosis*, fibromuscular dysplasia, Kawasaki's, systemic lupus erythematosus*, sarcoidosis*.
10. **Idiopathic** – in many cases, a cause is not found.

Further Reading
Ball WS. Cerebrovascular occlusive disease in childhood. Neuroimaging Clin North Am 1994;4:393–421.
Provenzale JM, Barboriak DP. Brain infarction in young adults: etiology and imaging. Am J Roentgenol 1997;169:1161–8.

14.65 LARGE HEAD IN INFANCY

1. **Hydrocephalus.**
2. **Chronic subdural haematoma.**
3. **Neurofibromatosis*.**
4. **Mucopolysaccharidoses.**
5. **Megalencephaly.**
6. **Alexander's disease** – leukodystrophy that typically involves the frontal lobes early in its course.
7. **Canavan's disease** – leukodystrophy that typically affects the subcortical arcuate fibres, but often involves the entire cerebral white matter.
8. **Hydranencephaly.**

14

14.66 WIDE CRANIAL SUTURES

>10mm at birth; >3mm at 2 years; >2mm at 3 years.

Normal

Raised intracranial pressure
Only seen in children <10 years.

1. Intracranial tumour.
2. Subdural haematoma.
3. Hydrocephalus.

Infiltration of sutures
1. Neuroblastoma – ± skull vault lucencies and 'sunray' spiculation (a reaction to subpericranial deposits).
2. Leukaemia.
3. Lymphoma*.

Metabolic disease
1. Rickets*.
2. Hypoparathyroidism.
3. Lead intoxication.
4. Bone dysplasias with defective mineralization.

Recovery from illness
Rapid rebound growth of the brain following:

1. Deprivational dwarfism.
2. Chronic illness.
3. Prematurity.
4. Hypothyroidism.

Trauma
Traumatic diastasis of the sutures.

14.67 HYPERECHOIC LESIONS IN THE BASAL GANGLIA ON CRANIAL ULTRASOUND OF NEONATES AND INFANTS

Single punctate, multiple punctate or stripe-like densities.

1. **Congenital infections** – CMV, toxoplasmosis, rubella, HIV and syphilis.
2. **Asphyxia/hypoxia.**
3. **Cardiac disease** – particularly hypoplastic left heart syndrome.
4. **Chromosome disorders.**
5. **Fetal alcohol and drug exposure.**
6. **Twin–twin transfusion.**
7. **Idiopathic.**

Further Reading

Coley BD, Rusin JA, Boue DR. Importance of hypoxic/ischemic conditions in the development of cerebral lenticulostriate vasculopathy. Pediatr Radiol 2000;30:846–55.

El Ayoubi M, de Bethmann O, Monset-Couchard M. Lenticulostriate echogenic vessels: clinical and sonographic study of 70 neonatal cases. Pediatr Radiol 2003;33(10):697–703.

Teele RL, Hernanz-Schulman M, Sorel A. Echogenic vasculature in the basal ganglia of neonates: a sonographic sign of vasculopathy. Radiology 1988;169:423.

14.68 MULTIPLE WORMIAN BONES

Intrasutural ossicles common in infancy (lambdoid, posterior sagittal and temporosquamosal). Considered abnormal if large (6×4mm or larger) and multiple (>10).

1. **Idiopathic.**
2. **Down's syndrome.**
3. **Pyknodysostosis.**
4. **Osteogenesis imperfecta*.**
5. **Rickets*.**
6. **Kinky hair (Menkes) syndrome.**
7. **Cleidocranial dysostosis.**
8. **Hypophosphatasia.**
9. **Hypothyroidism.**
10. **Otopalatodigital syndrome.**
11. **Primary acro-osteolysis (Hadju–Cheney).**
12. **Pachydermoperiostosis.**
13. **Progeria.**

14

Further Reading

Cremin B, Goodman H, Spranger J et al. Wormian bones in osteogenesis imperfecta and other disorders. Skeletal Radiol 1982;8:35–8.

Dahnert W. Radiology review manual, 5th edn. Williams and Wilkins, Baltimore, 2003.

Pryles CV, Khan AJ. Wormian bones. Am J Dis Child 1979;133:380–2.

14.69 CRANIOSYNOSTOSIS

Premature closure of one or more sutures. May occur as an isolated primary abnormality, as part of a more complex syndrome, or secondary to systemic disease. Fusion of a suture results in arrested growth of the calvarium. Raised intracranial pressure may occur with closure of multiple sutures. CT with 3D reformatting offers the best evaluation of the skull sutures and also demonstrates the intracranial contents (e.g. malformations, hydrocephalus, arrested brain growth).

Primary craniosynostosis

1. **Sagittal synostosis** – elongated narrow 'boat-shaped' skull (scaphocephaly/dolichocephaly).
2. **Unilateral coronal synostosis** – oblique appearance of the craniofacial structures with harlequin orbit (frontal plagiocephaly).
3. **Bilateral coronal synostosis** – 'short head', often seen with synostosis of other sutures (brachycephaly).
4. **Metopic synostosis** – triangular-shaped head (trigonocephaly).
5. **Unilateral lambdoid synostosis** – occipital plagiocephaly.
6. **Bilateral lambdoid synostosis** – occipital plagiocephaly with flattened occiput. Beware postural flattening of the occiput due to infants being placed to sleep on their backs to prevent sudden infant death syndrome. There is no sutural fusion in these cases.
7. **Cloverleaf skull (Kleeblattscheidel)** – synostosis of multiple paired sutures produces a 'trilobular skull'.

Syndromic craniosynostosis

The most frequently described syndromes are the acrocephalosyndactylies. This group of conditions includes Apert's, Carpenter's and Pfeiffer's syndromes. Each syndrome exhibits synostosis of multiple sutures with severe calvarial and facial malformations. Crouzon's syndrome differs in that there is no syndactyly.

Secondary

1. **Metabolic** – rickets, hyperthyroidism, hypophosphatasia.
2. **Inborn errors of metabolism** – Hurler's and Morquio's syndromes.
3. **Haematological disease** – thalassaemia, sickle-cell.
4. **Brain malformation** – holoprosencephaly, microcephaly.
5. **Iatrogenic** – shunted hydrocephalus.

Further Reading

Aviv RI, Rodger E, Hall CM. Craniosynostosis. Clin Radiol 2002;57:93–102.

Bensom ML, Oliverio PJ, Yue NC et al. Primary craniosynostosis: imaging features. Am J Roentgenol 1996;166:697–703.

Boyle CM, Rosenblum JD. Three-dimensional CT for pre- and post-surgical imaging of patients with craniosynostosis: correlation of operative procedure and radiologic imaging. Am J Roentgenol 1997;169:1173–7.

David DJ, Poswillo D, Simpson D. The craniosynostoses. Springer-Verlag, Berlin, 1982.

Fernbach SK. Craniosynostosis: concepts and controversies. Pediatr Radiol 1998;28:722–8.

14.70 CYSTIC LESIONS ON CRANIAL ULTRASOUND IN NEONATES AND INFANTS

Normal variants

1. **Coarctation of the lateral ventricle.** Synonym = connatal cysts: characteristic appearance on para-sagittal scan. On coronal scan located at or just below supero-lateral angle of frontal horn.
2. **Cavum septum pellucidum/vergae/veli interpositum.** Common, particularly in premature neonates.

Infratentorial cysts

1. **Mega cisterna magna.** Occurs in 1%. As isolated finding probably a normal variant.
2. **Dandy–Walker malformation.** Cystic dilatation of posterior fossa in communication with fourth ventricle, with associated vermian hypoplasia.
3. **Arachnoid cyst.** One-quarter occur in posterior fossa, most commonly retro-cerebellar.

Supratentorial cysts

1. **Subependymal cysts.** Located in subependymal region around caudo-thalamic notch. Most commonly represent previous germinal matrix haemorrhage. May be congenital, probably reflecting germinolysis, particularly in association with CMV infection.

14

2. **Choroid plexus cysts**. Usually located within body of choroids plexus. Weak markers of aneuploidy, particularly if large and bilateral. No clinical significance if detected after birth.
3. **Cystic periventricular leukomalacia**. White matter necrosis in preterm infant. Hyperechoic lesions dorsal and lateral to external angles of lateral ventricles, developing into cysts in severe cases.
4. **Porencephalic cyst**. An area of cystic encephalomalacia filled with CSF, commonly following haemorrhage or infection, with a communication with the ventricular system.
5. **Arachnoid cyst**. Most commonly in the sylvian fissure, and usually incidental. Suprasellar cysts more frequently symptomatic.
6. **Vein of Galen malformation**. Not a cyst, but may appear so on USS. Colour Doppler flow confirms.

Further Reading

Epelman M, Daneman A, Blaser SI et al. Differential diagnosis of intracranial cystic lesions at head US: correlation with CT and MR imaging. Radiographics 2006;26(1):173–96.

14.71 DISORDERS OF NEURONAL MIGRATION

The neuronal population of the normal cerebral cortex arrives by a process of outward migration from the periventricular germinal matrix between the 8th and 16th weeks of gestation. This complex process of cell migration can be interfered with by many causes, sporadic and unknown, chromosomal or genetic.

1. **Agyria–pachygyria** – poorly formed gyri and sulci, the former being more severe. Focal pachygyria may be the cause of focal epilepsy. Polymicrogyria (see below) may coexist with pachygyria. Extreme cases with a smooth brain may be termed lissencephaly. Complete lissencephaly ≡ agyria. Several distinct forms are recognized.
    (a) *Type I lissencephaly* – small brain with few gyri; smooth, thickened four-layer cortex resembling that of a 13-week fetus with diminished white matter and shallow vertical sylvian fissures ('figure-of-eight' appearance on axial images).
    ± agenesis of the corpus callosum. Severe mental retardation, diplegia, seizures, microcephaly and limited survival. Some infants have specific dysmorphic features: Miller–Dieker syndrome and Norman–Roberts syndrome. Pachygyria may also be observed in Zellweger syndrome and prenatal CMV infection.
    (b) *Type II lissencephaly* (Walker–Warburg syndrome) – smooth cortex, cerebellar hypoplasia and vermian aplasia and hydrocephalus (in 75%) due to cisternal obstruction by abnormal meninges or aqueduct stenosis.

2. **Polymicrogyria** – the neurons reach the cortex but are distributed abnormally. Macroscopically the surface of the brain appears as multiple small bumps. Localized abnormalities are more common than generalized and often involve arterial territories, especially the middle cerebral artery. The most common location is around the sylvian fissure. The cortex is isointense to grey matter but in 20% of cases the underlying white matter has high signal on T_2W. Linear flow voids due to anomalous venous drainage may be present. Polymicrogyrias may be present in the vicinity of a porencephalic cyst, be associated with heterotopic grey matter or agenesis of the corpus callosum or with evidence of fetal infection such as intracranial calcification. Symptoms and signs depend on the size, site and presence of associated abnormalities. The majority have mental retardation, seizures and neurological signs.

3. **Schizencephaly** – clefts which extend through the full thickness of the cerebral mantle from ventricle to subarachnoid space. The cleft is lined by heterotopic grey matter and microgyrias, indicating that it existed prior to the end of neuronal migration. Unilateral or bilateral (usually asymmetrical) and usually near the sylvian fissure. May be associated with absence of the septum pellucidum or, less commonly, dysgenesis of the corpus callosum. There are variable clinical manifestations, from profound retardation to isolated partial seizures.

4. **Heterotopic grey matter** – collections of neurons in a subependymal location, i.e. at the site of the germinal matrix or arrested within the white matter on their way to the cortex. Isointense to normal grey matter on all imaging sequences. Nodules or bands and may have mass effect. Frequently a part of complex malformation syndromes or, when isolated, may be responsible for focal seizures which are amenable to surgical treatment. Small heterotopias are probably asymptomatic.

5. **Cortical dysplasia** – focal disorganization of the cerebral cortex. A single enlarged gyrus resembling focal pachygyria. Usual presentation is with partial epilepsy.

Further Reading

Aicardi J. Clinics in developmental medicine. Diseases of the nervous system in childhood, 2nd edn. Ch. 3. MacKeith Press, London, 1992, p69–130.

Barkovich AJ. Pediatric neuroimaging, 4th edn. Lippincott Williams & Wilkins, Philadelphia, 2005, p320–64.

14

14.72 SUPRATENTORIAL TUMOURS IN CHILDHOOD

Primary CNS tumours are the second most common malignancy in children (leukaemia is the commonest). Overall, supratentorial and infratentorial tumours occur with equal incidence.

1. **Hemispheric astrocytoma** – solid, solid with a necrotic centre, or cystic with a mural nodule. Usually large at presentation and can involve the basal ganglia and thalami. Most are low grade. Enhancement with contrast medium does not correlate with histological grade. Associated with NF1.

2. **Craniopharyngioma** – more than half of all craniopharyngiomas occur in children (8–14 years). Cystic/solid partially calcified suprasellar mass presenting with headache, visual disturbance and endocrine abnormalities (see 12.37).

3. **Optic pathway glioma** – low grade, but infiltrating pilocytic astrocytomas associated with NF1. Solid enhancing tumours that extend along the length of the anterior optic pathways and may invade adjacent structures (e.g. hypothalamus) and extend posteriorly into the optic tracts and radiations.

4. **Giant cell subependymal astrocytoma** – slow-growing partially cystic, partially calcified tumour occurring in tuberous sclerosis. Located at the foramen of Monro and presents with obstructive hydrocephalus.

5. **Germ cell tumours** – germinomas, teratoma (see 12.39).

6. **Primitive neuroectodermal tumour (PNET)** – large heterogeneous hemispheric mass presenting in neonates and small infants. Necrosis, haemorrhage and enhancement are common.

7. **Dysembryoplastic neuroepithelial tumour (DNT)** – benign cortical tumour often presenting with seizures. Cortical (temporal) mass, usually small, that may demonstrate internal cyst formation and calcification.

8. **Ganglioglioma** – well-circumscribed peripheral tumour that often presents with seizures. Cystic tumour with mural nodule ± calcification.

9. **Choroid plexus papilloma** – presents in young children with hydrocephalus. Most occur in the atrium of the lateral ventricle (fourth ventricle in adults) and appear as a well-circumscribed multilobulated avidly enhancing intraventricular mass ± calcification. Invasion of brain suggests choroid plexus carcinoma.

10. **Ependymoma** – often in the frontal lobe adjacent to the frontal horn, but not usually within the ventricular system.

Further Reading
Barkovich AJ. Pediatric neuroimaging, 4th edn. Lippincott Williams & Wilkins, Philadelphia, 2005, p551–613.
Edwards-Brown MK. Supratentorial brain tumors. Neuroimaging Clin North Am 1994;4:437–55.
Griffiths PD. A neuroimaging protocol for imaging children with brain tumours. Clin Radiol 1999;54:558–62.

14.73 INFRATENTORIAL TUMOURS IN CHILDHOOD

These comprise 50% of paediatric cerebral tumours. The majority arise from the cerebellar parenchyma. Cerebellar astrocytomas, medulloblastomas and ependymomas present with symptoms of raised intracranial pressure and ataxia. Brainstem gliomas involve the cranial nerve nuclei and long tracts at an early stage.

1. **Cerebellar astrocytoma** – 20–25% of posterior fossa tumours. Vermis (50%) or hemispheres (20%) or both sites (30%) $\pm$ extension into the cavity of the fourth ventricle. Calcification in 20%.
   CT/MRI: Large lesion displacing the fourth ventricle $\rightarrow$ obstructive hydrocephalus. 80% are juvenile pilocytic astrocytomas with an excellent prognosis. Tumour can be cystic, solid or solid with central necrosis. 50% of all tumours are a cyst with an isodense enhancing mural nodule. The cyst contents have slightly > CSF attenuation on CT. 40–45% are solid with central necrosis. The solid component is isodense to hypodense to white matter on CT, low signal on T_1W MRI and high signal on T_2W MRI. The solid component enhances on CT and MRI. Larger tumour at diagnosis than the solid type. The solid type accounts for 10%.
2. **Medulloblastoma** – 30–40% of posterior fossa tumours. Short history. 80% located in the vermis; 30% extend into the brainstem.
   CT: Moderately well-defined, ovoid or spherical mass; slightly > surrounding cerebellum; rim of oedema. Usually uniform enhancement; non-enhancement rarely. Calcification (in 10%) is usually small, homogeneous and eccentric. Dystrophic calcification occurs after radiotherapy. Small cystic or necrotic areas are unusual.
   MRI: Low signal on T_1W; heterogeneous iso- to low signal on T_2W. Variable enhancement.
   Dissemination of tumour by: (a) seeding of the subarachnoid space; (b) retrograde ventricular extension; or (c) extracranial metastases to bone, lymph nodes or soft tissues. Recurrence of tumour is demonstrated by: (a) enhancement at the site of the lesion;

14

(b) enhancement of the subarachnoid space (basal cisterns, sylvian, fissures, sulci and ependymal surfaces of ventricles); or

(c) progressive ventricular enlargement.

3. **Ependymoma** – most commonly in the floor of the fourth ventricle. 8–15% of posterior fossa tumours. Usually a long clinical history. *CT:* Typically, an isodense to hyperdense fourth ventricular mass with punctate calcifications, small cysts and heterogeneous or homogeneous enhancement. Calcification within a fourth ventricular mass or adjacent to the fourth ventricle = ependymoma. *MRI:* Homogeneous or heterogeneous. Slightly hypointense on T_1W and isointense to grey matter on T_2W. Tumour extension through the foramen of Magendie, foramen magnum (behind the spinal cord) and foramen of Luschka (into the cerebellopontine angle) are important clues to the diagnosis.

4. **Brainstem glioma** – 20–30% of posterior fossa tumours. Insidious onset because of the location and tendency to infiltrate cranial nerve nuclei and long tracts without producing CSF obstruction until late. Four subgroups: (a) medullary, (b) pontine, (c) mesencephalic and (d) those associated with NF1. Tumours may also be diffuse (>50–75% of the brainstem in the axial plane) or focal (<50%). Calcification rare.

   (a) Medullary – least common. Young children. May be differentiated into focal dorsally exophytic and diffuse forms (with significantly worse prognosis). Low attenuation (CT), low signal (T_1W) and high signal (T_2W).

   (b) Pontine – most common. Diffuse tumours are low attenuation (CT), low signal (T_1W) and high signal (T_2W). Flattening of the floor of the fourth ventricle. Contrast enhancement is rare. Focal tumours are very uncommon but do exhibit heterogeneous enhancement.

   (c) Mesencephalic – focal tumours are more common than diffuse. Symptoms depend on the exact location of the mass.

   (d) Associated with NF1 – most commonly in the medulla. Similar imaging appearances to those without NF1, but patients may be asymptomatic and progression is slower.

Further Reading

Barkovich AJ. Pediatric neuroimaging, 4th edn. Lippincott Williams & Wilkins, Philadelphia, 2005, p514–551

Griffiths PD. A neuroimaging protocol for imaging children with brain tumours. Clin Radiol 1999;54:558–62.

Vezina L-G, Packer RJ. Infratentorial brain tumors of childhood. Neuroimaging Clin North Am 1994;4:423–36.

14.74 INTRAVENTRICULAR MASS IN CHILDREN

Lateral ventricles

1. **Glioma.**
2. **Primitive neuroectodermal tumour** – see 14.72.
3. **Choroid plexus papilloma** – see 14.72.
4. **Choroid plexus cyst.**
5. **Choroid plexus enlargement** – neurofibromatosis, Sturge–Weber.
6. **Subependymoma.**
7. **Meningioma.**
8. **Arteriovenous malformation** – enlarged draining veins.
9. **Subependymal heterotopia** – nodules of ectopic grey matter.
10. **Metastatic seeding** – e.g. medulloblastoma, ependymoma.

Foramen of Monro

1. **Subependymal giant cell astrocytoma** – see 14.72.

Third ventricle

1. **Craniopharyngioma** – see 12.37.
2. **Glioma** – hypothalamic, chiasmatic. See 14.72.
3. **Langerhans cell histiocytosis*** – see 12.36.
4. **Germinoma** – see 12.39.
5. **Choroid plexus papilloma** – see 14.72.
6. **Metastatic seeding.**

Fourth ventricle

1. **Medulloblastoma** – see 14.73.
2. **Ependymoma** – see 14.73.
3. **Choroid plexus papilloma** – see 14.73.
4. **Exophytic brainstem glioma** – see 14.73.

14

15

Evaluating statistics – explanations of terminology in general use

1. **Reliability**: reproducibility of results. (These may be from the same observer or from different observers.) Assessment of this can be built into a study of diagnostic accuracy of a technique, or evaluated beforehand.
2. **Accuracy**: 'proportion of results (positive and negative) which agree with the final diagnosis',

$$\text{i.e.} \quad \frac{\text{true positives} + \text{true negatives}}{\text{total number of patients in the study.}}$$

   NB. This does not take false positive and false negatives into account, and is therefore less meaningful than sensitivity and specificity.
3. **Sensitivity**: 'proportion of diseased patients who are reported as positive',

$$\text{i.e.} \quad \frac{\text{true positives}}{\text{total number of final diagnosis positive.}}$$

4. **Specificity**: 'proportion of disease-free patients who are reported as negative',

$$\text{i.e.} \quad \frac{\text{true negatives}}{\text{total number of final diagnosis negative.}}$$

5. **Positive predictive value**: 'proportion of patients reported positive who have the disease',

$$\text{i.e.} \quad \frac{\text{true positives}}{\text{true positives} + \text{false positives.}}$$

6. **Negative predictive value**: 'proportion of patients reported negative who do not have the disease',

$$\text{i.e.} \quad \frac{\text{true negatives}}{\text{true negatives} + \text{false negatives.}}$$

Differences in the prevalence of the disease in different studies can affect sensitivity and specificity. For example, if a study is conducted in a tertiary referral hospital the patients will be highly selected and this can alter the way that subtle abnormalities are interpreted as there is a high likelihood of disease being present.

Predictive values are now in common use to indicate the usefulness of an imaging test. However, these depend on sensitivity, specificity and prevalence and therefore only apply to settings with a similar prevalence. Formulae are available for calculation of predictive values for different prevalences – see Further reading.

7. **Receiver operating characteristic (ROC) curves**: In many situations it is not possible to be definitely positive or definitely negative when reporting. With this method approximately five or six levels of certainty may be used in reporting (e.g. 1 = definitely positive, 2 = probably positive, etc.). Using each of these levels in turn as the point of cut-off between a 'definitely positive' and a 'definitely negative' result, the sensitivity and specificity for each level are then plotted in the form of a graph of sensitivity against 1 – specificity. The area under the curve will be 1.0 for a perfect technique (or observer) and 0.5 for an absolutely useless technique (or observer!) (see Figure).

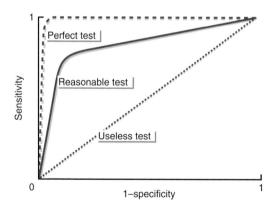

Further Reading

Freedman LS. Evaluating and comparing imaging techniques: a review and classification of study designs. Br J Radiol 1987;60:1071–81.

15

Part 2

ACHONDROPLASIA

A primary defect of enchondral bone formation. AD (but 80% are spontaneous mutations).

Skull

1. Large skull. Small base. Small sella. Steep clivus. Small funnel-shaped foramen magnum.
2. Hydrocephalus – of variable severity.

Thorax

1. Thick, stubby sternum.
2. Short ribs with deep concavities to the anterior ends.

Axial skeleton

1. Decreasing interpedicular distance caudally in the lumbar spine.
2. Short pedicles with a narrow sagittal diameter of the lumbar spinal canal.
3. Posterior scalloping.
4. Anterior vertebral body beak at T12/L1/L2.

Pelvis

1. Square iliac wings.
2. 'Champagne-glass' pelvic cavity.
3. Short, narrow sacrosciatic notch.
4. Horizontal sacrum articulating low on the ilia.

Appendicular skeleton

1. Rhizomelic micromelia with bowing of long bones.
2. Widened metaphyses.
3. Ball-and-socket epiphyseal/metaphyseal junction.
4. Broad and short proximal and short proximal and middle phalanges.
5. Trident-shaped hands.

ACQUIRED IMMUNE DEFICIENCY SYNDROME

Widespread use of highly active anti-retroviral therapy (HAART) over the past decade has significantly changed the patterns of presentation of HIV-related disease in adults.

A. Chest

Most patients will suffer one or more acute chest presentations.

If sputum analysis is negative then bronchoscopy, lavage ± transbronchial biopsy should be considered since CXR and CT changes are rarely able to provide definitive diagnosis.

The presence of nodes or pleural effusions often indicates infection (TB, fungal) or tumour (lymphoma, Kaposi's). Mediastinal/ hilar nodes are not a common feature of pneumocystis.

1. **Opportunist infections**
   (a) *Pneumocystis jiroveci* (previously *carinii*) most common opportunistic infection.
   Chest radiograph is normal at presentation in one-third. Typically there is bilateral perihilar and/or basal reticulonodular infiltrates with rapid progression to alveolar consolidation in 3–5 days.
   Less commonly:
   - (i) Asymmetrical upper lobe disease – especially following inhaled pentamidine therapy.
   - (ii) 10–30% have cystic parenchymal changes which (in 30%) are complicated by pneumothorax.
   - (iii) Miliary nodules or solitary nodule (mimics rounded consolidation; may cavitate).
   - (iv) Pleural effusion, but more common in mycobacterial and bacterial infections and neoplasia.
   HRCT demonstrates extensive ground-glass attenuation ± thickened interlobular septa and focal consolidation.
   (b) CMV. Present in 80% of autopsies but rarely the only pathogen. CXR typically indistinguishable from *Pneumocystis* or fibrosis.
   (c) Mycobacterium affects 10%, and can occur long before other features of AIDS.
   (d) Bacterial pneumonia with the usual community acquired pathogens, now the commonest cause of acute chest infection in HIV.
2. **Neoplasms**
   (a) Kaposi's sarcoma – lung involvement occurs in 20% of Kaposi's, and is almost always preceded by cutaneous and/or visceral involvement.
   (b) Pulmonary lymphoma – increasingly common non-Hodgkin's > Hodgkin's.

B. Abdomen

Infections

Dependent on level of immunocompromise.

CD4 <400 – TB, candida; CD4 <200 – *Candida, Histoplasmosis, Cryptosporidium, Pneumocystis*; CD4 <100 – CMV, herpes simplex, MAI.

1. Primary HIV – oesophageal ulceration.
2. *Candida.* Usually oropharynx and oesophagus. AIDS defining. Mucosal plaques, fold thickening, 'shaggy' oesophagus on barium swallow.
3. Herpes – small discrete ulcers on barium swallow.
4. CMV – most common GI infection. Can occur anywhere but usually lower GI. Oesophagus –large mid-oesophageal ulcer; CMV gastritis, enteritis and colitis – superficial progressing to deep ulceration (mimic Crohn's), extensive bowel wall thickening on CT, USS; segmental or diffuse, lymphadenopathy not prominent.
5. TB – ileocaecal jejunoileum most common sites (upper GI less common). Segmental ulcers, wall thickening, strictures, and mass-like lesions of the caecum and TI. Regional low-attenuation necrotic lymphadenopathy. Hepatosplenomegaly (occ. focal lesions).
6. *Mycobacterium avium* complex. Usually small bowel. Mimics Whipple's (irregular fold thickening and mild dilatation). Prominent lymphadenopathy. Hepatosplenomegaly (occ. focal lesions).
7. Cryptosporidium – diffuse fold thickening, flocculation of barium (mimics sprue). No lymphadenopathy.
8. *Rochalimaea henselae* (Peliosis hepatis). Fever, sweats, RUQ pain. Sonographically liver inhomogeneous, with hyperechoic and hypoechoic regions. Cavities may be visible on CT (if large).
9. PCP – liver/spleen/kidneys – hypoechoic/hypoattenuating masses or multiple tiny echogenic/hyperattenuating foci (calcified).

Malignancy

1. **Kaposi's sarcoma**
   CD4 count typically <200.
   (a) Liver/spleen – multifocal hyperechoic nodules (5–12mm) adjacent to portal veins on USS. CT – hypoattenuating nodules, with delayed enhancement (mimic haemangiomas).
   (b) GI tract – usually with cutaneous involvement. Anywhere in GI tract but duodenum most common. Submucosal masses (0.5–3cm) ± ulceration at CT/barium. Hyperattenuating lymphadenopathy.
2. **Lymphoma**
   Usually aggressive form of non-Hodgkin's lymphoma. Peripheral nodes are present in 50% and extranodal involvement is common, particularly bowel, viscera and marrow.

Common symptoms/signs

1. Dysphagia – common. Usually due to candidiasis, but occasionally caused by viral oesophagitis or Kaposi's sarcoma.
2. Hepatosplenomegaly – non-specific. Seen in many infections (CMV, TB, MAI) and lymphoma.
3. Diarrhoea – common. Usually CMV colitis if mild, or *Cryptosporidium* (protozoa) if severe. *Giardia, Clostridium difficile* and *Mycobacterium* may also occur.
4. Retroperitoneal/mesenteric lymphadenopathy
   (a) Progressive generalized lymphadenopathy syndrome – i.e. two or more extrainguinal nodes persisting for more than 3 months with no obvious cause. Biopsy reveals benign hyperplasia, and CT shows clusters of small nodes <1cm in diameter in the mesentery and retroperitoneum.
   (b) Kaposi's sarcoma (KS).
   (c) Lymphoma.
   (d) Mycobacterium/TB.
   (e) Non-specific.
5. AIDS cholangiopathy – right upper quadrant pain, nausea, vomiting and fever. Due to infection by CMV or Cryptosporidium. Gallbladder wall thickening, pericholecystic fluid, intrahepatic and extrahepatic bile duct strictures, diverticula, intraluminal filling defects and strictures of the juxta-ampullary pancreatic duct.
6. HIV nephropathy – proteinuria and rapidly progressive renal failure. Usually, globally enlarged kidneys.
7. Pyelonephritis and renal abscesses.

C. CNS

See 12.11.

D. Musculoskeletal

1. **Infection.**
   Opportunistic and non-opportunistic. Commonest organism is *Staph. aureus*, but also TB, *M. avium, Nocardia, Cryptococcus, Toxoplasmosis, Salmonella*.
   (a) Cellulitis.
   (b) Necrotizing fasciitis.
   (c) Pyomyositis.
   (d) Osteomyelitis.
   (e) Septic arthritis.
2. **Inflammatory**
   (a) Arthritides.
       (i) HIV associated (1–6 weeks).
       (ii) Painful articular syndrome (48 hours).
       (iii) Seronegative e.g. Reiter's syndrome.

    (b) Polymyositis. Bilateral symmetrical proximal muscle weakness and increased creatine kinase.

3. **Neoplasm**
   - **(a)** Non-Hodgkin's lymphoma.
   - **(b)** Kaposi sarcoma.
4. **Miscellaneous**
   - **(a)** Osteonecrosis.
   - **(b)** Osteoporosis.
   - **(c)** Rhabdomyolysis.
   - **(d)** Hypertrophic pulmonary osteoarthropathy.
   - **(e)** Anaemia – bone marrow – low signal intensity on T_1.

Further Reading

Boiselle PM, Crans SA Jr, Kaplan MA. The changing face of *Pneumocystis carinii* pneumonia in AIDS patients. Am J Roentgenol 1999;172:1301–9.

Burns J, Shaknovich R, Lau J et al. Oncogenic viruses in AIDS: mechanisms of disease and intrathoracic manifestations. Am J Roentgenol 2007;189:1082–7.

Guihot A, Couderc LJ, Rivaud E et al. Thoracic radiographic and CT findings of multicentric Castleman disease in HIV-infected patients. J Thorac Imaging 2007;22:207–11.

Kuhlman JE. Imaging pulmonary disease in AIDS: state of the art. Eur Radiol 1999;9:395–408.

Logan PM, Finnegan MM. Pictorial review: pulmonary complications in AIDS: CT appearances. Clin Radiol 1998;53:567–73.

Major NM, Tehranzadeh J. Musculoskeletal manifestations of AIDS. Radiol Clin North Am 1997;35:1167–90.

Provenzale JM, Jinkins JR. Brain and spine imaging findings in AIDS patients. Radiol Clin North Am 1997;35:1127–66.

Redvanly RD, Silverstein JE. Intra-abdominal manifestations of AIDS. Radiol Clin North Am 1997;35:1083–126.

Reeders JW, Goodman PC. Radiology of AIDS. Springer, Heidelberg, 2001.

Reeders JW, Yee J, Gore RM et al. Gastrointestinal infection in the immunocompromised (AIDS) patient. Eur Radiol 2004;14(Suppl 3):E84–102.

Restrepo C, Lemos D, Gordillo H. Imaging findings in musculoskeletal complications of AIDS. Radiographics 2004;24:1029–49.

Restrepo CS, Martínez S, Lemos JA et al. Imaging manifestations of Kaposi sarcoma. Radiographics 2006;26:1169–85

Richards PJ, Armstrong P, Parkin JM et al. Chest imaging in AIDS. Clin Radiol 1998;53:554–66.

ACQUIRED IMMUNE DEFICIENCY SYNDROME (AIDS) IN CHILDREN

The majority of cases (~80%) are due to transmission from an infected mother, with a 25% risk of acquiring infection. Acquisition from transfusions (in the neonatal period or because of diseases such as thalassaemia and haemophilia) is rare in the West but still occurs in developing countries. 50% of those infected congenitally will present in the first year of life.

AIDS in children differs from AIDS in adults in the following ways:

1. Shorter incubation period.
2. Children are more likely to have serious bacterial infections or CMV.
3. They develop pulmonary lymphoid hyperplasia (PLH)/lymphocytic interstitial pneumonia (LIP), which is rare in adults.
4. They almost never develop Kaposi's sarcoma.
5. They are less likely to be infected with *Toxoplasma, Mycobacterium tuberculosis, Cryptococcus* and *Histoplasma*.
6. Two patterns of presentation and progression can be recognized:
   (a) In the first year of life with serious infections and encephalopathy. Poor prognosis.
   (b) Preschool and school age with bacterial infections and lymphoid tissue hyperplasia. Survival is longer, to adolescence.

Prognostic factors are severity of disease in the mother, the age of onset and the severity at onset.

Generalized features

Failure to thrive; weight loss; fever; generalized lymphadenopathy; hepatosplenomegaly; recurrent infections; chronic diarrhoea; parotitis (hypoechoic nodules, hyperechoic striae and lympho-epithelial cysts on USS).

Chest

1. *Pneumocystis carinii* pneumonia (PCP) – may be localized initially but typically there is rapid progression to generalized lung shadowing which is a mixed alveolar and interstitial infiltrate. 50% of infections occur at age 3–6 months. Two-thirds of infections are the first and only infective episode.
2. Cytomegalovirus (CMV) pneumonia.
3. LIP/PLH – in 50% of patients. Insidious onset of clinical symptoms. CXR shows a diffuse, symmetrical reticulonodular or nodular pattern (2–3mm in diameter) which is most easily seen at the bases and periphery of the lungs ± hilar or mediastinal lymphadenopathy.

The nodules consist of collections of lymphocytes and plasma cells without any organisms. Children with LIP are more likely to have generalized lymphadenopathy, salivary gland enlargement (particularly parotid) and finger clubbing than those whose CXR changes due to opportunistic infection, and the prognosis for LIP is better. Long-standing LIP may be complicated by lower lobe bronchiectasis or cystic lung disease (resembling that seen in histiocytosis).

4. Mediastinal or hilar adenopathy may be secondary to PLH, *M. tuberculosis, M. avium intracellulare,* CMV, lymphoma or fungal infection.
5. Cardiomyopathy, dysrhythmias and unexpected cardiac arrest.

Abdomen

1. Hepatosplenomegaly – due to chronic active hepatitis, hepatitis A or B, CMV, Epstein–Barr virus (EBV) and *M. tuberculosis,* generalized sepsis, tumour (fibrosarcoma of the liver) or congestive cardiac failure.
2. Oesophagitis – *Candida,* CMV or herpes simplex.
3. Chronic diarrhoea – in 40–60% of children. Infectious agents are only infrequently found but include *Candida,* CMV and *Cryptosporidium.* Radiological findings are non-specific and include a malabsorption type pattern with thickening of bowel wall and mucosal folds and dilatation. Fine ulceration may be seen.
4. Pneumatosis coli.
5. Mesenteric, para-aortic and retroperitoneal lymphadenopathy – due to *M. avium intracellulare,* lymphocytic proliferation (lymph node syndrome), Non-Hodgkin's lymphoma or Kaposi's sarcoma (rare in childhood).
6. HIV nephropathy – children may present with proteinuria, fluid and electrolyte imbalances and/or acute or chronic renal failure. Ultrasound shows enlarged echogenic kidneys and CT shows enlarged pyramids. Simple cysts may be present.
7. Urinary tract infection – in up to 50% of AIDS patients. May be due to common organisms or unusual agents e.g. CMV, *Cryptococcus, Candida, Aspergillus, Mycobacteria* and *Pneumocystis.*

Head

1. HIV encephalopathy is divided into two types:
   (a) Progressive encephalopathy comparable to adult AIDS dementia complex. There is step-wise deterioration of mental status and higher functions. It is associated with severe immune deficiency.
   (b) Static encephalopathy, associated with better higher functions but failure to reach appropriate milestones.

Imaging may show:

(a) Cerebral atrophy – worse with progressive encephalopathy.
(b) Non-enhancing white matter of ↓ attenuation (CT) or ↑ T_2W signal (MRI) in the frontal lobes, periventricular regions and centrum semiovale.

2. Intracranial calcifications – in up to 33% of HIV-infected children. Usually bilateral and symmetrical and most commonly seen in the globus pallidus and putamen; less commonly in the subcortical frontal white matter and cerebellum. Usually not seen before 10 months of age; early calcifications are more likely because of congenital infections.
3. Malignancy – most commonly high-grade B cell lymphoma associated with EBV infection.
4. Cerebrovascular accidents.
5. Infections:
    (a) Progressive multifocal leukoencephalopathy – difficult to distinguish from HIV encephalopathy, but tends to be more focal, asymmetrical and commoner in the posterior parietal lobe.
    (b) Toxoplasmosis – enhancing mass lesions with surrounding oedema in the basal ganglia and corticomedullary junction of the periventricular white matter.
    (c) Meningitis – due to fungi, Mycobacteria spp. and Nocardia, in addition to the more usual causes of meningitis.
    (d) CMV.
6. Chronic otitis media and sinusitis.

Further Reading

Haller JO. AIDS-related malignancies in pediatrics. Radiol Clin North Am 1997;35 (6):1517–38.

Haller JO, Cohen HL. Pediatric HIV infection: an imaging update. Pediatr Radiol 1994;24:224–30.

Martinoli C, Pretolesi F, Del Bono V et al. Benign lymphoepithelial parotid lesions in HIV-positive patients: spectrum of findings at gray-scale and Doppler sonography. Am J Roentgenol 1995;165(4):975–9.

Miller CR. Pediatric aspects of AIDS. Radiol Clin North Am 1997;35:1191–222.

Stoane JM, Haller JO, Orentlicher RJ. The gastrointestinal manifestations of pediatric AIDS. Radiol Clin North Am 1996;34(4):779–90.

Safriel YI, Haller JO, Lefton DR et al. Imaging of the brain in the HIV-positive child. Pediatr Radiol 2000;30:725–32.

Zinn HL, Haller JO. Renal manifestations of AIDS in children. Pediatr Radiol 1999;29:558–61.

ACROMEGALY

The effect of excessive growth hormone on the mature skeleton.

Skull

1. Thickened skull vault.
2. Enlarged paranasal sinuses and mastoids.
3. Enlarged pituitary fossa because of the eosinophilic adenoma.
4. Prognathism (increased angle of mandible).

Thorax and spine

1. Increased sagittal diameter of the chest with a kyphosis.
2. Vertebral bodies show an increase in the AP and transverse dimensions with posterior scalloping.

Appendicular skeleton

1. Increased width of bones but unaltered cortical thickness.
2. Tufting of the terminal phalanges, giving an 'arrow-head' appearance.
3. Prominent muscle attachments.
4. Widened joint spaces – especially the metacarpophalangeal joints: due to cartilage hypertrophy.
5. Premature osteoarthritis.
6. Increased heel pad thickness (>21.5mm in female; >23mm in male).
7. Generalized osteoporosis.

ALKAPTONURIA

The absence of homogentisic acid oxidase leads to the accumulation of homogentisic acid and its excretion in sweat and urine.
The majority of cases are AR.

Axial skeleton

1. Osteoporosis.
2. Intervertebral disc calcification – predominantly in the lumbar spine.
3. Disc-space narrowing with vacuum phenomenon.
4. Marginal osteophytes and end-plate sclerosis.
5. Symphysis pubis – joint-space narrowing, chondrocalcinosis, eburnation and, rarely, bone ankylosis.

Appendicular skeleton

1. Large joints show joint-space narrowing, bony sclerosis, articular collapse and fragmentation, and intra-articular loose bodies.
2. Calcification of bursae and tendons.

Extraskeletal

Ochronotic deposition in other organs may have the following results:

1. Cardiovascular system – atherosclerosis, myocardial infarction, calcification of aortic and mitral valves.
2. Genito-urinary system – renal calculi, nephrocalcinosis, prostatic enlargement with calculi.
3. Upper respiratory tract – hoarseness and dyspnoea.
4. Gastrointestinal tract – dysphagia.

ANEURYSMAL BONE CYST

1. Age – 10–30 years (75% occur before epiphyseal closure).
2. Sites – ends of long bones (70–80%), especially in the lower limbs. Also flat bones and vertebral appendages.
3. Appearances:
   (a) Arises in unfused metaphysis or in metaphysis and epiphysis after fusion.
   (b) Well-defined lucency with thin but intact cortex.
   (c) Marked expansion (ballooning).
   (d) Thin internal strands of bone/ trabeculation
   (e) ± New bone in the angle between original cortex and the expanded part.
   (f) Fluid/fluid level(s) on CT and MRI.
   (g) In the spine they involve the posterior elements.

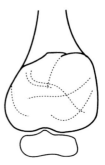

ANKYLOSING SPONDYLITIS

A seronegative spondyloarthropathy manifest as an inflammatory arthritis affecting the sacroiliac joints and entire spine, leading ultimately to fusion.

Axial skeleton

1. Involved initially in 70–80%. Initial changes in the sacroiliac joints followed by the thoracolumbar and lumbosacral regions. The entire spine may be involved eventually.
2. The radiological changes in the sacroiliac joints (see 3.12) are present at the time of the earliest spinal changes. MRI most sensitive technique for early disease and all changes except syndesmophytes.
3. Spondylitis – anterior and posterior erosion of vertebral end plates (Romanus). Enthesitis of annulus fibrosis. Then sclerosis causing 'shiny corner'.
4. Spondylodiscitis – inflammatory involvement of intervertebral disc (Andersson).
5. Syndesmophytes – bony outgrowths from vertebral margins.
6. Arthritis – facet, costovertebral and costotransverse joints (synovitis, erosion, ankylosis).

7. Enthesitis – interspinous ligaments with osteitis.
8. Ankylosis – fusion of spine from 5–7 plus bony extension through 4. Leads to 'bamboo spine'.
9. Fracture – insufficiency in ankylosed spine (esp. cervico-thoracic and thoraco-lumbar junctions).
10. Osteoporosis – with long-standing disease.
11. Kyphosis.
12. Arachnoiditis – rare and late. Arachnoid diverticulae, laminar erosions, dural calcification.

Appendicular skeleton

1. Hip – axial migration, concentric joint space narrowing, cuff-like femoral osteophytes, acetabular protrusion. Symptoms may be dominant leading to flexion contracture and ankylosis.
2. Shoulder – narrowing of glenohumeral and acromioclavicular joints. Hatchet erosion at greater tuberosity.
3. Knee – tricompartment narrowing and erosion.
4. Hand and foot – asymmetric involvement; small erosion and osseous proliferation.

Extraskeletal

1. Iritis in 20% – more frequent with a peripheral arthropathy.
2. Pulmonary disease
   (a) Restrictive defect due to costotransverse and costosternal joint involvement.
   (b) Bronchiolitis obliterans organizing pneumonia (BOOP).
3. Heart disease – aortic incompetence, conduction defects and pericarditis.
4. Amyloidosis.

Further Reading

Bennett DL, Ohashi K, El Khoury GY. Spondyloarthropathies: ankylosing spondylitis and psoriatic arthritis. Radiol Clin North Am 2004;42;121–34.
Hermann KA, Althoff CE, Schneider U et al. Spinal changes in patient with spondyloarthritis: comparison of MR imaging and radiographic appearances. Radiographics 2005;25:559–70.

ASBESTOS INHALATION

Lung and/or pleural disease caused by the inhalation of asbestos fibres (a group of fibrous silicates; different morphological forms – crocidolite, amosite, tremolite and chrysotile). Widely utilized in industry. Long latency (>20–30 years) between exposure and lung/pleural disease. Disease is more common with crocidolite (blue asbestos) than chrysotile (white asbestos). Pleural disease alone 50%; pleura and lung parenchyma 40%; lung parenchyma alone 10%.

Pleura

1. Pleural plaques – commonest manifestation of asbestos exposure developing 20–30 after exposure. Typically seen on parietal pleural on undersurface of ribs, diaphragmatic pleura and adjacent to spine; virtually pathognomonic. Sharply angulated, 'holly-leaf' opacities on chest radiography and sharply demarcated. Discrete 'punched-out' appearance at CT.
2. Benign pleural effusion – most common 'early' (<10 years) manifestation; occurs in <10%. Exudative fluid. May be unilateral or bilateral and might be followed by residual benign diffuse pleural thickening in around 50% or regions of rounded atelectasis ('folded lung').
3. Diffuse pleural thickening – less specific for asbestos exposure than plaques.
4. Rounded atelectasis – (a.k.a. folded lung, Blesovsky syndrome). Rounded mass, adjacent pleural thickening and parenchymal bands/distortion ('comet tail' appearance). Can be seen with other exudative effusions.
5. Malignant pleural mesothelioma – long latency (30–40 years). Lobulated pleural thickening involving mediastinal pleura ± large pleural effusion but minimal mediastinal shift. NB Can occur in peritoneum.

Lung parenchyma

1. Asbestosis – long latency (30–40 years). Crocidolite most fibrogenic, chrysotile least. Histological and radiological appearances almost identical to those seen in patients with cryptogenic fibrosing alveolitis/idiopathic pulmonary fibrosis.
2. Lung cancer – increased incidence even in the absence of a smoking history or asbestosis.

Other associations

1. Peritoneal mesothelioma.
2. Gastrointestinal carcinomas.
3. Laryngeal carcinoma.

Further Reading
Peacock C, Copley SJ, Hansell DM. Asbestos-related benign pleural disease. Clin
  Radiol 2000;55:422–32.

CALCIUM PYROPHOSPHATE DIHYDRATE DEPOSITION DISEASE

1. Three manifestations which occur singly or in combination:
   (a) Crystal-induced acute synovitis (pseudogout).
   (b) Cartilage calcification (chondrocalcinosis).
   (c) Structural joint abnormalities (pyrophosphate arthropathy).
2. Associated conditions are hyperparathyroidism and
   haemochromatosis (definite) and gout, Wilson's disease and
   alkaptonuria (less definite).
3. Chondrocalcinosis involves:
   (a) Fibrocartilage – especially menisci of the knee, triangular
       cartilage of the wrist, symphysis pubis and annulus fibrosus of
       the intervertebral disc.
   (b) Hyaline cartilage – especially the wrist, knee, elbow and hip.
4. Synovial membrane, joint capsule, tendon and ligament
   calcification.
5. Pyrophosphate arthropathy is most common in the knee,
   wrist, metacarpophalangeal joint and acromioclavicular joint.
   It has similar appearances to osteoarthritis but with several
   differences:
   (a) Unusual articular distribution – the wrist, elbow and shoulder
       are uncommon sites for osteoarthritis.
   (b) Unusual intra-articular distribution – the patellofemoral
       compartment of the knee and the radiocarpal compartment of
       the wrist.
   (c) Numerous, prominent subchondral cysts.
   (d) Marked subchondral collapse and fragmentation with multiple
       loose bodies simulating a neuropathic joint.
   (e) Variable osteophyte formation.

CHONDROBLASTOMA

1. Age – 5–20 years. M:F 2:1.
2. Sites – proximal humerus, distal femur and proximal tibia (50% occur in the lower limb).
3. Appearances:
   (a) Arises in the epiphysis prior to fusion and may expand to involve the metaphysis.
   (b) Well-defined lucency with a thin sclerotic rim.
   (c) Internal calcification in 60%.
   (d) Florid surrounding marrow oedema on MRI.

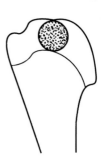

Further Reading

Robbin MR, Murphey MD. Benign chondroid neoplasms of bone. Semin Musculoskelet Radiol 2000;4(1):45–58.

CHONDROMYXOID FIBROMA

1. Age – 10–30 years.
2. Sites – proximal tibia (50%); also femur and ribs.
3. Appearances:
   (a) Metaphyseal ± extension into epiphysis, but never only in the epiphysis.
   (b) Round or oval, well-defined lucency with a sclerotic rim.
   (c) Eccentric expansion.
   (d) Internal calcification is uncommon, occasional septation.

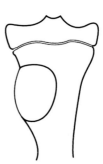

Further Reading

Robbin MR, Murphey MD. Benign chondroid neoplasms of bone. Semin Musculoskelet Radiol 2000;4(1):45–58.

CHONDROSARCOMA

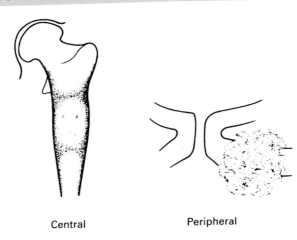

Central   Peripheral

Central

1. Age – 30–60 years. M:F 2:1.
2. Sites – femur, humerus, pelvis.
3. Appearances
   - (a) Metaphyseal or diaphyseal.
   - (b) Lucent, expansile lesion ± chondroid matrix.
   - (c) Endosteal cortical thickening or thinning.
   - (d) ± Cortical destruction and a soft-tissue mass.
   - (e) 'Pop-corn', 'ring and arc' or 'dot and comma' internal calcification.

Peripheral

1. Age – 30–60 years.
2. Sites – pelvic and shoulder girdle, upper femur and humerus.
3. Appearances:
   - (a) Soft-tissue mass, often arising from the cartilage tip of an osteochondroma. A cartilage cap >2cm in thickness, as measured by ultrasound, CT or MRI, is considered suspicious of malignant change.
   - (b) Multiple calcific densities.
   - (c) Ill-defined margins.
   - (d) In the later stages, destruction of underlying bone.

Further Reading
Flemming DJ, Murphey MD. Enchondroma and chondrosarcoma. Semin Musculoskelet Radiol 2000;4(1):59–71.

CLEIDOCRANIAL DYSPLASIA

AD. One-third are new mutations.

Skull

1. Brachycephaly. Wormian bones. Frontal and parietal bossing.
2. Wide sutures and fontanelles with delayed closure.
3. Broad mandible. Small facial bones. Delayed eruption and supernumerary teeth.
4. Basilar invagination.

Thorax

1. Aplasia or hypoplasia of the clavicles, usually the lateral portion but occasionally the middle portion.
2. Small, high scapulae.
3. Neonatal respiratory distress because of thoracic cage deformity.

Pelvis

1. Absent or delayed ossification of the pubic bones, producing apparent widening of the symphysis pubis.

Appendicular skeleton

1. Short or absent fibulae.
2. Coxa vara or coxa valga.
3. Congenital pseudarthrosis of the femur.
4. Hand
   (a) Long second and fifth metacarpals; short second and fifth middle phalanges.
   (b) Cone-shaped epiphyses.
   (c) Tapered distal phalanges.
   (d) Supernumerary ossification centres.

COAL MINER'S PNEUMOCONIOSIS

The effect of the inhalation of coal dust in coal workers.

Simple

1. Small round opacities, 1–5mm in size. Widespread throughout the lungs but sparing the extreme bases and apices.
2. Less well defined than silicosis.
3. Generally less dense than silicosis, but calcification occurs in at least a few of the nodules in 10% of older coal workers.
4. 'Egg-shell' calcification of lymph nodes in 1%.

Complicated, i.e. progressive massive fibrosis

See Silicosis.

Complications

See Silicosis.

CROHN'S DISEASE

Colon and small bowel are affected equally. Gastric involvement is uncommon and is usually affected in continuity with disease in the duodenum. Oesophageal involvement is rare.

Small bowel

1. Terminal ileum is the commonest site.
2. Asymmetrical involvement and skip lesions are characteristic. The disease predominates on the mesenteric border.
3. Aphthoid ulcers – the earliest sign in the terminal ileum and colon. May be invisible on CT and MRI.
4. Fissure ulcers – typically they are distributed in a longitudinal and transverse fashion. They may progress to abscess formation, sinuses and fistulae.
5. Blunting, thickening or distortion of the valvulae conniventes – the earliest sign in the small bowel proximal to the terminal ileum. Caused by hyperplasia of lymphoid tissue, producing an obstructive lymphoedema of the bowel wall. May give a granular appearance on barium studies.
6. 'Cobblestone' pattern – two possible causes
   (a) A combination of longitudinal and transverse fissure ulcers bounding intact mucosa.
   (b) The bulging of oedematous mucosal folds that are not closely attached to the underlying muscularis.
7. Separation of bowel loops – due to thickened bowel wall and/or fat hypertrophy

8. Strictures – may be short or long, single or multiple. Acute clinical obstruction is less commonly observed than subacute.
9. Pseudosacculation.

Colon

1. Asymmetrical involvement and skip lesions. The rectum is involved in 30–50%.
2. Aphthoid ulcers.
3. Deeper fissure ulcers which may produce a 'cobblestone' pattern.
4. Strictures.
5. Pseudosacculation.
6. Inflammatory pseudopolyps – more common in ulcerative colitis.
7. The ileocaecal valve may be thickened, narrowed and ulcerated.

Complications

1. Fistulae.
2. Perforation – usually localized and results in abscess formation.
3. Toxic megacolon – more common in ulcerative colitis.
4. Carcinoma
   (a) Colon – less common than in ulcerative colitis, but this may be because more patients with Crohn's disease undergo colectomy at an early stage.
   (b) Small bowel – 300× increased incidence.
5. Lymphoma.
6. Associated conditions
   (a) Erythema nodosum.
   (b) Arthritis
       (i) Spondyloarthritis mimicking ankylosing spondylitis. It follows a course independent of the bowel disease and precedes it in 25% of cases.
       (ii) Enteropathic synovitis, the activity of which parallels the bowel disease. The weight-bearing joints of the lower limbs, wrist and fingers are affected.
   (c) Cirrhosis.
   (d) Chronic active hepatitis.
   (e) Gallstones.
   (f) Oxalate urinary tract calculi.
   (g) Pericholangitis.
   (h) Cholangiocarcinoma.
   (i) Sclerosing cholangitis.

Further Reading

Ali S, Carty HM. Paediatric Crohn's disease: a radiological overview. Eur Radiol 2000;10:1085–94.
Wills JS, Lobis IF, Denstman FJ. Crohn disease. State of the art. Radiology 1997;202:597–610.

CUSHING'S SYNDROME

Cushing's syndrome results from increased endogenous or exogenous cortisol.

Spontaneous Cushing's syndrome is rare and due to:

1. Pituitary disease (Cushing's disease)   80%
   (90% of these are due to adenoma and 20% have radiological evidence of an intrasellar tumour)
2. Adrenal disease   – adenoma
                           – carcinoma } 20%
3. Ectopic ACTH, e.g. from a carcinoma of the bronchus.

Iatrogenic Cushing's syndrome is common and due to high doses of corticosteroids. The effects of excessive amounts of corticosteroids are:

1. Growth retardation in children.
2. Osteoporosis.
3. Pathological fractures which show excessive callus formation during healing; vertebral end-plate fractures, in particular, show prominent bone condensation.
4. Avascular necrosis of bone.
5. Increased incidence of infection – including osteomyelitis and septic arthritis (the knee is affected most frequently).
6. Hypertension.
7. Water retention resulting in oedema.

CYSTIC FIBROSIS

AR condition, with carrier rate of 1:25 in Caucasian population, affecting 1:2000 live births. Basic defect is of highly viscid secretions. Main complications are pulmonary. Life expectancy is improving with median survival now 35–40 years.

Thoracic findings

1. Peribronchial thickening.
2. Bronchial dilatation.
3. Mucus plugging. In central bronchi this may appear as nodules or filling in of airways. In peripheral bronchi this appears as centri-lobular nodules, often with the 'tree-in-bud' pattern.
4. Air-trapping. May result in generalized over-inflation of the lungs with diaphragmatic flattening. Mosaic attenuation on inspiratory CT which is accentuated on expiratory sections.

5. Cystic changes. Unusual in early disease. Not true cysts, but represent either areas of localized emphysema or cystic bronchiectasis.
6. Pulmonary hypertension.
7. Hilar enlargement: may be due to lymphadenopathy, which is common, or pulmonary arterial dilatation.

Gastrointestinal findings

1. Meconium ileus: in 10%. Distal intestinal obstruction (meconium ileus equivalent) may occur in later life.
2. Rectal prolapse.

Hepatobiliary/pancreatic

1. Pancreatic changes and exocrine insufficiency. Pancreas may demonstrate various abnormalities
   (a) Fatty replacement: may appear enlarged with lobulations and septations, or atrophic with partial fatty replacement.
   (b) Features of chronic pancreatitis (calcifications, atrophy, cyst formation).
   (c) Pancreatic fibrosis: low signal on T_1 and T_2W.
2. Liver disease
   (a) Hepatomegaly.
   (b) Fatty liver, periportal echogenicity, cirrhosis and portal hypertension.
   (c) Gallstones, biliary obstruction.

Skeletal

1. Retarded skeletal maturation.
2. Clubbing and hypertrophic osteoarthrophty.

Head and neck

1. Chronic sinusitis.
2. Nasal polyps.
3. Mucocoeles.

Further Reading

Aziz ZA, Davies JC, Alton EW et al. Computed tomography and cystic fibrosis: promises and problems. Thorax 2007;62(2):181–6.

King LJ, Scurr ED, Murugan N et al. Hepatobiliary and pancreatic manifestations of cystic fibrosis: MR imaging appearances. Radiographics 2000;20 (3):767–77.

Ruzal-Shapiro C. Cystic fibrosis. An overview. Radiol Clin North Am 1998;36(1):143–61.

DOWN'S SYNDROME (TRISOMY 21)

Craniofacial

1. Brachycephaly and microcephaly.
2. Hypoplasia of facial bones and sinuses.
3. Wide sutures and delayed closure. Multiple wormian bones.
4. Hypotelorism.
5. Dental abnormalities.

Central nervous system

1. Bilateral basal ganglia calcification ($>11\%$).
2. Spinal cord compression (due to atlanto-axial subluxation).

Axial skeleton

1. Increased height and decreased AP diameter of lumbar vertebrae.
2. Atlantoaxial subluxation (10–20%).
3. Atlanto-occipital subluxation.
4. Hypoplasia of the posterior arch of C1.
5. Incomplete fusion of vertebral arches of the lumbar spine.

Pelvis

1. Flared iliac wings with small acetabular angles resulting in an abnormal iliac index (iliac angle + acetabular angle).

Chest

1. Congenital heart disease (40%) – endocardial cushion defects, ventricular septal defects, aberrant right subclavian artery.
2. Eleven pairs of ribs.
3. Two ossification centres for the manubrium (90%).
4. Congenital chylous pleural effusion.
5. Subpleural pulmonary cysts.

Hands

1. Short tubular bones, clinodactyly (50%) and hypoplasia of the middle phalanx of the little finger (60%).

Gastrointestinal

1. Duodenal atresia/stenosis/annular pancreas.
2. Hirschsprung disease.
3. Anorectal malformation.

Further Reading

James AE Jr, Merz T, Janower ML et al. Radiological features of the most common autosomal disorders: trisomy 21-22 (mongolism or Down's syndrome), trisomy 18, trisomy 13-15, and the cri-du-chat syndrome. Clin Radiol 1971;22(4):417–33.

Stein SM, Kirchner SG, Horev G et al. Atlanto-occipital subluxation in Down syndrome. Pediatr Radiol 1991;21:121–4.

ENCHONDROMA

1. Age – 10–50 years.
2. Sites – hands and wrists predominate (50%). Any other bones formed in cartilage.
3. Appearances
   (a) Diaphyseal or diametaphyseal.
   (b) Well-defined lucency with a thin sclerotic rim.
   (c) Expansion of the cortex without cortical breach, scalloping of inner cortex.
   (d) Internal ground-glass appearance ± calcification/ chondroid matrix.
   (e) Pathological fracture – a frequent presenting complaint of enchondromas of the hands or feet.

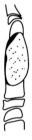

Syndromes

Ollier's disease – multiple enchondromas.
Maffucci's syndrome – enchondromas + soft-tissue haemangiomas

Further Reading

Flemming DJ, Murphey MD. Enchondroma and chondrosarcoma. Semin Musculoskelet Radiol 2000;4(1):59–71.

EOSINOPHILIC GRANULOMA

See Langerhans cell histiocytosis.

EWING'S SARCOMA

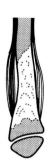

1. Age – 5–15 years.
2. Sites – femur, pelvis, shoulder girdle and ribs.
3. Appearances
   (a) Diaphyseal or, less commonly, metaphyseal.
   (b) Ill-defined medullary destruction.
   (c) ± Small areas of new bone formation.
   (d) Periosteal reaction – lamellated (onion skin), Codman's angle or 'sunray' speculation.
   (e) Saucerization of the cortex due to periosteal destruction.
   (f) Soft-tissue extension (best appreciated on MRI).
   (g) Metastases to other bones and lungs.

Further Reading
Hoffer FA. Primary skeletal neoplasms: osteosarcoma and Ewing sarcoma. Top Magn Reson Imaging 2002;13(4):231–9.

EXTRINSIC ALLERGIC ALVEOLITIS (EAA; HYPERSENSITIVITY PNEUMONITIS)

Immunological lung disease secondary to repeated exposure, of susceptible individuals, to a large variety of particulate organic antigens which might be animal/plant proteins, certain chemicals and various micro-organisms (including thermophilic actinomycetes, bacteria and fungi). Hence, many synonyms (e.g. farmer's lung, mushroom worker's lung, cheese washer's lung and Japanese summer type hypersensitivity pneumonitis). Pathogenesis of EAA thought to be related to deposition of particulate material in alveoli leading to Type III and IV immunological reactions. Histologically, there is a predominant lymphocytic infiltrate initially centred on small airways and adjacent interstitium accompanied by histiocytes and plasma cells. In subacute phase, loosely-formed, bronchiolocentric, non-caseating granulomata are formed which disappear in chronic disease where there is fibrosis. Cigarette smoking thought to confer some protection against EAA.

Acute EAA

1. Symptoms (dyspnoea, dry cough, fever, malaise and myalgia) frequently mimic a viral-type illness, and develop 4–8 hours after exposure. Thus, imaging tests rarely performed but if undertaken chest radiograph is either normal or demonstrates subtle findings (small nodules, ground-glass opacification).

Subacute EAA

1. Characterized clinically by acute episodes but with progressive decline in lung function.
2. On chest radiography profusion of fine nodules and ground-glass opacification bilaterally with sparing of lung bases.
3. At HRCT there is variably extensive ground-glass opacification (due to lymphocytic pneumonitis), centrilobular nodules (reflecting a cellular bronchiolitis) and lobular foci of decreased attenuation (with air trapping on expiratory CT; reflecting the bronchiolocentric nature). A few scattered thin-walled cysts are seen in some patients.

Chronic exposure

1. Usually due to persistent low-level exposure to organic antigen.
2. Reticular/reticulonodular pattern on chest radiography with a predilection for the upper zones. Lung volumes may be relatively preserved (possibly due to associated small airways [obstructive] disease).
3. At HRCT: reticular pattern, lobular areas of decreased attenuation, ground-glass opacification and tractional dilatation of bronchi and bronchioles; relative sparing of lower zones. Appearances may mimic those seen in cryptogenic fibrosing alveolitis. Emphysema in farmer's lung – even in lifelong non-smokers.

Further Reading
Silva CIS et al. Hypersensitivity pneumonitis: spectrum of high-resolution CT and pathologic findings. Am J Roentgenol 2007;188:334–44.

FIBROUS DYSPLASIA

Unknown pathogenesis. Medullary bone is replaced by fibrous tissue.

1. Diagnosis usually made between 3 and 15 years.
2. May be monostotic or polyostotic. In polyostotic cases the lesions tend to be unilateral; if bilateral then asymmetrical.
3. Most frequent sites are femur, pelvis, skull, mandible, ribs (most common cause of a focal expansile rib lesion) and humerus. Other bones are less frequently affected.
4. Radiological changes include:
   (a) A cyst-like lesion in the diaphysis or metaphysis with endosteal scalloping ± bone expansion. No periosteal new bone. The epiphysis is only involved after fusion. Thick sclerotic border: 'rind' sign. Internally the lesion shows a ground-glass appearance ± irregular calcifications together with irregular sclerotic areas.
   (b) Bone deformity, e.g. shepherd's crook deformity of the proximal femur.
   (c) Growth disparity.
   (d) Accelerated bone maturation.
   (e) Skull shows mixed lucencies and sclerosis, mainly on the convexity of the calvarium and the floor of the anterior fossa.
   (f) Leontiasis ossea is a sclerosing form affecting the face ± the skull base and producing leonine facies. In such cases extracranial lesions are rare. Involvement may be asymmetrical.
5. Associated endocrine abnormalities include:
   (a) Sexual precocity (+ skin pigmentation) – in 30% of females with the polyostotic form. This constitutes the McCune–Albright syndrome.
   (b) Acromegaly, Cushing's syndrome, gynaecomastia and parathyroid hyperplasia (all rare).

GIANT CELL TUMOUR

1. Age – 20–40 years (only 3% occur before epiphyseal closure).
2. Sites – long bones (75–90%), distal femur especially; occasionally the sacrum or pelvis. Spine rarely.
3. Appearances

    (a) Epiphyseal and metaphyseal, i.e. subarticular.

    (b) A lucency with an ill-defined endosteal margin.

    (c) Eccentric expansion ± cortical destruction and soft-tissue extension.

    (d) Cortical ridges or internal septa produce a multilocular appearance.

    (e) Fluid levels on CT or MRI.

    (f) 30% local recurrence rate and, rarely, pulmonary metastases.

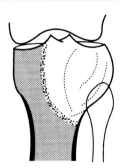

Further Reading
Lee MJ, Sallomi DF, Munk PL et al. Pictorial review: giant cell tumours of bone. Clin Radiol 1998;53: 481–9.

Murphey MD, Nomikos GC, Flemming DJ et al. Imaging of giant cell tumour and giant cell reparative granuloma of bone: radiologic-pathologic correlation. Radiographics 2001;21:1283–309.

GOUT

Caused by monosodium urate monohydrate or uric acid crystal deposition. Idiopathic (in the majority of patients) or associated with many other disorders, e.g. myeloproliferative diseases, drugs and chronic renal disease. Idiopathic gout may be divided into three stages.

Asymptomatic hyperuricaemia

1. No radiological signs but renal calculi or arthritis will develop in 20%.

Acute gouty arthritis

1. Monoarticular or oligoarticular; occasionally polyarticular.
2. Predilection for joints of the lower extremities, especially the first metatarsophalangeal joint (70%), intertarsal joints, ankles and knees. Other joints are affected in long-standing disease.
3. Soft-tissue swelling and joint effusion during the acute attack, with disappearance of the abnormalities as the attack subsides.

Chronic tophaceous gout

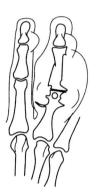

1. In 50% of patients with recurrent acute gout.
2. Eccentric, asymmetrical nodular deposits of calcium urate (tophi) in the synovium, subchondral bone, helix of the ear and in the soft tissues of the elbow, hand, foot, knee and forearm. Calcification of tophi is uncommon; ossification is rare.
3. Joint space is preserved until late in the disease.
4. Little or no osteoporosis until late, when there may be disuse osteoporosis.
5. Bony erosions are produced by tophaceous deposits and may be intra-articular, periarticular or well away from the joint. The latter two may be associated with an obvious soft-tissue mass. Erosions are round or oval, with the long axis in line with the bone. They may have a sclerotic margin. Some erosions have an overhanging lip of bone, which is strongly suggestive of the condition.
6. Severe erosive changes result in an arthritis mutilans.

Complications

1. Urolithiasis – in 10% of gout patients (higher in hot climates).
2. Renal disease
   (a) Acute urate nephropathy – precipitation of uric acid in the collecting ducts. Usually follows treatment with cytotoxic drugs.
   (b) Chronic urate nephropathy – rare.

HAEMANGIOMA OF BONE

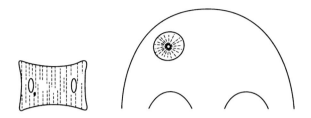

1. Age – 10–50 years.
2. Sites – vertebra (dorsal lumbar) or skull vault.
3. Appearances
    (a) Vertebra – coarse vertical striations, usually affecting only the body but the appendages are, uncommonly, also involved.
    (b) Skull – radial spiculation ('sunburst') within a well-defined vault lucency. 'Hair-on-end' appearance in tangential views.
    (c) High signal on T_1W and T_2W MRI because of high fat content.

HAEMOCHROMATOSIS

A genetically determined primary abnormality of iron metabolism secondary to disorder of Hepcidin, a polypeptide hormone produced in the liver. Linked to haemochromatosis gene (*HFE*; chromosome 6p21.3) and DNA-based blood test aids diagnosis.

May be secondary to alcohol, cirrhosis or multiple blood transfusions, e.g. in thalassaemia or chronic excessive oral iron ingestion.

Clinically – cirrhosis, skin pigmentation, diabetes (bronze diabetics; secondary to insulin resistance and cirrhosis), arthropathy and, later, ascites and cardiac failure.

Useful role for liver biopsy is the assessment of patients without typical haemochromatosis-associated HFE genotypes who have serum ferritin concentrations higher than 1000µg/L, because many such patients have an inflammatory disease, not iron overload.

Bones and joints

1. Osteoporosis.
2. Chondrocalcinosis – due to calcium pyrophosphate dihydrate deposition (q.v.).
3. Arthropathy – resembles the arthropathy of calcium pyrophosphate deposition disease (q.v.), but shows a predilection for the metacarpophalangeal joints (especially the second and third), the midcarpal joints and the carpometacarpal joints. It also exhibits distinctive beak-like osteophytes and is less rapidly progressive.

Liver and spleen

1. Liver fibrosis and cirrhosis. Increased risk of hepatoma.
2. Mottled increased density of liver and spleen (CT) and reduced signal intensity (MRI) due to the deposition of iron.

Others

1. Hypogonadism.
2. Cardiomyopathy.

Further Reading
Adams PC, Barton JC. Haemochromatosis. Lancet 2007;370:1855–60.

HAEMOPHILIA

Classical (Factor VIII deficiency) or Christmas disease (Factor IX deficiency). Both are X-linked recessive traits, i.e. manifest in males and carried by females.

Joints

1. Knee, elbow, ankle, hip and shoulder are most frequently affected.
2. Soft-tissue swelling due to haemarthrosis which may appear to be unusually dense owing to the presence of haemosiderin in the chronically thickened synovium.
3. Periarticular osteoporosis.
4. Erosion of articular surfaces, with subchondral cysts.
5. Preservation of joint space until late.
6. Accelerated maturation and growth of epiphyses resulting in disparity of size between epiphysis and diaphysis.
7. Contractures.

Bones

1. Osteonecrosis – especially in the femoral head and talus.
2. Haemophilic pseudotumour – in the ilium, femur and tibia most frequently.
   (a) Intraosseous – a well-defined medullary lucency with a sclerotic margin. It may breach the cortex. ± Periosteal reaction and soft-tissue component.
   (b) Subperiosteal – periosteal reaction with pressure resorption of the cortex and a soft-tissue mass.
3. Fractures – secondary to osteoporosis.

Soft tissues

1. Pseudotumour – slow-growing.
2. Ectopic ossification.

Further Reading
Stoker DJ, Murray RO. Skeletal changes in haemophilia and other bleeding disorders. Semin Roentgenol 1974;9:185–93.

HOMOCYSTINURIA

AR, inborn error of metabolism. A lack of cystathionine synthetase results in the accumulation of homocystine and methionine, with a deficiency of cystathionine and cystine.

1. Mental defect (60%).
2. Tall stature, slim build and arachnodactyly, with a morphological resemblance to Marfan's syndrome.
3. Pectus excavatum or carinatum, kyphoscoliosis, genu valgum and pes cavus.
4. Osteoporosis.
5. Medial degeneration of the aorta and elastic arteries.
6. Arterial and venous thromboses.
7. Lens subluxation – usually downward.

HURLER'S SYNDROME

A mucopolysaccharidosis transmitted as an AR trait. Clinical features become evident at the end of the first year: dwarfism, mental retardation, coarse facial features, corneal opacification, deformed teeth and hepatosplenomegaly. Respiratory infections and cardiac failure usually lead to death in the first decade.

Craniofacial

1. Scaphocephalic macrocephaly.
2. J-shaped sella (prominent sulcus chiasmatus).

Central nervous system

1. Hydrocephalus due to cystic arachnoiditis in the hypothalamic region.
2. Symmetrical low attenuation of white matter on CT (high signal on T_2W, MRI).

Axial skeleton

1. Oval vertebral bodies with an antero-inferior beak.
2. Kyphosis and a thoracolumbar gibbus.
3. Posterior scalloping with widened interpedicular distance.
4. Short neck.

Appendicular skeleton

1. Thickened diaphyses.
2. Angulated, oblique growth plates, e.g. those of the distal radius and ulna are angled toward each other.
3. Coxa valga (common). Genu valgum (always).
4. Trident hands with a coarse trabecular pattern. Proximal tapering of metacarpals.

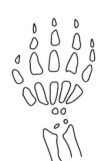

Cardiovascular system

1. Cardiac failure due to intimal thickening of coronary arteries or valves.

NB Hunter's syndrome is very similar clinically and radiologically, but the differences are:

(a) X-linked recessive transmission (i.e. no affected females).
(b) Later onset (2–6 years) and slower progression (death in the second or third decade).
(c) No corneal clouding.

HYPERPARATHYROIDISM, PRIMARY

Causes

1. Adenoma of one gland (90%) (2% of adenomas are multiple).
2. Hyperplasia of all four glands (5%) (more likely if there is a family history).
3. Carcinoma of one gland.
4. Ectopic parathormone – e.g. from a carcinoma of the bronchus.
5. Multiple endocrine adenopathy syndrome (type 1) – hyperplasia or adenoma associated with pituitary adenoma and pancreatic tumour.

Bones

1. Osteopenia – uncommon. When advanced there is loss of the fine trabeculae and sometimes a ground-glass appearance.
2. Subperiosteal bone resorption – particularly affecting the radial side of the middle phalanx of the middle finger, medial proximal tibia, lateral and occasionally medial end of clavicle, symphysis pubis, ischial tuberosity, medial femoral neck, dorsum sellae, superior surface of ribs and proximal humerus. Severe disease produces terminal phalangeal resorption and, in children, the 'rotting fence-post' appearance of the proximal femur.
3. Diffuse cortical change – cortical tunnelling eventually leading to a 'basketwork' appearance. 'Pepper-pot skull'.
4. Brown tumours – the solitary sign in 3% of cases. Most frequent in the mandible, ribs, pelvis and femora.
5. Bone softening – basilar invagination, wedged or codfish vertebrae, kyphoscoliosis, triradiate pelvis. Pathological fractures.

Soft tissues

1. Calcification in soft tissues, pancreas, lung and arteries.

Joints

1. Marginal erosions – predominantly the distal interphalangeal joints, the ulnar side of the base of the little-finger metacarpal and the hamate. No joint-space narrowing.
2. Weakened subarticular bone, leading to collapse.
3. Chondrocalcinosis (calcium pyrophosphate dihydrate deposition disease) and true gout.
4. Periarticular calcification, including capsular and tendon calcification.

Kidney

1. Nephrocalcinosis.
2. Calculi (in 50%).

Hypercalcaemia

1. Asymptomatic (in 15%) or overt (in 8%).

Gastrointestinal tract

1. Peptic ulcer.
2. Pancreatitis.

Further Reading

Hayes CW, Conway WF. Hyperparathyroidism. Radiol Clin North Am 1991;29(1):85–96.

HYPOPARATHYROIDISM

1. Short stature, dry skin, alopecia, tetany $\pm$ mental retardation.
2. Skeletal changes affecting the entire skeleton.
3. Minimal, generalized increased density of the skeleton, but especially affecting the metaphyses.
4. Calcification of paraspinal ligaments (secondary to elevation of plasma phosphate, which combines with calcium, resulting in heterotopic calcium phosphate deposits).
5. Basal ganglia calcification – uncommon.

HYPOPHOSPHATASIA

AR. Deficiency of serum and tissue alkaline phosphatase, with excessive urinary excretion of phosphoethanolamine. 50% die in early infancy.

Neonatal form

1. Most severely affected. Stillborn or die within 6 months.
2. Clinically – hypotonia, irritability, vomiting respiratory insufficiency, failure to thrive, convulsions and small stature with bowed legs.
3. Radiologically
   (a) Profoundly deficient mineralization with increased liability to fractures.
   (b) Irregular lack of metaphyseal mineralization affecting especially the wrists, knees and costochondral junctions.

Infantile form

1. Initially asymptomatic, but between 2 weeks and 6 months shows the same symptoms as the neonatal form. Most survive.

2. Radiologically
   (a) Cupped and frayed metaphyses with widened growth plates.
   (b) Demineralized epiphyses.
   (c) Defective mineralization of skull, including sutures which appear widened.
   (d) Premature sutural fusion; → craniostenosis with brachycephaly.

Childhood form

1. Presents 6 months to 2 years with bowed legs, genu valgum, delayed walking, bone pain, dental caries and premature loss of teeth.
2. Radiologically
   (a) Mild rickets.
   (b) No craniostenosis.

Adult form

1. Osteomalacia – both clinically and radiologically.

HYPOTHYROIDISM, CONGENITAL

Appendicular skeleton

1. Delayed appearance of ossification centres which may be
   (a) Slightly granular.
   (b) Finely stippled.
   (c) Coarsely stippled.
   (d) Fragmented.
   The femoral capital epiphyses may be divided into inner and outer halves.
2. Delayed epiphyseal closure.
3. Short long bones with slender shafts, endosteal thickening and dense metaphyseal bands.
4. Coxa vara with shortened femoral neck and elevated greater trochanter.

Skull

1. Brachycephaly.
2. Multiple wormian bones.
3. Delayed development of vascular markings and diploic differentiation.
4. Delayed sutural closure.
5. Poorly developed sinuses and mastoids.

Axial skeleton

1. Kyphosis at the thoracolumbar junction, usually associated with a hypoplastic or 'bullet-shaped' body of LV1 or LV2.

   The bone changes may have completely regressed in adults.

JUVENILE IDIOPATHIC ARTHRITIS

A heterogeneous group of conditions which begin in childhood (age <16 years) and involve persistent inflammation of one or more joints (for at least 6 weeks).

Oligoarticular or monoarticular onset (45%)

1. Most commonly presents at 1–5 years.
2. Four or fewer joints involved at the onset – knees, ankles and hips most commonly.
3. ± Iridocyclitis.

Polyarticular onset (23%)

1. Rh F negative – 21% of total. Rh F positive – 2% of total. F>M; onset >11 years.
2. Arthritis predominates with a similar distribution to the systemic onset, but also including the small joints of the fingers and toes. The cervical spine is involved frequently and early.
3. Prolonged disease leads to growth retardation and abnormal epiphyseal development.

Systemic onset

1. Most common at 1–5 years. M = F.
2. Severe extra-articular clinical manifestations include pyrexia, rash, lymphadenopathy and hepatosplenomegaly.
3. Joint involvement is late, but eventually a polyarthritis affects especially the knees, wrists, carpi, ankles and tarsi.

Psoriatic arthritis (13%)

1. M>F.

Enthesitis-related arthritis (10%)

1. Distal > proximal joints; lumbar spine, sacroiliac joints.
2. HLA B27 positive.
3. M>F. >8 years.

Radiological changes

1. Joint effusion – early finding.
2. Periarticular soft-tissue swelling – early finding.
3. Osteopenia – juxta-articular, diffuse or band-like in the metaphyses, the latter particularly in the distal femur, proximal tibia, distal radius and distal tibia.

4. Periostitis – common. Mainly periarticular in the phalanges, metacarpals and metatarsals, but when diaphyseal will eventually result in enlarged rectangular tubular bones.

5. Growth disturbances – epiphyseal overgrowth; premature fusion of growth plates; short broad phalanges, metacarpals and metatarsals; hypoplasia of the temporomandibular joint; micrognathia; leg length discrepancy.

6. Subluxation and dislocation – common in the wrist and hip. Atlantoaxial subluxation is most frequent in seropositive juvenile onset rheumatoid arthritis. Protrusio acetabuli of the hip.

7. Bony erosions – late manifestation; predominantly knees, hands and feet.

8. Joint-space narrowing – late manifestations due to cartilage loss.

9. Bony ankylosis – late finding; especially carpus, tarsus and cervical spine.

10. Epiphyseal compression fractures.

11. Lymphoedema.

Further Reading

Cohen PA, Job-Deslandre CH, Lalande G. Overview of the radiology of juvenile idiopathic arthritis (JIA). Eur J Radiol 2000;33:94–101.

Johnson K, Gardner-Medwin J. Childhood arthritis: classification and radiology. Clin Radiol 2002;57:47–58.

Johnson K (2007). Imaging of juvenile idiopathic arthritis. Paediatr Radiol 2007;36:743–58.

LANGERHANS CELL HISTIOCYTOSIS (LCH)

A disease of unknown aetiology characterized by intense proliferation of reticulohistiocytic elements. Younger patients have more disseminated disease. There are three clinical subgroups, with indistinguishable histology but marked differences in presentation, morbidity and mortality.

Eosinophilic granuloma

1. Accounts for 60–80% of LCH.

2. Benign disease limited to bone or lung.

3. Commonest in 4–7-year olds, who present with bone pain, local swelling and irritability.

3. 50–75% have solitary lesions. When multiple, usually only two or three. Long bones, pelvis, skull and flat bones are the most common sites involved. 20% of solitary lesions become multiple.

4. Radiological changes in the skeleton include

   (a) Well-defined lucency in the medulla ± thin sclerotic rim.
± Endosteal scalloping. True expansion is uncommon except in ribs and vertebral bodies. ± Overlying periosteal reaction.

   (b) Multilocular lucency, without expansion, in the pelvis.

   (c) Punched-out lucencies in the skull vault with little or no surrounding sclerosis. May coalesce to give a 'geographical skull'.

   (d) Destructive lesions in the skull base, mastoids, sella or mandible ('floating teeth').

   (e) Vertebra plana, with intact intervertebral discs.

5. Lung involvement in children, part of multisystem disease
   (a) Multiple nodules which cavitate.
   (b) May be complicated by pneumothorax and pleural effusion.
   (c) Not associated with a worse prognosis – in children <10 years may regress spontaneously.

6. Lung involvement in adults associated with a worse prognosis
   (a) Hilar lymphadenopathy.
   (b) Miliary shadowing.
   (c) 'Honeycomb lung'.

Hand–Schüller–Christian disease

1. Generally occurs <10 years but may appear in 20s–30s. Commonest in 1–3-year olds.
2. Osseous lesions together with mild to moderate visceral involvement which includes lymphadenopathy, hepatosplenomegaly, skin lesions, diabetes insipidus, exophthalmos and pulmonary disease, including pulmonary fibrosis.
3. Bone lesions are similar to eosinophilic granuloma, but more numerous, more destructive and widely distributed, with a predilection for the skull base.

Letterer–Siwe disease

1. Rarest and most aggressive form. Usually <2 years of age.
2. Major visceral involvement with less prominent bone involvement.
3. Widespread haemorrhagic rash, associated with neutropenia and thrombocytopenia.
4. Bone lesions are poorly defined.

Further Reading
Hoover KB, Rosenthal DI, Mankin H. Langerhans cell histiocytosis. Skeletal Radiol 2007;36(2):95–104.

LYMPHOMA

Intrathoracic lymphadenopathy

1. 66% of patients with Hodgkin's disease have intrathoracic disease and 99% of these have intrathoracic lymphadenopathy.
2. 40% of patients with non-Hodgkin's lymphoma have intrathoracic disease and 90% of these have intrathoracic lymphadenopathy.
3. Nodes involved are (in order of frequency) anterior mediastinal, paratracheal, tracheobronchial, bronchopulmonary and subcarinal. Involvement tends to be bilateral and asymmetrical, although unilateral disease is not uncommon.
4. Nodes show a rapid response to radiotherapy, and 'egg-shell' calcification of lymph nodes may be observed following radiotherapy.

Pulmonary disease

1. More common in Hodgkin's disease than non-Hodgkin's lymphoma.
2. Very unusual without lymphadenopathy, but may be the first evidence of recurrence after radiotherapy.
3. Most frequently one or more large opacities with an irregular outline. ± Air bronchogram.
4. Collapse due to endobronchial lymphoma or, less frequently, extrinsic compression (collapse is less common than in bronchial carcinoma).
5. Lymphatic obstruction → oedema or lymphangitis carcinomatosa.
6. Miliary or larger opacities widely disseminated throughout the lungs.
7. Cavitation – eccentrically within a mass and with a thick wall (more common than in bronchial carcinoma).
8. Calcification following radiotherapy.
9. Soft-tissue mass adjacent to a rib deposit.
10. Pleural and pericardial effusions.

Gastrointestinal tract

Involvement may be the primary presentation (5% of all lymphomas) or be a part of generalized disease (50% at autopsy). In descending order of frequency, solid organs, stomach, small intestine, rectum and colon may be involved.

Solid organs

1. In general may be focal, multifocal or diffuse.
2. Liver and spleen
    (a) Hypoattenuating nodules (HU > water); may resemble cysts on USS.
    (b) Diffuse involvement may result in organ enlargement only with no focal lesion.
    (b) May be more prominent on MRI (low on T_1, moderately high on T_2).
    (c) Difficult to differentiate from fungal infection (fungal microabscesses tend to be smaller with more heterogeneous enhancement).
    (c) Usually secondary; primary hepatic/splenic lymphoma very rare.
3. Pancreas
    (a) Involved in 30% of non-Hodgkin's lymphoma.
    (b) Diffuse involvement may mimic pancreatitis (organ enlargement, peripancreatic fat infiltration, reduced contrast enhancement).
    (c) Focal involvement may mimic adenocarcinoma but duct dilatation, gland atrophy and vascular invasion is rare with lymphoma).
4. Renal
    (a) Mainly late stage disease, more frequently with non-Hodgkin's.
    (b) Diffuse involvement results in organ enlargement and areas of reduced enhancement.
    (c) Most frequent pattern is multiple masses (1–3cm).

Gastrointestinal lumen

1. In general may cause mild to moderate wall thickening, luminal constriction of dilatation and/or cavitation. Usually homogeneous and hypoattenuating after contrast.
2. Bulky lymph nodes typically present.
3. Infiltration may cause tube-like aperistatic segment and/or aneurysmal dilatation of bowel

Stomach

1. Primary lymphoma accounts for 2.5% of all gastric neoplasms, and 2.5% of lymphomas present with a stomach lesion. Non-Hodgkin's lymphoma accounts for 80% (most common is mucosa-associated lymphoid tissue [MALT], related to *H. pylori*).

2. The radiological manifestations comprise
   - **(a)** Diffuse mucosal and fold thickening and irregularity ±
     decreased distensibility and peristaltic activity. ± Multiple
     ulcers.
   - **(b)** Smooth nodular mass ± central ulceration. Surrounding
     mucosa may be normal or show thickened folds.
   - **(c)** Single or multiple ulcers with irregular margins.
   - **(d)** Thickening of the wall with narrowing of the lumen. If the distal
     stomach is involved there may be extension into the
     duodenum.
   - **(e)** Duodenal ulcer associated with a gastric mass.

Small intestine

1. Usually secondary to contiguous spread from mesenteric lymph
   nodes. Primary disease only in non-Hodgkin's lymphoma. 20% of
   small bowel tumours are lymphoma.
2. Usually more than one of the following signs is evident
   - **(a)** Irregular mucosal infiltration → thick folds ± nodularity.
   - **(b)** Irregular polypoid mass ± barium tracts within it or central
     ulceration.
   - **(c)** Annular constriction – usually a long segment.
   - **(d)** Aneurysmal dilatation, with no internal mucosal pattern.
   - **(e)** Polyps – multiple and small or solitary and large. The latter may
     induce an intussusception.
   - **(f)** Multiple ulcers.
   - **(g)** Non-specific malabsorption pattern.
   - **(h)** Fistula.
   - **(i)** Perforation.

Colon and rectum

1. Rarely involved. Caecum and rectum more frequently involved than
   the rest of the colon.
2. Radiologically the disease may show
   - **(a)** Polypoidal mass – which may induce an intussusception.
   - **(b)** Diffuse infiltration of the wall.
   - **(c)** Constricting annular lesion.

Nodal disease

1. Normal lymph nodes are usually 3–10mm in diameter. Abdominal
   lymph nodes are likely abnormal if >10mm diameter. A localized
   cluster of lymph nodes 6–10mm in diameter should be considered
   highly suspect.

2. PET/CT improves accuracy of local staging and response assessment compared to conventional CT.
3. Negative PET imaging does not exclude viable disease, and a positive PET scan does not necessarily indicate viable tumour.

Skeleton

1. Radiological involvement in 10–20% of patients with Hodgkin's disease (50% at autopsy).
2. Involvement arises either from direct spread from contiguous lymph nodes or infiltration of bone marrow (spine, pelvis, major long bones, thoracic cage and skull are sites of predilection).
3. Patterns of bone involvement are
   (a) Predominantly osteolytic.
   (b) Mixed lytic and sclerotic.
   (c) Predominantly sclerotic – de novo or following radiotherapy to a lytic lesion.
   (d) 'Moth-eaten' – characteristic of round cell malignancies.
4. In addition, the spine may show
   (a) Anterior erosion of a vertebral body caused by involvement of an adjacent paravertebral lymph node.
   (b) Solitary dense vertebral body (ivory vertebra).
5. Hypertrophic osteoarthropathy.
6. Plain film may be negative with extensive disease on MRI.

Muscle

1. Primary muscle disease rare.
2. Patterns of primary muscle involvement
   (a) Focal mass.
   (b) Diffuse infiltration with preservation of myofascial planes.
   (c) Myofascial mantle of tumour in muscle compartment on surface of muscle.

Soft tissue

1. Subcutaneous – nodular or diffuse.

Central nervous system

1. Primary lymphoma (usually non-Hodgkin's B cell) shows increased incidence in HIV/AIDS and immunodeficiency states (Wiskott–Aldrich syndrome, IgA deficiency, X-linked lymphoproliferative syndrome and following organ transplantation). The cerebrum (deep hemispheric periventricular white matter), corpus callosum,

brainstem and cerebellum are affected (in order of frequency). Two patterns may be recognized:

(a) In immunocompetent patients there is a large, round or oval space-occupying lesion showing increased attenuation (CT), intermediate- to low-signal (T_1W MRI), isointense or hyperintense signal relative to grey matter (T_2W MRI) and surrounding oedema. Marked homogeneous enhancement (although avascular at angiography).

(b) In patients with HIV, a supratentorial mass frequently involves the corpus callosum, basal ganglia and other deep cerebral nuclei. Enhancement is variable and often bizarre. Multifocal lesions in 50%. Ependymal seeding in one-third, but meningeal disease is infrequent.

2. Systemic lymphoma typically presents as leptomeningeal disease.

Further Reading

Craig O, Gregson R. Primary lymphoma of the gastrointestinal tract. Clin Radiol 1981;32:63–71.

Erdag N, Bhorade RM, Alberico RA et al. Primary lymphoma of the central nervous system: typical and atypical CT and MR imaging appearances. Am J Roentgenol 2001;176:1319–26.

Felson B (ed). The lymphomas and leukaemias. Part 1. Semin Roentgenol 1980;15(3).

Felson B (ed). The lymphomas and leukaemias. Part 2. Semin Roentgenol 1980;15(4).

Ghai S, Pattison J, Ghai S et al. Primary gastrointestinal lymphoma: spectrum of imaging findings with pathologic correlation. Radiographics 2007;27:1371–88.

Leite NP, Kased N, Hanna RF et al. Cross-sectional imaging of extranodal involvement in abdominopelvic lymphoproliferative malignancies. Radiographics 2007;27:1613–34.

Libshitz HI (ed). Imaging the lymphomas. Radiol Clin North Am 1990;28(4).

Parker BR. Leukaemia and lymphoma in childhood. Radiol Clin North Am 1997;35:1495–516.

Rehm PK. Radionuclide evaluation of patients with lymphoma. Radiol Clin North Am 2001;39(5):957–78.

Ruzek KA, Wenger DE. The multiple faces of lymphoma in the musculoskeletal system. Skeletal Radiol 2004;33:1–8.

MARFAN'S SYNDROME

A connective tissue disorder transmitted as an AD trait, but with variable expression. 25% spontaneous mutations. Multisystem defects due to defective fibrillin, a component of microfibrils which is found in mesenchymal tissues.

Skeletal system

1. Scoliosis (>20°) or spondylolisthesis.
2. Pectus carinatum.
3. Pectus excavatum.
4. Acetabular protrusion.
5. Tall stature (upper:lower segment <0.86; or arm span to height ratio >1.05).
6. Pes planus – medial displacement of medial malleolus.
7. Joint hypermobility.
8. High arched palate with crowding of teeth.
9. Abnormal facies – dolichocephaly, malar hypoplasia, enophthalmos, retrognathism.
10. Arachnodactyly (metacarpal index 8.4–10.4).
11. Dislocations of sternoclavicular joint and hip and perilunate dislocation.
12. Rib notching.

Ocular system

Ectopia lentis – usually upwards.

Cardiovascular system

1. Ascending aortic dilatation ± aortic regurgitation.
2. Descending thoracic or abdominal aorta dilatation ± dissection.
3. Pulmonary artery dilatation.
4. Mitral valve prolapse; calcification of mitral annulus.

Dura

1. Lumbosacral dural ectasia.

Lungs

1. Pulmonary emphysema and bullae.
2. Spontaneous pneumothorax.

Further Reading
Ha HI, Seo JB, Lee SH et al. Imaging of Marfan syndrome: multisystemic manifestations. Radiographics 2007;27:989–1004.

MORQUIO'S SYNDROME

A mucopolysaccharidosis transmitted as an AR trait. Clinical presentation during the second year, with decreased growth, progressive skeletal deformity, corneal opacities, lymphadenopathy, cardiac lesions and deafness.

Axial skeleton

1. Universal vertebra plana. Wide discs.
2. Hypoplastic dens.
3. Hypoplastic dorsolumbar vertebra which may be displaced posteriorly.
4. Central anterior vertebral body beaks.
5. Short neck.
6. Dorsal scoliosis and dorsolumbar kyphosis.

Appendicular skeleton

1. Defective irregular ossification of the femoral capital epiphyses leading to flattening.
2. Genu valgum.
3. Short, wide tubular bones with irregular metaphyses. Proximal tapering of the metacarpals.
4. Irregular carpal and tarsal bones.

Cardiovascular system

1. Late-onset aortic regurgitation.

MULTIPLE ENDOCRINE NEOPLASIA (MEN) SYNDROMES

Multiple endocrine neoplasia is an autosomal dominant syndrome where there is an occurrence of two or more endocrine tumours associated with hyperfunction and neoplasia.

MEN I (Werner's syndrome)
1. Hyperparathyroidism (90%).
2. Pancreatic islet cell tumours (60%)
    (a) Gastrinomas (60%) – usually slow-growing: → Zollinger–Ellison syndrome.
    (b) Insulinomas – symptoms of hypoglycaemia.
    (c) VIPomas – secreting vasoactive intestinal peptide → explosive, watery diarrhoea with hypokalaemia and achlorhydria.
    (d) Glucagonomas – produce a syndrome of diabetes mellitus, necrolytic migratory erythema, anaemia, weight loss and thromboembolic complications.
3. Pituitary tumours (5%) – hormone-secreting and non-secreting.
4. Thyroid adenoma.
5. Adrenal adenoma.
6. Carcinoid tumour – originate in foregut.
7. Multiple facial angiofibromas (85%).

MEN IIA (Sipple's syndrome)
1. Medullary carcinoma of the thyroid (100%).
2. Phaeochromocytoma (50%).
3. Hyperparathyroidism (10%).

MEN IIB
1. Marfanoid appearance (100%).
2. Multiple mucosal neuromas (100%).
3. Medullary carcinoma of the thyroid (100%).
4. Phaeochromocytoma (50%).

Further Reading
Scarsbrook AF, Thakker RV, Wass JAH et al. Multiple endocrine neoplasia: spectrum of radiologic appearances and discussion of a multitechnique imaging approach. Radiographics 2006;26:433–51.

MULTIPLE MYELOMA/PLASMACYTOMA

Plasma cell neoplasms of bone are solitary (plasmacytoma; 3% of all plasma cell tumours) or multiple (multiple myeloma; 94% of all plasma cell tumours). 3% of all plasma cell tumours are solely extraskeletal.

Plasmacytoma

1. A well-defined, grossly expansile bone lesion arising, most commonly, in the spine, pelvis or ribs.
2. It may also exhibit soft-tissue extension, internal septa or pathological fracture.
3. Extramedullary plasmacytomas rare.
4. Absence of hypercalcaemia, renal insufficiency, anaemia; normal skeletal survey and normal paraprotein levels.

Multiple myeloma

Radiological manifestations are skeletal and extraskeletal.

Skeletal
Four forms of skeletal involvement

1. Solitary lesion (plasmacytoma) – see above.
2. Diffuse skeletal involvement (myelomatosis). Multiple osteolytic lesions usually
   (a) Widely disseminated at the time of diagnosis (spine, pelvis, skull, ribs and shafts of long bones).
   (b) Uniform in size (cf. metastases, which are usually of varying size).
   (c) Well-defined, subcortical with a narrow zone of transition.
   (d) Vertebral body collapse, occasionally with disc destruction. ± Paravertebral shadow. Involvement of pedicles is late.
   (e) Rib lesions tend to be expansile and associated with extrapleural soft-tissue masses.
   (f) Pathological fractures occur and healing is accompanied by much callus.
   (g) Show a permeating, mottled pattern of bone destruction similar to other round cell malignancies, e.g. Ewing's sarcoma, anaplastic metastatic carcinoma, leukaemia and reticulum cell sarcoma.
3. Diffuse skeletal osteopenia. Usually thoracic or lumbar spinal often with multiple compression fractures. CT and MRI more sensitive at staging.
4. Sclerosing myeloma. Rare. Multiple sclerotic lesions. Associated with POEMS (polyneuropathy, organomegaly, endocrinopathy, monoclonal gammopathy and skin changes).

Extraskeletal
1. Hypercalcaemia (30%).
2. Soft-tissue tumours in sinuses, the submucosa of the pharynx and trachea, cervical lymph nodes, skin and gastrointestinal tract.
3. Hepatosplenomegaly. Hepatic involvement focal or diffuse.
4. Leptomeningeal spread (rare).

Further Reading
Antuaco EJ, Fassas AB, Walker R et al. Multiple myeloma: clinical review and diagnostic imaging. Radiology 2004;231:11–23.

MYASTHENIA GRAVIS

An autoimmune disorder characterized by muscle weakness and fatiguability. Confirmed clinically by a positive response to intravenous edrophonium chloride (Tensilon test) and the presence of acetylcholine receptor antibodies.

1. Thymus is normal or involuted in 20%, hyperplastic in 65%, and 15% have a thymoma. Hyperplasia is more common in the young; thymoma more common after the fourth decade.
2. 60% of thymomas are benign and well-encapsulated; 40% are locally invasive and show subpleural deposits.

Further Reading
Moore NR. Imaging in myasthenia gravis. Clin Radiol 1989;40:115–6.

NEUROFIBROMATOSIS

Neurofibromatosis 1 (NF-1; von Recklinghausen disease)
90% of all cases. Prevalence 1 in 4000 persons. 50% are new mutations, 30% are AD. Gene is located on chromosome 17. May be diagnosed if two or more of the following criteria are present

(a) Six or more café-au-lait spots >5mm in diameter in prepubertal patients and >15mm in postpubertal patients.
(b) Two or more neurofibromas.
(c) Axillary or groin freckling.
(d) One plexiform neurofibroma.
(e) Two or more iris hamartomas (Lisch nodules).
(f) Optic glioma.

(g) Typical bone lesions such as sphenoid dysplasia or tibial pseudarthrosis.

(h) One or more first-degree relatives with NF-1.

Neurofibromatosis 2 (NF-2)

10% of all cases. Rare in childhood. Prevalence 1 in 50,000 persons. AD with the gene located on chromosome 22. Manifestations include VIIIth nerve tumours or schwannomas, other intracranial or spinal tumours such as neurinomas and meningiomas. May be diagnosed if one of the following criteria is present

(a) Bilateral VIIIth nerve tumours.

(b) Unilateral VIIIth nerve tumour in association with any two of the following: meningioma, neurofibroma, schwannoma, juvenile posterior subcapsular cataracts.

(c) Unilateral VIIIth nerve tumour with other spinal or brain tumour as above in a first-degree relative.

Skull

1. Dysplastic sphenoid – absent greater wing $\pm$ lesser wing (empty orbit), absent posterolateral wall of the orbit. May result in proptosis.
2. Lytic defects in the calvarium, especially in or near the lambdoid suture.
3. Enlargement of foramina.
4. Mandibular abnormalities.
5. Enlarged internal auditory meati – due to acoustic neuromas or dural ectasia without associated neuroma.

Brain (see also 12.30)

1. Focal or multifocal $\downarrow T_1W$ and/or $\uparrow T_2W$ signal without mass effect, most often in the basal ganglia, cerebellum and cerebral peduncles. No enhancement. ?Due to hamartomas. More common in younger patients and in those with an optic glioma. Tendency to regress after teenage years.
2. Tumours
   (a) Optic tract, chiasm and nerve gliomas (common). 10–30% of optic gliomas are associated with NF-1. The association is higher with optic nerve gliomas, and bilateral optic nerve gliomas are found almost exclusively in NF-1. Optic nerve glioma is not found in NF-2.
   (b) Optic nerve sheath meningiomas (rare).
   (c) Cranial nerve (V–XII) schwannomas. Frequently multiple and bilateral in NF-2. Acoustic neuromas (schwannomas) are bilateral in at least 90% of NF-2.
   (d) Brainstem and supratentorial gliomas.
   (e) Intracranial meningiomas – often multiple in NF-2.

3. Macrocephaly.
4. Hydrocephalus, of insidious onset – usually due to aqueduct stenosis caused by gliosis but may be secondary to a tumour.
5. Cerebral and cerebellar calcification. Heavy calcification of the choroid plexuses is rare but classic.
6. Arachnoid cyst.
7. Arterial occlusive disease, including moya-moya.

Spine
1. Scoliosis (typically acute and thoracic) and kyphosis.
2. Dural ectasia with posterior scalloping.
3. Absent or hypoplastic pedicles.
4. Spondylolisthesis.
5. Lateral meningocoele (rare).
6. Multiple neurofibromas (enhancing) ± dumbbell. Enlargement of intervertebral foramina. Most common in the cervicothoracic region.
7. Paraspinal plexiform neurofibromas.

Thorax
1. Rib notching, 'twisted ribbon' ribs and splaying of ribs.

Gastrointestinal
1. Neurogenic neoplasms – neurofibroma (inc. plexiform), malignant nerve sheath tumour.
2. Neuroendocrine neoplasms – carcinoid, phaeochromocytoma, paraganglionoma.
3. Non-neurogenic gastrointestinal mesenchymal neoplasms – GIST, leiomyosarcoma.
4. Embryonal tumours – rhabdomyosarcoma, neuroblastoma, Wilms' tumour.
5. Miscellaneous tumours – GI adenocarcinoma, pancreatic and biliary adenocarcinoma.

Appendicular skeleton
1. Overgrowth or, less commonly, undergrowth of long bones.
2. Overtubulation or undertubulation (due to cortical thickening).
3. Anterior and lateral bowing of the tibia with irregular periosteal thickening is common and is usually evident in the first year. It frequently progresses to no. 4.
4. Pseudarthrosis.
5. Intraosseous neurofibromas present as subperiosteal or cortical lucencies with a smooth expanded outer margin.
6. Cortical pressure resorption from an adjacent soft-tissue neurofibroma.
7. Cortical defects may also be due to dysplastic periosteum.
8. Association of non-ossifying fibromas and neurofibromatosis.

Other

1. Soft-tissue neurofibromas and plexiform neurofibromas. The latter may be associated with partial gigantism.
2. Renal artery stenosis or aneurysm.
3. Osteomalacia.

Further Reading

Levy AD, Patel N, Dow N. Abdominal neoplasms in patients with neurofibromatosis type 1. Radiographics 2005;25:455–80.

Menor F, Martí-Bonmatí L, Mulas F et al. Imaging considerations of central nervous system manifestations in paediatric patients with neurofibromatosis type 1. Pediatr Radiol 1991;21:389–94.

Murphey MD, Smith WS, Smith SE et al. Imaging of musculoskeletal neurogenic tumors: radiologic-pathologic correlation. Radiographics 1999;19:1253–80.

Rossi SE, Erasmus JJ, McAdams HP et al. Thoracic manifestations of neurofibromatosis-1. Am J Roentgenol 1999;173:1631–8.

NEUROPATHIC ARTHROPATHY

Disease	Sites of involvement
Diabetes mellitus	Metatarsophalangeal, tarsometatarsal and intertarsal joints
Steroid treatment	Hips and knees
Syringomyelia	Shoulder, elbow, wrist and cervical spine
Tabes dorsalis	Knee, hip, ankle and lumbar spine
Congenital insensitivity to pain	Ankle and intertarsal joints
Myelomeningocoele	Ankle and intertarsal joints
Leprosy	Hands (interphalangeal), feet (metatarsophalangeal) and lower limbs
Chronic alcoholism	Metatarsophalangeal and interphalangeal joints
Spinal trauma	Spine – lower thoracic and lumbar

Radiological changes include

1. Sclerosis and fragmentation.
2. Joint destruction and disorganization. Subluxation and dislocation.
3. Ligament laxity.
4. Joint effusion.
5. Osteophyte formation – may be large in hypertrophic subtype.
6. Bone resorption – predominates in atrophic subtype.

7. Bone density preserved.
8. Fractures – e.g. posterior calcaneum and second metatarsal in diabetes.
9. Callus tissue excessive.
10. Variable progression, but often rapid. In the early stages can resemble osteoarthritis.
11. Spinal neuropathic arthropathy requires distinction from osteomyelitis and metastasis.

Further Reading

Aliabadi P, Nikpoor N, Alparslan L. Imaging of neuropathic arthropathy. Semin Musculoskeletal Radiol 2003;7(3):217–25.

Jones EA, Manamaster BJ, May DA et al. europathic osteoarthropathy: diagnostic dilemmas and differential diagnosis. Radiographics 2000;20:5279–93.

NON-ACCIDENTAL INJURY

Skeletal

1. **Fractures** in 11–55% and significantly more common in the younger child. Typically multiple, in varying stages of healing and explained by an implausible history.
2. **Shaft fractures** are more common than metaphyseal fractures although the latter are characteristic.
3. **Metaphyseal fractures** are due to tractional and torsional stresses on limbs and histologically there is a transmetaphyseal disruption of the most immature metaphyseal primary spongiosa. The most subtle indication of injury is a transverse lucency within the subepiphyseal region of the metaphysis. It may be visible in only one projection and its appearance is influenced by the severity of the bony injury, the degree of displacement of the fragments and the chronicity of the process. Peripherally the fracture line may undermine and isolate a thicker fragment of bone and it is this thick peripheral margin of bone that produces the corner fractures and bucket handle configurations.
4. **Rib fractures** comprise 5–27% of all fractures in abused children. Posterior rib fractures have a higher specificity for abuse than anterolateral fractures. In the absence of prematurity, birth injury, metabolic disorders, bone dysplasias and major trauma, e.g. road traffic accidents, rib fractures may be considered specific for abuse. The majority are occult.
5. **Skull fractures** which are linear and in the parietal bone are most common; features suggesting NAI include multiple or complex

fractures, diastased fractures, fracture crossing a suture and non-parietal fractures.

6. In infants and young children certain fractures have a high specificity for abuse owing to their unusual locations. These include scapular injuries, injuries involving the small bones of the hands and feet and spinal injuries.

7. **Dislocations** are rarely encountered in abused children. Malalignment of bones sharing an articulation usually indicates a growth plate injury rather than dislocation. When dislocations do occur they are likely to be secondary to massive injury and are accompanied by adjacent fracture.

Intracranial injuries – brain

Shaking is the most important mechanism in the production of intracranial injury in non-accidental injury. Intracranial injury may be detected when the skeletal survey is normal and in the setting of a normal neurological examination.

In cases of suspected NAI, head CT should be performed as soon as the child is stabilized. Plain skull radiographs should also be performed to confirm the presence and extent of skull fractures. If the initial brain CT is abnormal, or if a child has neurological symptoms despite a normal or equivocal CT, brain MRI should be performed and interpreted by a neuroradiologist. Delayed CT at days 8–10 may clarify the presence and extent of any abnormality seen on the initial CT. MRI at 3 months documents the extent of permanent damage.

1. Subdural haematoma – haematomas of different ages are highly suspicious of NAI. Posterior interhemispheric and occipital SDHs are common and occur following laceration of bridging veins. Chronic SDHs with CSF signal must be differentiated from benign enlargement of the subarachnoid space. The latter is most often seen overlying the anterior frontal lobes. MRI may aid diagnosis in difficult cases since haematomas should not be isointense with CSF on PD and FLAIR sequences.

2. Skull fracture – complex, bilateral, depressed, multiple and non-parietal fractures are suggestive of NAI.

3. Cortical contusions/shearing injuries – see 12.13.

4. Cerebral oedema – effacement of the cerebral sulci and basal cisterns plus loss of normal grey-white matter differentiation.

5. Hypoxia – the cerebellum and thalami appear relatively hyperdense in comparison with the low-density cerebral hemispheres as a result of asphyxia (reversal sign).

6. Subarachnoid and intraventricular haemorrhage.

7. Subdural hygromas – tears in the arachnoid may allow CSF to collect within the subdural space.

8. Cerebral laceration – best identified by ultrasound and MRI. Virtually pathognomonic of shaking injury in the first 6 months.
9. Vascular injuries – dissection of intracranial or cervical vessels. May lead to pseudoaneurysm formation.
10. Late sequelae – hydrocephalus, atrophy, gliosis and growing fractures.
11. Coexistent non-CNS injuries – retinal haemorrhages, skeletal fractures, visceral injuries.

Visceral trauma

Commonly occurs after the child is able to move about. Mortality of 50% for visceral injuries associated with child abuse. The most likely mechanism of injury is a direct blow or the effect of rapid deceleration after being hurled. The most common injuries involve the hollow viscera, mesenteries, liver and pancreas.

Skeletal survey for NAI

The skeletal survey should be reviewed by a radiologist before the child leaves the department.

1. Neuroimaging
    (a) CT brain in all pre-mobile children in whom NAI is suspected.
    (b) Consider in ambulant small children in whom NAI is suspected, if thought not to be appropriate this should be documented in the hospital notes.
2. Skull (SXR)
    (a) AP and lateral, plus Towne's view for occipital injury.
    (b) SXRs should be taken with a skeletal survey even if a CT scan has been performed, as in plane horizontal fractures can be missed on CT.
3. Body
    (a) AP/frontal chest (including clavicles).
    (b) Oblique views of the ribs (left and right).
    (c) AP abdomen with pelvis and hips.
4. Spine
    Lateral spine – cervical and thoraco-lumbar.
5. Limbs
    – AP humeri
    – AP forearms
    – AP femora
    – AP tib/fib
    – PA hands
    – AP feet

Supplemented by, at the discretion of radiologist reviewing the films

(a) Lateral views of any suspected shaft fracture.
(b) Lateral coned views of the elbows/wrists/knees/ankles – may demonstrate metaphyseal injuries in greater detail than AP views of the limbs alone.

Further Reading

Chapman S. Radiological aspects of non-accidental injury. J R Soc Med 1990;83:67–71.

Harwood-Nash DC. Abuse to the pediatric central nervous system. Am J Neuroradiol 1992;13:569–75.

Hymel KP, Rumack CM, Hay TC et al. Comparison of intracranial computed tomographic (CT) findings in pediatric abusive and accidental head trauma. Pediatr Radiol 1997;27:743–7.

Jaspan T, Narborough G, Punt JA et al. Cerebral contusional tears as a marker of child abuse – detection by cranial sonography. Pediatr Radiol 1992;22:237–45.

Kleinman P. Diagnostic imaging of child abuse, 2nd edn. CV Mosby, St Louis, 1998.

Merten, DF, Radkowski MA, Leonidas JC. The abused child: a radiological reappraisal. Radiology 1983;148:377–81.

Rao P, Carty H. Non-accidental injury: review of the radiology. Clin Radiol 1999;4:11–24.

Stoodley N. Neuroimaging in non-accidental head injury: if, when, why and how. Clin Radiol 2005;60(1):22–30.

Strouse PJ, Close BJ, Marshall KW et al. CT of bowel and mesenteric trauma in children. Radiographics 1999;19:1237–50.

Worlock P, Stower M, Barbor P. Patterns of fractures in accidental and non-accidental injury in children: a comparative study. Br Med J 1986;293:100–3.

NON-OSSIFYING FIBROMA (FIBROUS CORTICAL DEFECT)

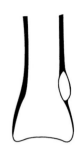

1. Age – 10–20 years.
2. Sites – femur and tibia.
3. Appearances
   (a) Diametaphyseal, becoming diaphyseal as the bone grows.
   (b) Well-defined lucency with a sclerotic margin. Increasing sclerosis as lesion matures.
   (c) Eccentric ± slight expansion; in thin bones, e.g. fibula, it occupies the entire width of the bone.

OCHRONOSIS

See Alkaptonuria.

OSTEOBLASTOMA

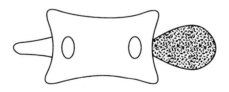

1. Age – 10–20 years. M:F 2:1.
2. Sites – vertebra (neural arch predominantly) and, less commonly, in the long bones.
3. Appearances
   (a) Well-defined lucency with a sclerotic rim.
   (b) May be expansile, but the cortex is preserved.
   (c) ± Internal calcification.
   (d) May be purely sclerotic in the spine.
   (e) In long bones it is metaphyseal or diaphyseal.

Further Reading
White LM, Kandel R. Osteoid-producing tumors of bone. Semin Musculoskelet Radiol 2000;4(1):25–43.

OSTEOCHONDROMA (EXOSTOSIS)

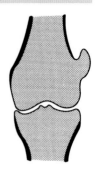

1. Age – 10–20 years. M<F.
2. Sites – distal femur, proximal tibia, proximal humerus, pelvis and scapula. When there are multiple osteochondromas the condition is termed diaphyseal aclasis (AD).
3. Appearances
    (a) Metaphyseal.
    (b) Well-defined eccentric protrusion with the parent cortex and trabeculae continuous with that of the tumour.
    (c) Tumour is usually directed away from the end of the bone and migrates away from the end as growth proceeds.
    (d) The cartilage cap is not visible in childhood, but becomes calcified in the adult.
    (e) If large → failure of correct modelling.
4. Complications
    (a) Cosmetic deformity.
    (b) Bony deformity.
    (c) Fracture.
    (d) Vascular compromise.
    (e) Peripheral nerve and spinal cord compression.
    (f) Bursa formation.
    (g) Malignant transformation. Rapid growth of a stable lesion suggests transformation to a chondrosarcoma (less than 1% of solitary, 5–25% of multiple osteochondromas).

Further Reading
Lee KCY, Davies AM, Cassar-Pullicino VN. Imaging the complications of osteochondromas. Clin Radiol 2002;57:18–28.

OSTEOGENESIS IMPERFECTA

A clinically heterogeneous condition with bone fragility. There are several distinct genetic entities and the current classification is shown below (Expanded Sillence classification). Extraskeletal features include blue sclerae, hearing impairment, dentinogenesis imperfecta, hyperlaxity of joints and wormian bones. Most forms are autosomal dominant inheritance, although spontaneous mutations also occur. Most cases have a mutation in one of the genes encoding the α chain of type 1 collagen – COL1A1 or COL1A2.

Type 1

1. Premature stop codon in COL1A1 gene.
2. Mild with no major bone deformities.
3. Vertebral fractures may lead to scoliosis.
4. Blue sclera.
5. No dentinogenesis imperfecta.

Type II

1. Glycine substitution in COL1A1 or COL1A2.
2. Lethal perinatal.
3. Extremely severe osseous fragility.
4. Severely deforming.
5. Multiple rib and long bone fractures at birth.
6. Marked osteopenia of skull bones.
7. Dark sclera.

Type III

1. Rare.
2. Glycine substitution in COL1A1 or COL1A2.
3. Severe deformity of long bones and spine result in severe dwarfing.
4. Severe scoliosis.
5. Respiratory difficulty with high morbidity and mortality.
6. Greyish sclera.
7. Dentinogenesis imperfecta.

Type IV

1. Rare.
2. Glycine substitution in COL1A1 or COL1A2.
3. Moderate deformity.
4. Variable short stature.

5. Grey/white sclera.
6. Dentinogenesis imperfecta.

The following groups describe patients who do not fit into the above classification and who do not have COL1A1 or COL1A2 mutations.

Type V

1. Seems to be autosomal dominant inheritance pattern.
2. Mutation not identified.
3. Moderately deforming.
4. Calcification of radio-ulnar interosseous membrane → radial head dislocation.
5. Hyperplastic callus, which can mimic osteosarcoma.
6. White sclera.
7. No dentinogenesis imperfecta.

Type VI

1. Unknown pattern of inheritance.
2. Mutation not identified.
3. Moderate to severely deforming.
4. Based on bone biopsy findings of increased osteoid and abnormal lamellation ('fish-scale').

Type VII

1. Autosomal recessive.
2. Mutation of the CRTAP (cartilage-associated protein) gene.
3. Moderately deforming.
4. Short humeri and femora.
5. Coxa vara.
6. White sclera.
7. No dentinogenesis imperfecta.

Type VIII

1. Autosomal recessive.
2. Caused by a deficiency of P3H1 (prolyl 3-hydroxylase 1) due to a mutation to the LEPRE1 gene.
3. Resembles lethal Type II or Type III OI in appearance and symptoms except that infants have white sclera.
4. Severe growth deficiency.
5. Extreme skeletal under mineralization.

Further Reading

Martin E, Shapiro JR. Osteogenesis imperfecta: epidemiology and pathophysiology. Curr Osteoporos Rep 2007;5:91–7.

Marini JC, Cabral WA, Barnes AM et al. Components of the collagen prolyl 3-hydroxylation complex are crucial for normal bone development. Cell Cycle 2007;6:1675–81.

Rauch F, Glorieux FH. Osteogenesis imperfecta. Lancet 2004;363 (9418):1377–85.

Sillence DO. Osteogenesis imperfecta. An expanding panorama of variants. Clin Orthop 1981;159:11–25.

Sillence DO, Senn A, Danks DM. Genetic heterogeneity in osteogenesis imperfecta. J Med Genet 1979;16:101–16.

Smith R, Francis MJO, Houghton GR. The brittle bone syndrome: osteogenesis imperfecta. Butterworth, London, 1983.

Thompson EM, Young ID, Hall CM et al. Recurrence risk and prognosis in severe sporadic osteogenesis imperfecta. J Med Genet 1987;24:390–405.

OSTEOID OSTEOMA

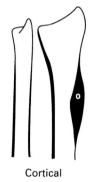 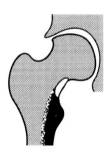

Cortical   Cancellous

1. Age – 10–30 years.
2. Sites – most commonly femur and tibia.
3. Appearances:
   Cortical
   (a) Central lucent nidus (<1cm) ± dense calcified centre.
   (b) Dense surrounding bone.
   (c) Eccentric bone expansion ± periosteal reaction.
   Cancellous
   (a) Usually femoral neck.
   (b) Lucent lesion with bone sclerosis a distance away. The head and neck may be osteoporotic.

OSTEOMALACIA

Increased uncalcified osteoid in the mature skeleton.

1. Decreased bone density.
2. Looser's zones – bilaterally symmetrical transverse lucent bands of uncalcified osteoid which, later in the disease, have sclerotic margins. Common sites are the scapulae, femoral necks and shafts, pubic rami and ribs.
3. Coarsening of the trabecular pattern with ill-defined trabeculae.
4. Bone softening – protrusio acetabuli, bowing of long bones, biconcave vertebral bodies and basilar invagination.

Further Reading
Pitt MJ. Rickets and osteomalacia are still around. Radiol Clin North Am 1991;29(1):97–118.

OSTEOPETROSIS

A defect of bone resorption caused by decreased osteoclastic activity. A number of forms have been recognized.

Benign or tarda, AD

1. Often asymptomatic individuals in whom a chance diagnosis is made on radiographs taken for some other purpose. Some have a mild anaemia and there may be cranial nerve compressions. Predisposition to fractures. Tooth extraction may be complicated by osteomyelitis.
2. Increasing bone sclerosis during childhood, with some sparing of the peripheral skeleton.
3. 'Bone-within-bone' appearance – usually disappearing by the end of the second decade.
4. 'Rugger jersey' spine.

Malignant or congenita, AR

1. Manifestations during infancy – failure to thrive and evidence of marrow failure due to bone overgrowth, i.e. anaemia, thrombocytopenia and hepatosplenomegaly. Pathological fractures. Cranial nerve palsies due to bony compression. Death in the first decade.
2. Generalized bone sclerosis with transverse metaphyseal bands.
3. 'Bone-within-bone' appearance.
4. 'Rugger jersey' spine.
5. Later, flask-shaped ends of the long bones.

Intermediate, AR
With renal tubular acidosis, AR

1. Presents in early childhood with failure to thrive and hypotonia due to renal tubular acidosis. Anaemia, cranial nerve lesions and fractures are variable features.
2. Radiology is similar to the benign form but tends to normality in later childhood. Basal ganglia and periventricular calcification are consistent findings which differentiate this form from the others.

Further Reading

Beighton P. Inherited disorders of the skeleton. Churchill Livingstone, Edinburgh, 1988, p163–9.

Beighton P, Cremin BJ. Sclerosing bone dysplasias. Springer-Verlag, Berlin, 1980, p19–31.

Herman TE, Siegel MJ. Infantile autosomal-recessive malignant osteopetrosis. J Perinatol 2007;27(7):455–6.

OSTEOSARCOMA

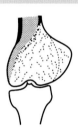

1. Age – 10–25 years with a second peak in the seventh decade (flat bones).
2. Sites – distal femur, proximal tibia, proximal humerus and pelvis.
3. Predisposing factors – Paget's disease, radiotherapy, osteochondroma, fibrous dysplasia, retinoblastoma, osteopetrosis and bone infarct.
4. Association – bilateral retinoblastoma.
5. Appearances
    (a) Metaphyseal; epiphyseal (<1%) and diaphyseal (10%) are unusual.
    (b) May be predominantly lytic, sclerotic or mixed.
    (c) Wide zone of transition with normal bone.
    (d) Cortical destruction with soft-tissue extension.
    (e) ± Internal calcification of bone.
    (f) Periosteal reaction – 'sunray' spiculation, lamellated and/or Codman's triangle.
6. Unusual variants
    (a) Telangiectatic – 5% of osteosarcomas. Aggressive. Characterized by large blood-filled cavities and thin septations within the tumour. Similar presentation to conventional osteosarcoma but pathological fracture is more common.

Diaphyseal > metaphyseal. Majority in femur and tibia. Usually entirely osteolytic. Fluid/fluid levels on CT and MRI.

(b) Small cell – 1% of osteosarcomas. Similar appearance and presentation to conventional osteosarcoma but prognosis is much worse.

(c) Low grade or intraosseous well-differentiated – 1–2%. Older age at presentation and more chronic history. More benign-looking radiological appearance.

(d) Parosteal – 5%. Attached to the surface of the bone by a stalk (early) or a broad base (late) with a tendency to encircle it. Older age group, 20–40 years. Femur is most common site.

(e) Extraskeletal – buttocks and thighs. Ossification or calcification in a soft-tissue mass.

(f) Multicentric – rapidly fatal.

Further Reading

Bloem JL, Kroon HM. Osseous lesions. Radiol Clin North Am 1993;31(2):261–78.
Murphey MD, Robbin MR, McRae GA et al. The many faces of osteosarcoma. Radiographics 1997;17:1205–31.

PAGET'S DISEASE

A condition characterized by excessive abnormal remodelling of bone. Increasing prevalence with age: rare in patients less than 40 years old, 3% of the population in middle age and 10% of the population in old age. The disease predominates in the axial skeleton – spine (75%), skull (65%), pelvis (40%) – and proximal femur (75%). (The percentages represent patients with Paget's disease in whom these sites are affected.) Monostotic disease does occur. There are three stages.

Active (osteolytic)

1. Skull – osteoporosis circumscripta, especially in the frontal and occipital bones.
2. Long bones – a well-defined, advancing radiolucency with a V-shaped margin which begins subarticularly.

Osteolytic and osteosclerotic

1. Skull – osteoporosis circumscripta with focal areas of bone sclerosis.
2. Pelvis – mixed osteolytic and osteosclerotic areas.
3. Long bones – epiphyseal and metaphyseal sclerosis with diaphyseal lucency.

Inactive (osteosclerotic)

1. Skull – thickened vault. 'Cotton wool' areas of sclerotic bone. The facial bones are not commonly affected (cf. fibrous dysplasia).
2. Spine – especially the lumbar spine. Enlargement of vertebrae and coarsened trabeculae. Cortical thickening produces the 'picture frame' vertebral body. Ivory vertebra.
3. Pelvis – widening and coarsened trabeculation of the pelvic ring, with splitting of the iliopectineal line may progress to widespread changes in the pelvis which are commonly asymmetrical.
4. Long bones – sclerosis due to coarsened, thickened trabeculae. Cortical thickening with encroachment on the medullary canal. The epiphyseal region is nearly always involved.

Complications

1. Bone softening – bowed bones, basilar invagination and protrusio acetabuli.
2. Fractures – transverse with a predilection for the convex aspect of the bone and which usually only partially traverse the bone.
3. Sarcomatous change – in 1% of patients (5–10% if there is widespread involvement). Femur, pelvis and humerus most commonly affected. Osteogenic sarcoma (50%), fibrosarcoma (25%) and chondrosarcoma (10%) are the most common histological diagnoses. They are predominantly lytic.
4. Degenerative joint disease – most frequent in the hip and knee.
5. Neurological complications – nerve entrapment and spinal cord compression.
6. High output cardiac failure.
7. Extramedullary haemopoiesis.
8. Osteomyelitis.

PARANEOPLASTIC SYNDROMES

Non-metastatic systemic or remote effects of tumours.

Endocrine disorders

1. Cushing's syndrome – carcinoma of the bronchus, malignant epithelial thymoma, islet cell carcinoma, small cell carcinoma, medullary thyroid carcinoma, ovarian carcinoma.
2. Hypercalcaemia – osseous metastases; carcinoma of lung, oesophageal carcinoma, squamous carcinomas of the head and neck, lymphoma and leukaemia.
3. Hypocalcaemia and osteomalacia – non-ossifying fibroma, giant cell tumour, osteoblastoma (and fibrous dysplasia, neurofibromatosis and melorrheostosis bone).
4. Hypoglycaemia – sarcomas, mesothelioma, lymphoma, gastrointestinal carcinomas, adrenal cortical carcinoma.
5. Hyperglycaemia – glucagon-producing islet cell tumour, enteroglucagon-producing renal carcinoma.
6. Inappropriate antidiuretic hormone – carcinoma of bronchus, adenocarcinomas of the gastrointestinal tract.
7. Carcinoid syndrome – adenocarcinoma of pancreas, islet cell tumours, small cell carcinoma of the lung, medullary carcinoma of the thyroid, APUD (amine precursor uptake and decarboxylation) tumours.
8. Gynaecomastia – non-seminomatous tumours of the testis, liver and renal cell carcinomas, carcinoma of bronchus.
9. Hyperthyroidism – hydatidiform mole or choriocarcinoma, non-seminomatous tumours of testis.
10. Hypertension – phaeochromocytoma, neuroblastoma, aldosterone-secreting tumours, renal tumours (Wilms' tumour, renal cell carcinoma, haemangiopericytoma).

Haematological disorders

1. Polycythaemia – renal tumours (Wilms' tumour, renal cell carcinoma), liver cell carcinoma, cerebellar haemangioblastoma, uterine fibroids, renal cystic disease.
2. Red cell aplasia – thymoma, carcinomas of the bronchus, stomach or thyroid.
3. Haemolytic anaemia – lymphoid malignancies, carcinomas of the ovary, stomach, colon, bronchus, cervix and breast.
4. Thrombocytosis and leukocytosis – bone marrow metastases.

Digestive disorders

1. Zollinger–Ellison syndrome – non-beta cell adenomas or carcinomas of the pancreas or duodenum, mucinous adenocarcinoma of the ovary.
2. Multiple endocrine neoplasia (MEN) (q.v.).
3. Tumour-related diarrhoea – Zollinger–Ellison syndrome, carcinoid syndrome, non-beta cell tumour of the pancreas, vasoactive intestinal peptide-secreting tumours (VIPomas).

Renal dysfunction

1. Nephrotic syndrome – lymphoma, carcinomas of the bronchus, stomach, colon and ovary.
2. Tubular dysfunction – multiple myeloma.

Musculoskeletal disorders

1. Hypertrophic osteoarthropathy (see 1.27) – carcinoma of bronchus, metastases, lymphomas, pleural fibroma.
2. Dermatomyositis – carcinomas of the breast, bronchus, ovary or stomach, leukaemia, lymphoma and sarcomas.
3. Oncogenic osteomalacia.

Skin disorders

1. Acanthosis nigricans – adenocarcinoma of the stomach.
2. Pellagra-like lesions – carcinoid syndrome.
3. Porphyria cutanea tarda – liver cell carcinoma or adenoma.
4. Pemphigus vulgaris – adenocarcinoma of the pancreas.

Neurological disorders

1. Progressive multifocal leukoencephalopathy – leukaemia, lymphoma, myeloma.
2. Cerebellar atrophy – carcinomas of the lung, breast, ovary and kidney; lymphomas.
3. Central pontine myelinolysis – leukaemia.
4. Myelopathy – visceral carcinomas.
5. Myasthenia gravis – thymoma, thymic hyperplasia.
6. Myasthenic syndrome – small cell carcinoma of the lung (Lambert–Eaton syndrome).
7. Opsimyoclonus (dancing eyes) – neuroblastoma (usually cervicothoracic).

Further Reading
Taybi H, Lachman RS. Radiology of syndromes, metabolic disorders, and skeletal dysplasias, 4th edn. CV Mosby, St Louis, 1996, p693–5.

PERTHES' DISEASE (LEGG–CALVÉ–PERTHES DISEASE)

1. Idiopathic childhood avascular necrosis of the femoral head.
2. M>F. Age 4–8 years.
3. The epiphysis appears small and sclerotic and the joint space may be widened. Demineralization is seen, particularly in the metaphyseal area of the neck, which may appear rarefied. There is no articular cortex destruction.
4. Later a subchondral fracture may be seen as a radiolucent crescent. A subcortical fracture may be seen on the anterior articular surface (frog lateral view).
5. Femoral neck cysts may be seen.
6. Fragmentation develops and this may lead to coxa plana.
7. Femoral head remodelling leads to coxa magna.
8. Delayed bony maturation may occur.
9. As with other causes of avascular necrosis MRI is more sensitive, particularly in the early stage of the disease process when plain films are normal.

PIGMENTED VILLONODULAR SYNOVITIS

1. Benign proliferative disorder of synovium.
2. Knee (80%) > hip > ankle > shoulder.
3. Young adults (third and fourth decades).
4. Also known as giant cell tumour of tendon sheath when it affects tendons in the hands and feet. It is the second commonest soft-tissue mass of the hands and feet after ganglion.
5. Radiographs
   (a) Normal or periarticular soft-tissue swelling.
   (b) Bone density preserved.
   (c) Joint space preserved until late in the disease.
   (d) Well-defined erosions on both sides of the joints.
   (e) Erosions are more prominent when joint capsule is tight (e.g. hip).
6. MRI
   (a) Diffuse nodular thickening of the synovium with low signal intensity due to haemosiderin deposition.
   (b) Localized intra-articular variant typically affects Hoffa's fat.

Further Reading
Llauger J, Palmer J, Rosón N et al. PVNS and giant cell tumor of the tendon sheath. Am J Roentgenol 1999;172:1087–91.

PLASMACYTOMA

See Multiple myeloma/plasmacytoma.

POLYCYSTIC DISEASE, AUTOSOMAL RECESSIVE

Polycystic kidneys, with periportal hepatic fibrosis and bile duct obstruction. In general, the relative severity of renal and liver disease is inversely proportional to each other in individual patients: this probably reflects the later development of liver problems. Those with severe renal disease do not live long enough to develop liver disease. Four subgroups: perinatal, neonatal, infantile and juvenile, based on age at presentation, kidney size and clinical course. Infants presenting in the perinatal period have renal failure and/or respiratory distress because of elevated diaphragms and pulmonary hypoplasia due to oligohydramnios. The majority die in a few days. Disease in the neonatal group is milder. Children present in the first month and most die within the first year. The infantile group have both renal and hepatic disease. The juvenile form presents between 6 months and 5 years with portal hypertension, but little renal impairment.

Renal disease

1. In neonates and infants, bilateral, large, smooth kidneys. Abdominal distension on AXR with bowel gas displaced medially. Severe disease is associated with pulmonary hypoplasia. Normal size kidneys at birth effectively excludes the diagnosis.
2. Markedly enlarged hyperechoic kidneys on ultrasound with loss of corticomedullary differentiation. There may be a thin rim of compressed normal parenchyma. May be some small macrocysts, best visualized with linear high resolution probe.
3. Dense striated nephrograms (because of dilated tubules) on IVU (rarely performed today) and CT. Calyces are not usually demonstrated but are normal.
4. Increased signal on T_2W MRI.
5. In older children kidneys may be normal or show changes similar to, but milder than, the neonatal form.

Liver disease

1. Heterogeneous or diffuse increased echogenicity on ultrasound ± periportal echogenicity.
2. Variable biliary dilatation, occasionally appears indistinguishable from Caroli disease.
3. Signs of portal hypertension – varices, splenomegaly, etc.

Further Reading

Avni E, Guissard G, Hall M et al. Hereditary polycystic kidney diseases in children: changing sonographic patterns through childhood. Pediatr Radiol 2002;32:169–74.

Lonergan GJ, Rice RR, Suarez ES. Autosomal recessive polycystic kidney disease: radiologic-pathologic correlation. Radiographics 2000;20:837–55.

POLYCYSTIC DISEASE, AUTOSOMAL DOMINANT

Multi-system disease that presents in the third/fourth decade and is responsible for 10–15% of all patients on renal dialysis. Mutations of two genes, PKD1 and PKD2, account for approximately 85% and 15% of cases, respectively. The clinical manifestations of these two genotypes overlap completely but patients with PKD1 have much more severe renal disease compared with those with PKD, as evidenced by end-stage renal failure occurring approximately 15 years earlier. Diagnosed by screening family members (antenatally and postnatally) or identified as an incidental finding.

Kidneys

1. Bilateral, but asymmetrical, enlarged lobulated kidneys. Unilateral in 8%.
2. Multiple smooth defects in the nephrogram with elongation and deformity of calyces giving a 'spider leg' appearance. Cysts may produce filling defects in the renal pelvis.
3. Multiple cysts on ultrasound, CT and MRI.
4. Calcifications in the walls of the cysts are common and stones develop in 20–35% of patients.
5. Increased incidence of renal cell carcinoma (may be bilateral) when on dialysis.

6. There are a number of criteria for positive ultrasound screening examinations. The most widely used is still that proposed by Ravine et al (1994)
    (a) Two renal cysts (unilateral or bilateral) in patients with a family history and age <30 years.
    (b) At least two renal cysts in each kidney in patients with a family history and age 30–59 years.
    (c) At least four renal cysts in each kidney in patients with a family history and age >60 years.

The sensitivity in individuals aged >30 years with either PKD1 or PKD2 is 100%, but if there is a clinical suspicion of ADPKD type 2 in individuals <30 years, genetic linkage analysis should also be considered as sensitivity of ultrasound is less.

Other organs

1. Cystic changes in the liver (in 75% by 60 years of age) and, less commonly, in the pancreas (10%) and spleen.
2. Colonic diverticula.
3. Subarachnoid haemorrhage (2–11%) due to intracranial aneurysm (18–26%). Cerebrovascular accidents unrelated to aneurysms are more common.
4. Structural abnormalities of cardiac valves.

Further Reading

Nicolau C, Torra R, Badenas C et al. Autosomal dominant polycystic kidney disease Types 1 and 2: assessment of US sensitivity for diagnosis. Radiology 1999;213:273–6.

Pei Y. Diagnostic approach in autosomal dominant polycystic kidney disease. Clin J Am Soc Nephrol 2006;1:1108–14.

Ravine D, Gibson RN, Walker RG. Evaluation of ultrasonographic diagnostic criteria for autosomal dominant polycystic kidney disease 1. Lancet 1994;343:824–7.

PSEUDOHYPOPARATHYROIDISM

End organ unresponsiveness to parathormone. X-linked dominant transmission.

1. Short stature, round face, thickset features, mental retardation and hypocalcaemia.
2. Short fourth and fifth metacarpals and metatarsals.
3. Basal ganglia calcification (50%).
4. Soft-tissue calcification.

PSEUDOPSEUDOHYPOPARATHYROIDISM

Similar clinical and radiological features to
pseudohypoparathyroidism but with a normal plasma calcium.

PSORIATIC ARTHROPATHY

Occurs in 5% of psoriatics and may antedate the skin changes in
15%. There are three clinical and radiological types. The hallmarks
are erosion and bone proliferation.

1. Monoarthritis or oligoarthritis with enthesitis.
2. Polyarthritis – symmetrical and resembling rheumatoid.
3. Axial disease – rare <5% – like ankylosing spondylitis ± peripheral
   joint disease.

The radiological changes comprise

1. Bone erosion
   (a) Surface erosion – erodes along articular surface.
   (b) Enthesitic erosion – away from joint along joint capsule.
2. Bone proliferation
   (a) Adjacent to erosions.
   (b) Periosteal reaction along diaphysis.
3. Preservation of bone density.
4. Sacroiliitis – bilateral and asymmetrical. Large erosions with bone
   proliferation but ankylosis rare.
5. Spondylitis – prominent asymmetrical paravertebral ossification.
6. Joints involved – knee, PIP (feet and hands), metatarsophalangeal,
   ankle, metacarpophalangeal and distal interphalangeal (feet and
   hands).
7. Dactylitis – sausage digit – digital oedema, arthritis of
   interphalangeal joint and tenosynovitis.
8. Pencil-in-cup and cup-and-saucer appearances are a consequence of
   severe erosive changes. Severe erosions give rise to 'arthritis
   mutilans'.
9. Distal phalangeal tuft resorption – associated with psoriatic nail
   changes.

Further Reading
Bennett DL, Ohashi K, El Khoury GY. Spondyloarthropathies: ankylosing
spondylitis and psoriatic arthritis. Radiol Clin North Am 2004;42;121–34.

PULMONARY EMBOLIC DISEASE

Clinical conditions which predispose to venous thromboembolism are

1. Surgical procedures, especially major abdominal and gynaecological surgery and hip operations.
2. Trauma.
3. Prolonged bed-rest.
4. Neoplastic disease.
5. Pregnancy and the puerperium.
6. Oestrogens.

Pulmonary embolism is massive if there is cardiorespiratory collapse. Duration of embolism in the pulmonary arteries may be acute (<48 hours), subacute (several days or weeks) or chronic (months or years).

Imaging acute PE

1. The CXR is rarely normal but not usually helpful. If changes are minimal it is likely perfusion scanning will be diagnostic.
2. Asymmetrical oligaemia – often best diagnosed by comparison with a previous CXR. The main pulmonary artery may be enlarged.
3. CT pulmonary angiography shows an intraluminal well-defined filling defect.
4. Although segmental oligaemia ± dilatation of the segmental artery proximal to the obstruction may be observed, this is uncommon.
5. Pulmonary infarction follows in about 33%. The signs are non-specific but include
   (a) Subpleural consolidation – segmental or subsegmental. Single or multiple.
   (b) Segmental collapse and later linear (plate) atelectasis.
   (c) Pleural reaction with a small effusion.
   (d) Elevation of the hemidiaphragm on the affected side.
   (e) Cavitation of the infarct.
6. Infarction is more common on the right side and in the lower zones.

Despite the popularity of CT, the ventilation-perfusion radionuclide lung scan is an extremely useful investigation, especially if the CXR is normal or nearly normal. The characteristic abnormality is a segmental perfusion defect at the periphery of the lung with no corresponding ventilation defect, i.e. a mismatched defect. When the CXR shows collapse or infarction the lung scan often shows a corresponding matched ventilation and perfusion defect and this is a non-specific finding.

Chronic PE

1. 'Plump' hila with peripheral arterial pruning, i.e. the signs of pulmonary arterial hypertension.
2. ± Multiple areas of linear atelectasis.

Further Reading

Gefter WB (ed). Pulmonary thromboembolic disease. Semin Ultrasound CT MRI 1997;18(5).
Kerr IH, Simon G, Sutton GC. The value of the plain radiograph in acute massive pulmonary embolism. Br J Radiol 1971;44:751–7.
Padley SP. Lung scintigraphy vs spiral CT in the assessment of pulmonary emboli. Br J Radiol 2002;75:5–8.
Remy-Jardin M, Mastora I, Remy J. Pulmonary embolus imaging with multislice CT. Radiol Clin North Am 2003;41:507–19.
Worsley DF, Alavi A. Radionuclide imaging of acute pulmonary embolism. Radiol Clin North Am 2001;39(5):1035–52.

REITER'S SYNDROME

Sexually transmitted or following dysentery. Males predominate.

1. Urethritis ± cystitis ± prostatitis.
2. Circinate balanitis (30%).
3. Conjunctivitis (30%).
4. Keratoderma blenorrhagica.
5. Arthritis (radiological changes in 80% of cases)
   (a) Involvement of synovial and cartilaginous joints and entheses.
   (b) Asymmetrical involvement of the lower limbs – most commonly the knees, ankles, small joints of the feet and calcaneum. The spine and sacroiliac joints are involved less frequently.
   (c) Soft-tissue swelling.
   (d) Osteoporosis is a feature of the acute disease but not of recurrent or chronic disease.
   (e) Erosions which are initially periarticular and progress to involve the central portion of the articular surface.
   (f) Periosteal new bone.
   (g) New bone formation at ligament and tendon insertions.
   (h) Sacroiliitis and spondylitis with paravertebral ossification.

RENAL OSTEODYSTROPHY

Due to renal glomerular disease: most bilateral reflux nephropathy pyelonephritis and chronic glomerulonephritis. It consists of osteomalacia or rickets + secondary hyperparathyroidism + osteosclerosis.

Children

1. Changes most marked in the skull, pelvis, scapulae, vertebrae and metaphyses of tubular bones.
2. Vertebral sclerosis may be confined to the upper and lower thirds of the bodies – 'rugger jersey' spine.
3. Soft-tissue calcification – less common than in adults.
4. Rickets – the epiphyseal plate is less wide and the metaphysis is less cupped than in vitamin D-dependent rickets.
5. Secondary hyperparathyroidism – subperiosteal erosions and a 'rotting fence-post' appearance of the femoral necks. ± Slipped upper femoral epiphysis.
6. Delayed skeletal maturation.

Adults

1. Hyperparathyroidism (q.v.).
2. Soft-tissue calcification is common, especially in arteries.
3. Osteosclerosis, including 'rugger jersey' spine.
4. Osteomalacia is mainly evident as Looser's zones.

RHEUMATOID ARTHRITIS

1. A symmetrical arthritis of synovial joints, especially the metacarpophalangeal and proximal interphalangeal joints of the hands and feet, wrists, knees, ankles, elbows, glenohumeral and acromioclavicular joints and hips. The synovial articulations of the axial skeleton may also be affected, especially the apophyseal and atlantoaxial joints of the cervical spine. Less commonly the sacroiliac and temporomandibular joints are involved.
2. Cartilaginous joints, e.g. discovertebral junctions outside the cervical spine, symphysis pubis and manubriosternal joints, and entheses are less frequently and less severely involved (cf. seronegative spondyloarthropathies).
3. The sequence of pathological/radiological changes at synovial joints is
   (a) Synovial inflammation and effusion → soft-tissue swelling and widened joint space.
   (b) Hyperaemia and disuse → juxta-articular osteoporosis; later generalized.
   (c) Destruction of cartilage by pannus → joint-space narrowing.
   (d) Pannus destruction of unprotected bone at the insertion of the joint capsule → periarticular erosions.
   (e) Pannus destruction of subchondral bone → widespread erosions and subchondral cysts.
   (f) Capsular and ligamentous laxity → subluxation, dislocation and deformity.
   (g) Fibrous and bony ankylosis.
4. Periosteal reaction – uncommon.
5. Proliferative new bone formation – not present, a distinction from seronegative arthropathies.
6. Secondary degenerative arthritis in the major weight-bearing joints.
7. Pyogenic arthritis is a recognized complication.

Pararticular, extrarticular and systemic features in rheumatoid arthritis

Musculoskeletal
1. Subcutaneous rheumatoid nodules – over bony prominences; calcification rare.
2. Tendons – synovitis of sheath, tendinitis, tendon rupture. Especially extensor carpi ulnaris, flexor carpi ulnaris and extensor carpi radialis
3. Bursae – synovitis, erosion of adjacent bone. Retrocalcaneal, olecranon and subacromial bursae common sites.
4. Bones – osteopaenia, avascular necrosis.

Systemic

1. Anaemia, lymphadenopathy, hepatosplenomegaly, leukocytosis and fever.
2. Felty's syndrome – splenomegaly, leukopenia and rheumatoid arthritis.

Pulmonary

1. Interstitial pneumonitis and fibrosis (mid and lower zones).
2. Bronchiolitis obliterans.
3. Organizing pneumonia.
4. Follicular bronchiolitis.
5. Bronchiectasis.
6. Rheumatoid nodules.
7. Pleural effusion/thickening.
8. Caplan's syndrome – rheumatoid nodules plus pneumoconiosis.

Cardiac

1. Pericarditis ± effusion.

Ocular

1. Episcleritis.
2. Uveitis.
3. Sjögren's syndrome.

Vascular

1. Arteritis.
2. Raynaud's phenomenon.
3. Leg ulcers.
4. Visceral ischaemia.

Miscellaneous

1. Peripheral and autonomic neuropathy.
2. Amyloidosis.
3. Complications of therapy.

Further Reading

Sommer OJ, Kladosek A, Weiler V. Rheumatoid arthritis: a practical guide to state-of-the-art imaging, image interpretation and clinical implications. Radiographics 2005;25:381–98.

RICKETS

Increased uncalcified osteoid in the immature skeleton.

Changes at the growth plate and cortex

1. Widened growth plate (a).
2. Fraying, splaying and cupping of the metaphysis, which is of reduced density (b).
3. Thin bony spur extending from the metaphysis to surround the uncalcified growth plate (c).
4. Indistinct cortex because of uncalcified subperiosteal osteoid (d).
5. Rickety rosary – cupping of the anterior ends of the ribs and, on palpation, abnormally large costochondral junctions.
6. Looser's zones uncommon in children.

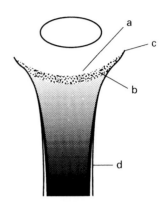

Changes due to bone softening (deformities)

1. Bowing of long bones.
2. Triradiate pelvis.
3. Harrison's sulcus – indrawing of the lower part of the chest wall because of soft ribs.
4. Scoliosis.
5. Biconcave vertebral bodies.
6. Basilar invagination.
7. Craniotabes – flattening of the occiput and accumulating osteoid in the frontal and parietal regions.

General changes

1. Retarded bone maturation and growth.
2. Decreased bone density – uncommon.

Further Reading
Pitt MJ. Rickets and osteomalacia are still around. Radiol Clin North Am 1991;29(1):97–118.

SAPHO

1. Acronym for **S**ynovitis, **A**cne, **P**ustulosis, **H**yperostosis, **O**steitis.
2. A spectrum of conditions related to chronic recurrent multifocal osteomyelitis (CRMO).
3. An inflammatory osteitis ± Dermatological features usually with negative bacterial cultures.

Adults

1. Anterior chest wall lesions – sternocostoclavicular joints
   (a) Stage I – enthesopathy – new bone and soft tissue mass.
   (b) Stage II – arthropathy, with erosions overlap with stage III.
   (c) Stage III – osteosclerosis, hyperostosis and hypertrophy esp medial clavicle.
   (d) Bone scintigraphy – buffalo sign caused by increased activity in the manubrium sternum (head) and medial clavicles (horns).
2. Spine
   (a) Segmental: thoracic > lumbar and cervical.
   (b) Non-specific spondylodiscitis.
   (c) Osteosclerosis.
   (d) Paravertebral ossification.
   (e) Sacroiliac – frequently unilateral, sclerosis and hyperostosis.
3. Long bones
   (a) Metadiaphyseal, esp. femur and tibia.
   (b) Sclerosis and periostitis.
4. Flat bones
   (a) Ilium and mandible – sclerosis and periostitis.
5. Peripheral arthritis
   (a) Axial and peripheral.
   (b) Juxta-articular osteoporosis; narrowing with central or marginal erosions.
6. Skin – palmoplantar pustulosis and acne.

Children

1. Disease usually presents as CRMO.
2. Long bone metaphyses in lower extremity > clavicles and spine.

Further Reading
Earwaker JWS, Cotton A. SAPHO: syndrome or concept? Imaging findings. Skeletal Radiol 2003;32:311–27.

SARCOIDOSIS

A multisystem disease of unknown aetiology characterized histologically by the presence of non-caseating granulomata. More common in black population. Differing modes of presentation between black and white populations: erythema nodosum and 'incidental' finding on chest radiography, uncommon in former. Survival also poorer in former. Equal sex incidence in white population but female preponderance in black population. Raised serum angiotensin converting enzyme levels in around 50% but not specific. Lymphocytosis in bronchoalveolar lavage fluid in 'active' disease.

Intrathoracic sarcoidosis

Thoracic disease at some stage in majority (>90%) of patients. Nodal enlargement on chest radiography is most common manifestation and almost always before lung infiltration.

1. Lymph node enlargement – symmetrical bilateral hilar (BHL) ± unilateral (right) or bilateral paratracheal nodal enlargement most common pattern. Anterior mediastinal lymph nodes also involved in 16% but isolated anterior node disease very rare (think lymphoma, metastatic malignancy). Unilateral hilar lymphadenopathy in 1–5%. 'Egg-shell' calcification occurs in 1–5% and takes about 6 years to develop.
2. Parenchymal disease manifests as
   (a) Bilateral micronodules (2–4mm in diameter) or reticulo-nodular opacities predominantly in the mid/upper zones, along subpleural surfaces (including fissures) and bronchovascular bundles.
   (b) Large nodules (0.5–5.0cm) generally ill-defined. Cavitation rare. May partially or completely regress
   (c) 'Air space' opacities (due to both air space filling and interstitial thickening) seen in up to 20% of cases.
   (d) Coarse linear/reticular pattern with mid/upper zone predilection. Bronchocentric distribution at CT; tendency to distort bronchovascular structures posteriorly.
   (e) Mosaicism – due to small airways obstruction.
3. Pleural involvement rare; 5–7%. Effusion in 2%.
4. Pneumothorax – secondary to chronic lung fibrosis.
5. Bronchial stenosis in 1–2% – extrinsic compression or endobronchial granuloma.

Skin sarcoidosis

1. Erythema nodosum – almost always in association with bilateral hilar lymphadenopathy.
2. Lupus pernio, plaques, subcutaneous nodules and scar infiltration.

Ocular sarcoidosis

1. Most commonly manifests as acute uveitis + bilateral hilar lymphadenopathy + erythema nodosum.

Hepatic and gastrointestinal sarcoidosis

1. Hepatic granulomas in 66%, but symptomatic hepatobiliary disease is rare.
2. Gastric and peritoneal granulomas occur but are asymptomatic.

Neurological sarcoidosis

1. Neuropathies – especially bilateral lower motor neurone VIIth nerve palsies.
2. Cerebral sarcoidosis is evident in 14% of autopsies of patients dying of sarcoidosis, but in only 1–5% clinically. Most commonly it produces nodular granulomatous masses in the basal meninges or adhesive meningitis, which result in cranial nerve palsies and/or hydrocephalus. Granulomas in the brain parenchyma present as space-occupying lesions. (On CT scanning they have a high attenuation, are homogeneously enhancing and peripherally situated.)

Joint sarcoidosis

1. A transient, symmetrical arthropathy involving knees, ankles and, less commonly, the wrists and interphalangeal joints.

Bone sarcoidosis

1. In 3% of patients and most frequently associated with skin lesions.
2. Hands and feet are most commonly affected
    (a) Enlarged nutrient foramina in phalanges and, occasionally, metacarpals and metatarsals.
    (b) Coarse trabeculation, eventually assuming a lacework, reticulated pattern. Initially metaphyseal and eventually affecting the entire bone.
    (c) Larger, well-defined lucencies.
    (d) Resorption of distal phalanges.
    (e) Terminal phalangeal sclerosis.
    (f) Periarticular calcification.

    (g) Subperiosteal bone resorption – simulating hyperparathyroidism.
    (h) Periosteal reaction.
    (i) Soft-tissue swelling – dactylitis.
3. In the remainder of the skeleton
    (a) Well-defined lucencies with a sclerotic margin.
    (b) Paraspinal masses with an extradural block at myelography.
    (c) Destructive lesions of the nasal and jaw bones.

Sarcoidosis elsewhere

1. Peripheral lymphadenopathy in 15%.
2. Hypercalcaemia (10%) and hypercalciuria (60%).
3. Splenomegaly in 6%.
4. Uveoparotid fever (uveitis, cranial nerve palsy, fever and parotitis).

Further Reading

Miller BH, Rosado-de-Christenson ML, McAdams HP et al. Thoracic sarcoidosis: radiologic-pathologic correlation. Radiographics 1995;15:421–37.

SCLERODERMA (PROGRESSIVE SYSTEMIC SCLEROSIS)

A relatively rare autoimmune connective tissue disorder characterized by microvascular injury and deposition of collagen and extracellular matrix. The most obvious clinical manifestation of the disease is induration and thickening of the skin. However, Raynaud's phenomenon (plus other vascular manifestations) and involvement of other organ systems (typically, lungs, heart, renal and gastrointestinal) is not uncommon. Elevated titres of various autoantibodies (classically, anticentromere and anti-DNA-topoisomerase I [formerly called anti-Scl-70]) may be found. Recent interest in increased circulating levels of anti-PDGF receptor antibody.

Skin

1. Thickening, tightness and non-pitting induration – extent of skin disease defines two important clinical subsets: *limited cutaneous scleroderma* (lcSSc; skin involvement distal to the elbows) and *diffuse cutaneous scleroderma* (dcSSc).

2. Raynaud's phenomenon – occurs in over 80% of patients and can precede skin changes by years.
3. Hyperpigmentation, hypopigmentation and depigmentation.
4. Telangiectasia.
5. Digital pitting scars.
6. Loss of soft tissue substance from finger pads.

Joints

1. Eventually 50% of patients have articular involvement. Fingers, wrists and ankles are commonly affected.
2. Terminal phalangeal resorption is associated with soft-tissue atrophy.
3. Erosions at the distal interphalangeal, first carpometacarpal, metacarpophalangeal and metatarsophalangeal joints.

Mandible

1. Thickening of the periodontal membrane ± loss of the lamina dura.

Ribs

1. Symmetrical erosions on the superior surfaces which predominate along the posterior aspects of the third to sixth ribs.

Cardiopulmonary

1. Lung disease most common cause of death (due to pulmonary hypertension and/or interstitial fibrosis). Prevalence between 40–80% (but crucially dependent on method of detection) and more common in patients with dcSSc and anti-DNA-topoisomerase I antibodies. Fibrosis more prevalent than in rheumatoid arthritis. *Non-specific interstitial pneumonia* more prevalent than *usual interstitial pneumonia* pattern of fibrosis. Other patterns of lung disease in systemic sclerosis include organizing pneumonia and diffuse alveolar damage.
2. Aspiration pneumonia – secondary to gastro-oesophageal reflux.
3. Cardiomegaly (30%) – due to myocardial ± pericardial involvement. ± Pericardial effusion.
4. Cor pulmonale.

Gastrointestinal system

1. Oesophageal abnormalities (50%) – dilatation, atonicity, poor or absent peristalsis and free gastro-oesophageal reflux through a widely open gastro-oesophageal junction.

2. Small bowel (75%) – dilated, atonic, thickened mucosal folds and pseudosacculation.
3. Colon (75%) – atonic with pseudosacculations on the antimesenteric border.

SCURVY

The result of vitamin C deficiency.

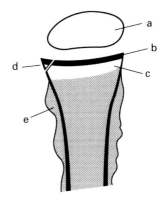

1. Onset at 6 months to 2 years. Rare in adults.
2. Earliest signs are seen at the knees.
3. Osteoporosis (usually the only sign seen in adults).
4. Loss of epiphyseal density with a pencil-thin cortex (Wimberger's sign) (a).
5. Dense zone of provisional calcification – due to excessive calcification of osteoid (b).
6. Metaphyseal lucency (Trümmerfeld zone) (c).
7. Metaphyseal corner fractures through the weakened lucent metaphysis (Pelkan spurs) resulting in cupping of the metaphysis (d).
8. Periosteal reaction due to subperiosteal haematoma (e).

SICKLE-CELL ANAEMIA

Skeletal

1. Marrow hyperplasia (red marrow persistence or reconversion) produces widening of medullary cavities, decreased bone density, coarsening of the trabecular pattern, and cortical thinning and expansion. The changes are most marked in the axial skeleton.
    (a) Skull – coarse granular osteoporosis with widening of the diploë which spares the occiput below the internal occipital protuberance. 'Hair-on-end' appearance (5%).
    (b) Spine – osteoporosis, exaggerated vertical trabeculae and biconcave vertebral bodies (but see also 2(c) below).
2. Vascular occlusion results in osteonecrosis.
    (a) Sickle-cell dactylitis (hand-foot syndrome) – in children aged 6 months to 2 years. Symmetrical soft-tissue swelling, patchy lucency and sclerosis of the shafts of metacarpals, metatarsals and phalanges, and periosteal reaction with bone shortening.

(b) Long bones – diaphyseal or epiphyseal infarcts.

(c) Spine – square-shaped compression infarcts of the vertebral end-plates produce characteristic 'H-shaped' vertebrae.

3. Growth disturbances – retarded growth, delayed closure of epiphyses and tibiotalar slant.

4. Osteomyelitis and pyogenic arthritis – due to Salmonella in over 50% of cases. However, infarction is 50× more common than infection.

Extraskeletal

1. Extramedullary haemopoiesis – paraspinal; also liver, spleen, adrenals, skin and breasts.

Thorax

1. Acute chest syndrome – a new focus of opacity on CXR, associated with fever, leucocytosis, hypoxia and chest pain. Peak incidence at 2–4 years and decreases with age.

2. Pneumonia.

3. Chronic interstitial lung disease.

4. Pulmonary embolism.

5. Pulmonary hypertension.

Spleen

1. Splenomegaly is rare in adults with sickle-cell anaemia, but is common in other sickle haemoglobinopathies, e.g. Hb SC and Hb S beta thalassaemia.

2. Splenic hypofunction in 30% by 1 year and 90% by 6 years, increasing the risk of septicaemia (commonest cause of death in sickle-cell disease with peak at 1–3 years of age).

3. Splenic sequestration – severe anaemia and hypovolaemia due to sudden accumulation of blood in the spleen, usually before the age of 6 years.

4. Focal abnormalities in the spleen on ultrasound, CT and MRI have imaging characteristics of residual normal splenic tissue.

Liver and biliary system

1. Biliary calculi – pigmented.

2. Viral hepatitis – post-transfusion.

3. Hepatic crisis – acute vaso-occlusive crisis; acute hepatic sequestration rare.

4. Cirrhosis.

5. Fibrosis.

6. Intrahepatobiliary duct stenoses.

Renal disease

1. Large kidneys in 50%.
2. Papillary necrosis.
3. Priapism.
4. Renal medullary carcinoma – mostly in patients with sickle-cell trait.
5. Renal infarction.

Central nervous system disease

1. Stroke is the commonest cause of death (12% of paediatric deaths).
2. Three patterns of vascular disease
   (a) Proximal branch occlusion or stenosis.
   (b) Distal branch occlusion.
   (c) Aneurysm.
3. Orbital haemorrhage.

Further Reading

Madani G, Papadopoulou AM, Holloway B. The radiological manifestations of sickle cell disease. Clin Radiol 2007;62:528–38.

SILICOSIS

Lung disease due to exposure to free silica (silicon dioxide). Occurs in miners, quarry workers, masons, pottery workers, sand blasters, foundry workers and boiler scalers. Deposition of particulate material (1–5μm diameter) in respiratory bronchioles followed by ingestion by and eventual death of macrophages. Key histopathological lesion is the fibrotic *hyalinized silicotic nodule*; more common in upper zones. Lung disease generally requires chronic (>20 years) exposure but a more accelerated form known to occur with very high exposure in significantly shorter period (e.g. 4–10 years). Acute silicoproteinosis related to heavy exposure, often in confined spaces, over a short period of time (sometimes only 6–8 months): can lead to acute respiratory failure and death.

Uncomplicated ('simple') silicosis

1. Multiple nodules, measuring less than 1 cm in diameter, most pronounced in the upper and posterior zones with tendency to increasing profusion over time. Sharply demarcated, dense nodules with exposure to pure silica dust but less well-defined, lower density radiographic nodules with mixed dusts; gold miners have very dense nodular shadows. Also nodule density tends to increase with

size. Calcification of nodules occasionally noted (especially gold miners).
2. Hilar and mediastinal lymph-node enlargement recognized but more obvious when calcification occurs (in 5%). Anterior and posterior mediastinal lymph nodes may also enlarge.
3. Reticular pattern (Kerley A and B lines).

Complicated silicosis (i.e. progressive massive fibrosis – PMF)

1. Defined as large (>1cm diameter) and dense nodules; due to coalescence of small nodules in upper/mid zones and initially in the periphery of both lungs but tending to migrate towards the hila.
2. Usually bilateral and roughly symmetrical, 'sausage-shaped' opacities.
3. Emphysematous lung destruction at the periphery.
4. May cavitate or calcify.

Acute silicoproteinosis

1. Widespread ground-glass opacification on plain chest radiography.
2. Crazy-paving pattern (geographical ground-glass opacification and thickened inter- and intralobular septa).

Complications

1. Infections – chronic bronchitis and tuberculosis.
2. Pneumothorax – but usually limited by thickened pleura.
3. Cor pulmonale – a common cause of death.
4. Caplan's syndrome – in patients with rheumatoid disease. Well-defined, peripheral nodules 0.5–5cm in diameter. Calcification and cavitation may occur.

SIMPLE BONE CYST

1. Age – 5–15 years.
2. Sites – proximal humerus and femur
   (75% of cases) and apophysis of the
   greater trochanter.
3. Frequently presents with a pathological
   fracture, especially proximal humerus.
4. Appearances
   (a) Metaphyseal, extending to the
       epiphyseal plate. It migrates away
       from the metaphysis with time.
   (b) Well-defined lucency with a thin
       sclerotic rim.
   (c) Usually central.
   (d) Thinned cortex with slight
       expansion (never more than the
       width of the epiphyseal plate).
   (e) Thin internal septa.
   (f) Pathological fracture may be associated with the 'fallen
       fragment' sign – a small fragment of bone in the dependent
       part of the cyst.

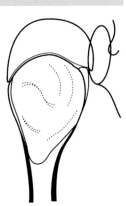

SLIPPED CAPITAL FEMORAL EPIPHYSIS

1. Commonest hip abnormality in adolescence and a major cause of
   early osteoarthritis.
2. M > F.
3. The child is often overweight.
4. Presentation with hip or knee pain. When it occurs before
   adolescence it may be associated with an underlying pathology
   such as malnutrition, endocrine disturbance or developmental
   dysplasia of the hip.
5. Radiology – AP and true lateral films. A frog lateral may exacerbate
   the slip. Initially widening of the physis is seen with or without
   demineralization. The femoral may then slip posteriorly so an early
   slip is best seen on a lateral view. With continued posterior slippage
   the femoral head may appear smaller with apparent narrowing of
   the physis. As the slip progresses the femoral head displaces
   medially and the Line of Klein becomes abnormal. The metaphyseal
   blanch sign may be seen before the slip itself is detected – it relates
   to an area of healing leading to a metaphyseal opacity.

6. Grading
   (a) Mild slip = displacement of femoral head <1/3 the metaphyseal diameter.
   (b) Moderate = displacement of femoral head 1/3–2/3 the metaphyseal diameter.
   (c) Severe = displacement of femoral head >2/3 the metaphyseal diameter.
7. Complications
   (a) Progression.
   (b) Chondrolysis – joint space less than 3mm or loss of greater than 50% of the cartilage thickness. Occurs on both sides of the joint.
   (c) Avascular necrosis – causing the same appearance as seen in other causes of AVN.
   (d) Late complications leading to further radiographic changes including pistol grip deformity, (femoral neck broadening, shortening with varus angulation), osteoarthritis and differences in limb length.

Further Reading
Boles CA, el-Khoury GY. Slipped capital femoral epiphysis. Radiographics, 1997;17:809–23.

STEROIDS

See Cushing's syndrome.

SYSTEMIC LUPUS ERYTHEMATOSUS

Musculoskeletal

1. Polyarthritis – bilateral and symmetrical, involving the small joints of the hand, knee, wrist and shoulder. Soft-tissue swelling and periarticular osteoporosis of the proximal interphalangeal and metacarpophalangeal joints simulate rheumatoid arthritis, but periarticular erosions are not a usual feature. In 10% deforming arthritis is present with ulna drift, boutonniere and swan neck deformities (Jaccoud arthritis).
2. Osteonecrosis – most frequently of the femoral head.
3. Terminal phalangeal sclerosis and resorption.

Respiratory

1. Pleural effusion (60%), which is often recurrent. Bilateral in 50%. Pleuritis and pleural fibrosis.
2. Pneumonia.
3. Acute lupus pneumonitis.
4. Diffuse interstitial disease – uncommon.
5. Pulmonary haemorrhage – rare.
6. Pulmonary artery hypertension.

Cardiovascular

1. Myocarditis – silent in 50%.
2. Pericarditis.
3. Valvular disease – valve leaflet thickening; endocarditis.
4. Vasculitis – an important feature giving rise to multisystem pathology.

Abdomen

1. Oesophageal hypomotility.
2. Vasculitis – bowel ischaemia, cholecystitis, pancreatitis.
3. Hepatosplenomegaly.
4. Renal disease eventually results in small, smooth, non-functioning kidneys.

Neurological

1. Dural venous sinus thrombosis.
2. Vasculitis – stroke.
3. Subarachnoid haemorrhage.
4. Lupus psychosis.

Antiphospholipid syndrome

1. 27–42% of SLE patients.
2. Arterial and veno-occlusive disease; recurrent vascular thromboses.
3. Thrombocytopaenia.
4. Recurrent miscarriages.
5. Present with recurrent strokes, Budd–Chiari, venous sinus thrombosis, ischaemic bowel and recurrent pulmonary embolism.

Further Reading
Lalani TA, Kanne JP, Hatfield GA et al. Imaging findings in systemic lupus erythematosus. Radiographics 2004;24:1069–86.

THALASSAEMIA

Skeletal

1. Marrow hyperplasia is more pronounced than in sickle-cell anaemia (q.v.). The changes in thalassaemia major are more severe than in thalassaemia minor. Initially both axial and appendicular skeleton are affected but as marrow regresses from the appendicular skeleton at puberty the changes in the latter diminish.
    (a) Skull – granular osteoporosis, widening of the diploë, thinning of the outer table and 'hair-on-end' appearance. Involvement of the facial bones produces obliteration of the paranasal sinuses, hypertelorism and malocclusion of the teeth. These changes are rarely a feature of other haemoglobinopathies and are important differentiating signs.
    (b) Spine – osteoporosis, exaggerated vertical trabeculae and fish-shaped vertebrae.
    (c) Ribs, clavicles and tubular bones of the hands and feet show the typical changes of marrow hyperplasia (see Sickle-cell anaemia).
2. Growth disturbances.
3. Fractures.

Extraskeletal

1. Extramedullary haemopoiesis – including hepatosplenomegaly.
2. Cardiomegaly.

Further Reading
Tunaci M, Tunaci A, Engin G et al. Imaging features of thalassaemia. Eur Radiol 1999;9:1804–9.

TUBEROUS SCLEROSIS

Tuberous sclerosis complex is a neurocutaneous syndrome. Clinical features include seizures, mental retardation and skin lesions.

Central nervous system

See 12.30.

Kidneys

1. Angiomyolipomas (AML) – asymptomatic or cause haematuria. Multiple, bilateral.
2. Cysts – in 50%. ± AML.
3. Increased incidence of renal cell carcinoma and Wilms' tumour.
4. Intratumoral and perirenal haemorrhage.
5. Aneurysms of intrarenal arteries.

Skeletal

1. Sclerotic lesions in the skull, vertebrae, pelvis and long bones.
2. Irregular periosteal new bone formation.
3. Distal phalangeal erosion by subungual fibroma.
4. Cyst-like defects in phalanges, metacarpals and metatarsals.
5. Rib expansion and sclerosis.

Lungs

See 4.16.

Heart

1. Cardiac rhabdomyomas. May be diagnosed in utero. Usually multiple. Presentation with cardiac failure, murmur and/or arrhythmias. Most regress spontaneously (within weeks of birth).

Further Reading
Evans JC, Curtis J. The radiological appearances of tuberous sclerosis. Br J Radiol 2000;73:91–8.

TURNER'S SYNDROME

Females with XO chromosome pattern.

1. Small stature with retarded bone maturation.
2. Mental retardation in 10%.
3. Osteoporosis.

Chest

1. Cardiovascular abnormalities – present in 20%, and 70% are coarctation.
2. Broad chest, mild pectus excavatum; widely spaced nipples.

Abdomen

1. Ovarian dysgenesis.
2. Renal anomalies – 'horseshoe kidney' and bifid renal pelvis are the most common.

Axial skeleton

1. Scoliosis and kyphosis.
2. Hypoplasia of the cervical spine.

Appendicular skeleton

1. Cubitus valgus in 70%.
2. Short fourth metacarpal and/or metatarsal in 50% ± short third and fifth metacarpals.
3. Madelung's deformity.
4. Enlargement of the medial tibial plateau ± small exostosis inferiorly.
5. Pes cavus.
6. Transient congenital oedema of the dorsum of the feet.

ULCERATIVE COLITIS

1. Diseased colon is affected in continuity with symmetrical involvement of the wall.
2. Rectum involved in 95%. The rectum may appear normal if steroid enemas have been administered.
3. Granular mucosa and mucosal ulcers.
4. 'Thumbprinting' due to mucosal oedema.
5. Mural thickening usually less than in Crohn's disease
6. Blunting of haustral folds progresses to a narrowed, shortened and tubular colon if the disease becomes chronic.
7. Widening of the retrorectal space.
8. Inflammatory pseudopolyps due to regenerating mucosa. Found in 10–20% of ulcerative colitics and usually following a previous severe attack. Filiform polyps occur in quiescent phase. May be difficult to differentiate from adenomatous polyps using imaging.
9. Patulous ileocaecal valve with reflux ileitis (dilated terminal ileum).

Complications

1. Toxic megacolon – in 7–10%
2. Strictures – much less common than in Crohn's disease and must be differentiated from carcinoma.
3. Carcinoma of the colon – 20–30× increased incidence if extensive colitis has been present for more than 10 years. Endoscopic surveillance indicated in chronic disease. Imaging insensitive to subtle pre-cursor colonic mucosal dysplasia. Risk remains in rectal remnant following sub-total colectomy.
4. Associated conditions
   (a) Erythema nodosum, aphthous ulceration and pyoderma gangrenosum.
   (b) Arthritis – similar to Crohn's disease (q.v.).
   (c) Cirrhosis.
   (d) Chronic active hepatitis.
   (e) Pericholangitis.
   (f) Sclerosing cholangitis.
   (g) Bile duct carcinoma.
   (h) Oxalate urinary calculi.

INDEX

Index

Index

Index

Index

Index

Index

Index

Index

Index